THE YEAR IN RHEUMATIC DISORDERS VOLUME 4

THE YEAR IN RHEUMATIC DISORDERS

VOLUME 4

Edited by

RAJAN MADHOK and **HILARY CAPELL**

CLINICAL PUBLISHING
OXFORD

Distributed worldwide by
CRC Press
Boca Raton London New York Washington, DC

Clinical Publishing

an imprint of Atlas Medical Publishing Ltd

Oxford Centre for Innovation
Mill Street, Oxford OX2 0JX, UK

Tel: +44 1865 811116
Fax: +44 1865 251550
Web: www.clinicalpublishing.co.uk

Distributed by:

CRC Press LLC
2000 NW Corporate Blvd
Boca Raton, FL 33431, USA
E-mail: orders@crcpress.com

CRC Press UK
23–25 Blades Court
Deodar Road
London SW15 2NU, UK
E-mail: crcpress@itps.co.uk

First published 2004

A catalogue record for this book is available from the British Library

ISBN 1 904392 29 6
ISSN 1476-2188

Project manager: Tina Allen
Typeset by Footnote Graphics Ltd, Warminster, Wiltshire, UK
Printed by Alden Press, Oxford, UK

Contents

Part III
Connective tissue disorders

Part IV
Osteoarthritis

Part V
Osteoporosis

Editors

HILARY A CAPELL, MD, FRCP, Centre for Rheumatic Diseases, Glasgow Royal Infirmary, Glasgow, UK

RAJAN MADHOK, MBChb, MD, FRCP, Centre for Rheumatic Diseases, Glasgow Royal Infirmary, Glasgow, UK

Contributors

GRACIELA S ALARCÓN, MD, MPH, Division of Clinical Immunology and Rheumatology, the University of Alabama at Birmingham, Birmingham, Alabama, USA

DANIEL ALETAHA, MD, Vienna Medical University, Department of Internal Medicine III, Division of Rheumatology, Vienna, Austria

HILARY A CAPELL, MD, FRCP, Centre for Rheumatic Diseases, Glasgow Royal Infirmary, Glasgow, UK

ERNEST CHOY, MD, FRCP, Sir Alfred Baring Garrod Clinical Trials Unit, Academic Department of Rheumatology, GKT School of Medicine, King's College Hospital, Denmark Hill, London, UK

WILLIAM D FRASER, BSc, MD, MRCP, FRCPath, Professor, Department of Clinical Chemistry, Royal Liverpool University Hospital, Liverpool, UK

ARIANE HERRICK, MD, FRCP, Senior Lecturer in Rheumatology, University of Manchester, Manchester, UK

ADRIAN JONES, BSc, DM, FRCP, AKC, Rheumatology Unit, Nottingham City Hospital, Nottingham, UK

RAASHID LUQMANI, DM, FRCP (Ed), Rheumatology Department, Western General Hospital, Crewe Road, Edinburgh, UK

KLAUS P MACHOLD, MD, Vienna Medical University, Department of Internal Medicine III, Division of Rheumatology, Vienna, Austria

RAJAN MADHOK, MBChb, MD, FRCP, Centre for Rheumatic Diseases, Glasgow Royal Infirmary, Glasgow, UK

IAIN B MCINNES, FRCP, PhD, Centre for Rheumatic Diseases, University of Glasgow, Glasgow, UK

FREDERICK W MILLER, MD, PhD, Environmental Autoimmunity Group, Office of Clinical Research, National Institute of Environmental Health Sciences, National Institutes of Health, Bethesda, Maryland, USA

ELAINE MORRISON, MB, ChB, Southern General Hospital, Glasgow, UK

NICOLÒ PIPITONE, MD, PhD, Sir Alfred Baring Garrod Clinical Trials Unit, Academic Department of Rheumatology, GKT School of Medicine, King's College Hospital, Denmark Hill, London, UK

NAVEED SATTAR, MBChB, MRCPath, PhD, Department of Vascular Biochemistry, Glasgow Royal Infirmary, Glasgow, UK

GURKIRPAL SINGH, MD, Institute of Clinical Outcomes Research and Education (ICORE), Woodside, California, USA

JOSEF S SMOLEN, MD, Vienna Medical University, Department of Internal Medicine III, Division of Rheumatology, Vienna, Austria

SERGIO M TOLOZA, MD, Division of Clinical Immunology and Rheumatology, the University of Alabama at Birmingham, Birmingham, Alabama, USA

GEORGE TRIADAFILOPOULOS, MD, Department of Medicine, Division of Hepatology and Gastroenterology, Stanford University School of Medicine, and Gastroenterology Section, Veterans Affairs Palo Alto Health Care System, Palo Alto, California, USA

AMÉRICA G URIBE, MD, Division of Clinical Immunology and Rheumatology, the University of Alabama at Birmingham, Birmingham, Alabama, USA

WALTHER J VAN VENROOIJ, PhD, Department of Biochemistry, University of Nijmegen, The Netherlands

ANIL VASISHTA, PhD, Axis-Shield Diagnostics Ltd, Dundee, UK

ERNESTO ZATARAIN, MD, Department of Medicine, Division of Immunology and Rheumatology, Stanford University School of Medicine, Stanford, California, and Rheumatology Section, Veterans Affairs Palo Alto Health Care System, Palo Alto, California, USA

Foreword

Someone once said that a week in political life is a very long time and it is certainly true that a year in the field of rheumatology research can yield remarkable developments in our understanding and therapy of rheumatic diseases.

This current volume focuses on advances in five main areas of rheumatology and for the busy clinician provides an excellent synthesis and discussion of the key literature published over the last two years. The exciting developments in anticytokine therapy in rheumatoid arthritis and also more recently in the seronegative diseases raise the prospect of altering the natural history of these challenging and disabling disorders.

Rheumatologists have known for a very long time that rheumatic diseases are multisystem disorders and that they have an impact on patients' cardiovascular morbidity and mortality. We now have good epidemiological and immunopathological data to support the clinical experience, and the section on cardiovascular disease in rheumatoid arthritis provides an excellent review of the burgeoning literature in this area.

Osteoarthritis and the connective tissue disorders still present major therapeutic challenges, and for those who need to know the strengths and weaknesses of the trials assessing the efficacy of hyaluronate, glucosamine and chondroitin in the most common chronic joint disease will find much to mull over in the osteoarthritis section.

I found the 2004 edition of the *Year in Rheumatic Disorders* a fascinating and stimulating read. Madhok and Capell have targeted the major growth points in rheumatology and have reinforced the adage *nemo solis satis sapet* (nobody knows enough alone).

Roger D Sturrock MD FRCP
McLeod/Arthritis Research Campaign
Professor of Rheumatology
University of Glasgow
Glasgow
Scotland

Part I

Advances in diagnosis and therapy

Advances in diagnosis and therapy

RAJAN MADHOK

Introduction

Rheumatologists now have at their disposable a sizeable armamentarium—but what remains unclear is how and when we should use each of these agents. Collected in this section are papers published over the last year and a half that we hope make the use of these agents a little clearer.

The mortality from non-steroidal anti-inflammatory drug use is high. The availability of selective and specific cyclooxygenase 2 inhibitors has improved their gastrointestinal toxicity profile, but what remains unclear is whether the long-term problems with their use can be avoided.

Disease-modifying antirheumatic drugs (DMARDs) not only reduce synovial inflammation but also reduce damage to articular cartilage and peri-articular bone. The benefit from conventional agents is similar except for auranofin and hydroxychloroquine which are less effective. The remainder of the drugs differ in their toxicity profiles and the duration that patients remain on each drug. Machold, Aletaha and Smolen review the recent evidence of new regimens and strategies of the so-called traditional DMARDs. Also reviewed are the accumulating data on the youngest of the DMARDs leflunomide (Arava). A number of previous observations have suggested that there is a window of opportunity in early disease for DMARD therapy that provides not only a short-term advantage in symptom relief but also the potential to modify disease severity in the long term. Recent studies have cast doubt on this hypothesis—it is clear that most clinical trials are short in rheumatoid arthritis (RA), whereas the disease is long and it is incumbent on us to undertake long-term trials having proven the efficacy of the drugs available to us.

Unlike traditional DMARDs, the biologics/anticytokine therapies are both accurate and precise in disabling single molecules. The availability of antitumour necrosis factor (anti-TNF)-α therapies has allowed rheumatologists to offer some patients with such treatments not only suppression of symptoms but also a much improved quality of life. What remains unclear is the cost both in terms of long-term toxicity and for most healthcare systems of the financial burden. In 2003, papers have clarified some of the medium-term toxicity. Also included are key papers on adalimumab

(Humira), a fully humanized monoclonal antibody against TNF-α. Like etanercept (Enbrel), it can be self-administered which is a considerable advantage. Although the pathogenetic pathways differ between RA and the seronegative spondyloarthropathies, TNF-α is understood to be the key mediator in the final common pathway of these diseases. Reviewed in this section for completeness and in the section on seronegative sponadarthropathies are some of the initial studies which have reported the benefits of anti-TNF-α antagonism in these disorders.

Premature cardiovascular disease is the main contributing factor to the reduced life span in RA. Previous studies have shown that of traditional risk factors only diastolic blood pressure is present in RA patients. Sattar reviews evidence that suggests RA itself may be a risk factor. In parallel, there is accumulating evidence that atheroma itself has a significant inflammatory component. Could it be that the inflammation in RA accelerates the process in the vessels? Some papers published in 2003 suggest that this may indeed be the case. As HMG CoA reductive inhibitors, statins also have an anti-inflammatory effect; their use may offer rheumatologists a single agent with the ability not only to reduce cardiovascular risk in RA but also to reduce the premature mortality.

The therapeutic arsenal available to us now is indeed an exciting one.

1

Non-steroidal anti-inflammatory drugs: cyclooxygenase 2 inhibition

GURKIRPAL SINGH, ERNESTO ZATARAIN, GEORGE TRIADAFILOPOULOS

Introduction

Non-steroidal anti-inflammatory drugs (NSAIDs) are one of the most widely used classes of medications worldwide. NSAIDs form the mainstay of therapy in osteoarthritis (OA), the most common rheumatic disease [1,2]. Although NSAIDs are generally well tolerated, gastrointestinal (GI) adverse events can occur in many patients causing significant morbidity and mortality [3–8]. NSAID-related GI complications can range from nuisance symptoms such as dyspepsia to fatal GI bleeds [3]. Nuisance symptoms such as heartburn, dyspepsia and abdominal pain can occur in 10–20% of patients taking an NSAID [3–8]. These symptoms are often quite debilitating and have a major impact on compliance with therapy. On the other hand, endoscopically visible mucosal lesions are common and can be seen in as many as 80% of patients [6]. Acute haemorrhages and erosions occur within several minutes to hours of taking NSAIDs. These lesions are generally asymptomatic, and will heal and redevelop over time. Serious GI complications such as perforations, obstructions and bleeding from gastric and duodenal ulcers occur annually in 1–2% of individuals taking NSAIDs regularly. In 1997, we estimated that there were approximately 103 000 hospitalizations and 16 500 deaths in the USA related to NSAID-associated serious GI complications (Fig. 1.1) [3–7]. However, the risk of NSAID-related hospitalizations and deaths has been steadily coming down in the USA in recent years, perhaps relating to *Helicobacter pylori* eradication, better patient selection, widespread use of proton pump inhibitors (PPIs) and cyclooxygenase (COX)-2 selective agents [9].

While dyspeptic symptoms are common in patients on NSAIDs, there is little correlation between these symptoms and serious GI complications. Therefore, it is important to identify and recognize risk factors that will predict the risk of serious complications in patients taking NSAIDs. Advanced age, higher NSAID doses, history of GI problems (e.g. peptic ulcer disease and GI bleeding), concomitant corticosteroid, anticoagulant and aspirin use, and serious coexisting morbidity have

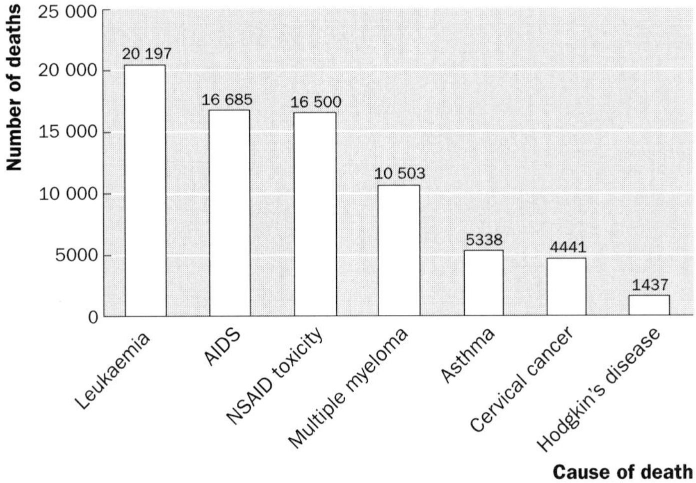

Fig. 1.1 US mortality data for seven selected disorders in 1997. Source: Wolfe *et al.* (1999) |**6**|.

all been linked to an increased risk of serious GI complications |**3–8**|. We recently developed a simple, point-based algorithm that patients and physicians can use to estimate the risk of an NSAID-related GI complication. This algorithm, called the Standardized Calculator of Risks for Events (SCORE) is available from the authors and allows stratification of patients into four risk categories, thus facilitating informed decisions regarding the prescription of NSAID therapy and the use of prophylactic therapy |**10**|.

In recent years, there has been considerable work in identifying the aetiology and pathogenesis of NSAID-induced GI damage. Simple concepts such as topical injury have evolved to theories involving multiple mechanisms with both local and systemic effects. The systemic effects appear to have the predominant role in producing mucosal injury and are largely believed to be the result of inhibition of endogenous prostaglandin synthesis. The synthesis of prostaglandins requires the catabolism of arachidonic acid by the COX enzyme pathway (Fig. 1.2). Two related isoenzymes, called COX-1 and COX-2 have been identified |**6**|. The COX-1 enzyme is constitutively present in most tissues and appears to function in a 'housekeeping role'. The COX-2 enzyme is mostly induced by inflammatory stimuli, and is not normally present in most tissues. The anti-inflammatory properties of NSAIDs are believed to be mediated through the inhibition of COX-2 while the adverse effects such as GI damage occur as a result of inhibition of COX-1. In the stomach, COX-1 promotes the synthesis of prostaglandin E_2 (PGE_2), which mediates cytoprotection of the gastric mucosa against gastric acid and pepsin by stimulating the secretion of bicarbonate and mucus. Normally, the mucous barrier and the secretion of bicarbonate

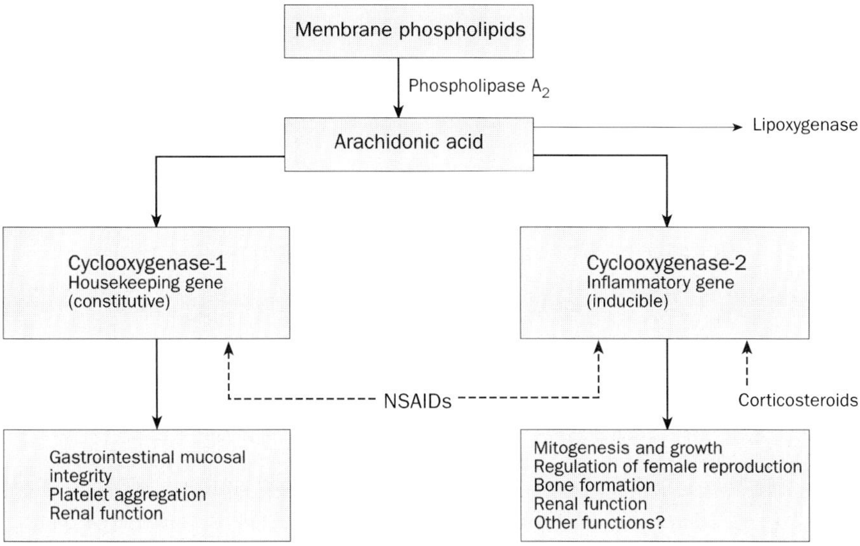

Fig. 1.2 Biosynthesis of prostaglandins through the COX pathways. The immediate precursor of prostaglandins, arachidonic acid, is derived from membrane phospholipids and is catalysed by the two COX isoenzymes (also designated as prostaglandin H synthase), COX-1 and COX-2. The gene for COX-1, the housekeeping enzyme, is expressed constitutively and maintains the homeostasis of organs, including gastric mucosal integrity. In contrast, the gene for COX-2, the inflammatory enzyme, is inducible. Although both pathways can be variably inhibited by different NSAIDs, only the gene for COX-2 contains a corticosteroid-responsive repressor element in its promoter region. The broken arrows indicate the inhibitory effects of pharmacological agents. Source: Wolfe *et al.* (1999) |**6**|.

prevent autodigestion of the gastric mucosa by acid and pepsin. If this cytoprotective mechanism is interfered with by an inhibition of the synthesis of PGE_2, autodigestion of the gastric mucosa may occur, and an ulcer may develop. This has led to the development of a new class of NSAIDs called COX-2-selective NSAIDs that preferentially inhibit COX-2 in the joints and have no effect on the constitutively present COX-1 enzyme in the GI tract. This selective inhibition of COX-2, with a sparing of COX-1, is presumably less likely to cause such problems |**6**|.

Cyclooxygenase-2-selective non-steroidal anti-inflammatories: efficacy

In the USA, there are three NSAIDs designated by the FDA as COX-2-selective: celecoxib, rofecoxib and valdecoxib. There is conflicting evidence about the comparative efficacy of these drugs in relieving symptoms of arthritis and pain [**11,12**]. As all of these drugs rely on the inhibition of the COX-2 enzyme for their efficacy, and this effect is dose dependent, it is likely that when used in appropriate doses, all of them would have equal efficacy. Pharmacokinetic differences, such as absorption kinetics, may influence the onset of action but in chronic diseases such as OA, once a steady state has been reached, there should not be any difference in perceived efficacy.

Comparing the efficacy of cyclooxygenase 2-specific inhibitors in treating osteoarthritis

Gibosky A, Williams GW, McKenna F, Fort JG. *Arthritis Rheum* 2003; **48**: 3102–11

BACKGROUND. Previous studies comparing the efficacy of COX-2-specific inhibitors have come to varying conclusions. McKenna *et al.* showed that there was no statistically significant difference between celecoxib 200 mg/day and rofecoxib 25 mg/day in the treatment of OA; both drugs were more effective than placebo [11]. However, this study had a small sample size and was not adequately powered to show a difference between the two drugs. Geba and colleagues [12] compared the efficacy of rofecoxib 12.5 mg/day and 25 mg/day, celecoxib 25 mg/day and acetaminophen 4000 mg/day in treating OA. The study concluded that rofecoxib at a dose of 25 mg/day was statistically superior in efficacy to celecoxib 200 mg/day. However, there were significant design issues with the study, including the use of inappropriate statistics and *P* values unadjusted for multiple comparisons. This is the third study comparing the two drugs.

INTERPRETATION. In this study, the authors compared celecoxib 200 mg/day and rofecoxib 25 mg/day in a randomized, double-blinded 6-week multicentre study of 475 patients with OA of the knee. A placebo arm was also included to validate the results. There were two co-primary end-points, a visual analogue scale for pain (0–100 mm) and the Western Ontario and McMaster Universities Osteoarthritis Index (WOMAC). Table 1.1 shows the primary results. The difference between celecoxib and rofecoxib was –2.5 mm on a 100 mm visual analogue scale for pain, which was well within the pre-specified criteria for non-inferiority. Both treatments were well tolerated.

Comment

There are several strengths in the trial design used in this study. Even though the primary aim was to compare two active treatments, the inclusion of a placebo arm provides the assurance that measurable differences could be detected. A minimal clinically significant difference was pre-specified and used in power calculations in order to avoid 'overpowering' the study, where small differences could become statistically significant. Minimal clinically significant difference is believed to be the smallest difference in efficacy that a patient would appreciate in routine clinical care and it is designed to assure that only clinically significant differences are evaluated. These issues of trial design are nicely explored in an accompanying editorial.

Table 1.1 Summary of effects of treatment at week 6 (or final visit) for the intent-to-treat cohort*

Measure	Celecoxib 200 mg/day (*n* = 189)	Rofecoxib 25 mg/day (*n* = 190)	Placebo (*n* = 96)
Pain on walking (by 100 mm VAS)			
Baseline	68.6 ± 1.4	66.4 ± 1.4	68.3 ± 1.8
Week 6	36.9 ± 1.8	38.4 ± 1.9	49.0 ± 2.9
Change from baseline	–31.5 ± 2.0†	–29.2 ± 2.0	–19.2 ± 2.7
WOMAC subscales			
Pain (range 0–20)			
Baseline	11.2 ± 0.3	10.8 ± 0.2	11.0 ± 0.3
Week 6	6.5 ± 0.3	6.5 ± 0.3	8.5 ± 0.5
Change from baseline	–4.7 ± 0.3†	–4.6 ± 0.3	–2.6 ± 0.4
Stiffness (range 0–8)			
Baseline	4.9 ± 0.1	4.9 ± 0.1	4.9 ± 0.1
Week 6	3.1 ± 0.1	3.2 ± 0.1	3.8 ± 0.2
Change from baseline	–1.8 ± 0.1†	–1.7 ± 0.1	–1.1 ± 0.2
Physical functioning (range 0–68)			
Baseline	38.8 ± 0.8	38.3 ± 0.7	38.4 ± 1.0
Week 6	34.2 ± 1.0	35.1 ± 1.0	30.5 ± 1.5
Change from baseline	–14.7 ± 1.0†	–13.6 ± 1.0	–8.2 ± 1.3
Patient's global assessment, no. (%) improved‡	91 (48)†	82 (43)	26 (27)
Physician's global assessment, no. (%) improved‡	92 (49)†	82 (43)	31 (32)

*Baseline and week 6 values for the visual analogue scale (VAS) and the Western Ontario and McMaster Universities Osteoarthritis Index (WOMAC) are expressed as the observed mean ± SEM; changes from baseline are expressed as the least square mean changes ± SEM.
† $P \leq 0.016$ versus placebo; differences between celecoxib and rofexcoxib were not significant. For global assessments, *P* values were based on odds ratios.
‡ Improved is defined as a reduction of at least 2 grades on the 5-point scale, or a change to 'very good' (grade 1).
Source: Gibosky *et al.* (2003).

Cyclooxygenase-2-selective non-steroidal anti-inflammatories: tolerability

Nuisance symptoms such as dyspepsia and abdominal pain are common with NSAID therapy and are a frequent cause of treatment discontinuation. The aetiology of dyspeptic symptoms is not well understood. There is little correlation between dyspepsia and endoscopically documented mucosal lesions |**3–8**|. Most patients with dyspepsia do not progress to serious complications such as GI bleeds and most patients (80%) with GI bleeding are asymptomatic |**3**|. There are few prospective studies that have been designed to look at the rate of dyspeptic symptoms in patients treated with COX-2-selective NSAIDs. The following article summarizes the largest

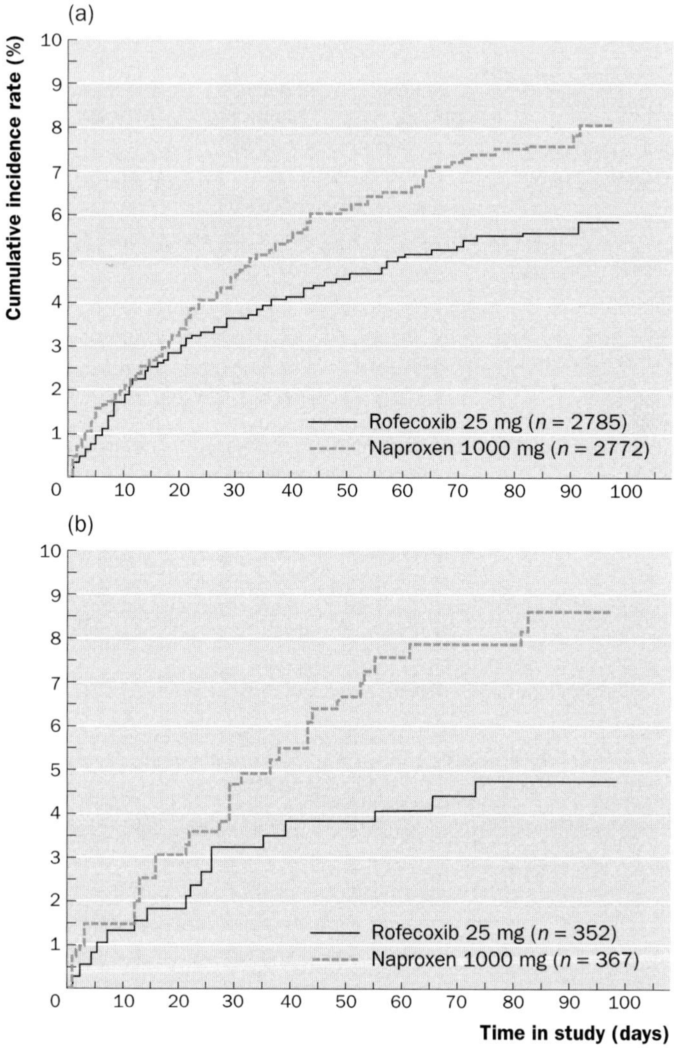

Fig. 1.3 Cumulative incidence of discontinuation due to GI adverse events. (a) The incidence among the overall study sample. (b) The incidence among patients who used low-dose aspirin. For both parts, Kaplan–Meier curves display the time course of cumulative incidence of discontinuations due to GI adverse events by treatment group. Source: Lisse *et al.* (2003).

study comparing GI symptoms in patients using COX-2-selective agents and conventional NSAIDs.

Gastrointestinal tolerability and effectiveness of rofecoxib versus naproxen in the treatment of osteoarthritis

Lisse JR, Perlman M, Johannson G, *et al. Ann Intern Med* 2003; **139**: 539–46

BACKGROUND. There have been calls for trials to report findings in patients that represent those encountered in daily practice. Clinical trials often sacrifice generalizability for homogeneity. Compared with patients in clinical trials, OA patients treated in clinical practice tend to be older, have significant comorbidity and are frequently using other medications. Rates of GI adverse events may be different in relatively unselected populations than in standard clinical trials utilizing strict inclusion criteria. In this randomized, double-blind, placebo-controlled trial, the primary end-point was GI tolerability. In a multicentre study involving 5557 patients typical of community practices, rofecoxib 25 mg/day, or naproxen 500 mg twice daily were compared in 2785 and 2772 patients, respectively, for 12 weeks. Mean age was 63 years, 71% were women, with generalized OA of longer than 1 year duration. Twenty-nine per cent reported a past history of GI event associated with NSAID use. Fifteen per cent had stopped NSAIDs because of past stomach or abdominal symptoms. Almost 50% of patients were using antihypertensive medication and 13% were receiving low-dose aspirin.

INTERPRETATION. Rofecoxib compared with naproxen was associated with a significantly lower incidence of discontinuation due to GI adverse events (5.9% vs 8.1%, respectively). Among low-dose aspirin users, 5.2% taking rofecoxib and 9.4% taking naproxen discontinued the use of the drugs (Fig. 1.3). There were two confirmed serious upper GI complications in the rofecoxib group and nine in the naproxen group. Five myocardial infarctions (MIs) occurred in the rofecoxib group, and one in the naproxen group ($P > 0.2$). Efficacy was similar for both agents.

Comment

A major strength of this study is the inclusion of patients typical of community practice. However, the study was short term (3 months) and it remains unclear if the benefits of rofecoxib therapy would persist for a longer time period. The study evaluated continuous NSAID therapy for 3 months. Most OA patients in the community are treated with long-term, intermittent doses for symptom relief. Future studies should evaluate safety and efficacy of these drugs in community patients treated chronically and/or intermittently for long periods of time.

Over-the-counter non-steroidal anti-inflammatories compared with cyclooxygenase-2-selective non-steroidal anti-inflammatories: gastrointestinal safety

Several NSAIDs are available over the counter (OTC) around the world and are widely used. In the USA in 1998, 16.1 billion tablets of OTC NSAIDs were sold compared with 2.9 billion of prescription NSAIDs |**8**|. Of the more than 30 million people who regularly take NSAIDs, 40% take both prescription and OTC NSAIDs at the same time. In a random population-based survey, it was seen that 75% of consumers who regularly used NSAIDs did not know or were unconcerned about NSAID-related GI complications |**6,8**|. The next paper is the first study that compares OTC ibuprofen with celecoxib.

A randomized, controlled comparison of Ibuprofen at the maximal over-the-counter dose compared with prescription-dose celecoxib on upper gastrointestinal mucosal injury

Scheiman JM, Cryer B, Kimmey MB, Rothstein RI, Riff DS, Wolfe MM. *Clin Gastroenterol Hepatol* 2004; **2:** 290–5

Background. Ibuprofen is generally considered as a safe NSAID, especially at OTC doses. The authors compared endoscopic injury related to non-prescription doses of ibuprofen (1200 mg/day) with prescription doses of celecoxib (200 mg/day) in a randomized, placebo-controlled double-dummy endoscopic evaluation. Naproxen and placebo were used as positive and negative controls respectively. A two-way crossover with a 4–5-week washout period was used. Ninety-five healthy subjects (average age 43.7 years, 53% men) were enrolled in the study, but only 79 completed both phases. Twenty per cent of patients were infected with *H. pylori*. Subjects were stratified by the presence or absence of *H. pylori* infection and were randomly assigned to one of the four sequences (phase 1/2) as follows: ibuprofen/celecoxib, celecoxib/ibuprofen, naproxen/placebo, or placebo/naproxen. Each treatment was given for 10 days, and endoscopy was performed on the 11th day. Primary end-points were the frequency of endoscopic ulcers and erosions in the groups administered (i) celecoxib versus ibuprofen, and (ii) naproxen versus placebo.

Interpretation. A total of 17.6% subjects treated with ibuprofen developed ulcers after 10 days of treatment, compared with only 2.6% of those treated with celecoxib ($P = 0.056$). As a study validation, significantly more naproxen-treated patients developed ulcers (25%) compared with those treated with placebo (2.5%, $P < 0.01$).

Comment

The observation that OTC doses of ibuprofen used for short periods cause significant GI damage is extremely important, given the millions of people who take this drug without prescription. The difference compared with celecoxib was striking—17.6% vs 2.6%—even though it just failed to reach statistical significance. The borderline statistical significance is probably related to the small sample size, as the authors designed the study with the assumption of equal endoscopic damage with both drugs. It is difficult to extrapolate results from this endoscopic study to clinically relevant significant GI events; however, previous work from our group has shown a significant increase of serious GI complications with OTC NSAIDs in patients with rheumatoid arthritis (RA) [8]. This study highlights once again that though OTC NSAIDs may be well tolerated for short-term use, a potential for significant GI damage exists even with OTC doses used for short periods. The authors urge appropriate caution for both patients and physicians when using OTC ibuprofen.

Another caution for ibuprofen: potential inhibition of cardioprotective benefit of aspirin

The clinical benefit of low-dose aspirin in the prophylaxis of acute MI (AMI) is well recognized. This effect is most likely mediated by an irreversible inhibition of platelet COX-1. Aspirin and non-selective NSAIDs share a common docking site on COX-1 [13,14], raising the potential for a competitive interaction between the two. The competitive inhibition of the active site by an NSAID may impede access of aspirin to its binding site on the COX-1 enzyme. Catella-Lawson and colleagues illustrated this effect in an elegant study in healthy human volunteers [15]. If 81 mg of aspirin is given to healthy volunteers followed 2 h later by 400 mg ibuprofen, maximum inhibition of platelet thromboxane generation and consequent inhibition of platelet aggregation is sustained for 24 h after dosing. However, if the drug order is switched, and ibuprofen is given before aspirin, the pharmacodynamic effect of aspirin is prevented, enzyme function is reversibly inhibited (by ibuprofen, which presumably reaches the active site first and blocks aspirin), and platelet aggregation declines by about 60% after 6 h. If ibuprofen 400 mg is administered three times a day, sufficient NSAID remains from the evening dose to cause the interaction even when aspirin is given before ibuprofen the next morning [15]. The next paper illustrates the potential clinical consequences of this interaction.

Effect of ibuprofen on cardioprotective effect of aspirin

MacDonald T, Wei L. *Lancet* 2003; **361**: 573–4

BACKGROUND. The authors investigated the potential clinical consequences of aspirin–NSAID interaction in an observational database study. The primary goal of the

study was to evaluate whether patients with known cardiovascular disease who take low-dose aspirin and ibuprofen or diclofenac have an increased risk of cardiovascular mortality. They studied 7107 patients who were discharged after first admission for cardiovascular disease between April 1989 and April 1997, and who were prescribed low-dose aspirin (<325 mg/day) and survived for at least 1 month. The study population was derived from a database of Tayside residents who registered with a family doctor between January 1989 and December 1997, or who died during the study period (we obtained death certificates from the general registry office).

Interpretation. Patients taking aspirin plus ibuprofen had an increased risk of all-cause mortality (adjusted hazard ratio [HR] 1.93; 95% confidence interval [CI] 1.30–2.87; $P = 0.0011$) and cardiovascular mortality (HR 1.73; 95% CI 1.05–2.84; $P = 0.0305$) compared with those taking ibuprofen alone. However, this interaction was not seen with diclofenac.

Comment

This study, along with a *post-hoc* analysis of the US Physicians Health Study |**16**|, lends credibility to the hypothesis that ibuprofen may interact with the cardioprotective effects of aspirin. The absence of an interaction with diclofenac may represent a differential physical positioning of diclofenac within the active site of COX-1 enzyme, or its relative preference for COX-2 inhibition. COX-2-selective inhibitors are not expected to show this interaction, although there are limited human data on this issue.

Cyclooxygenase-2-selective non-steroidal anti-inflammatories versus concomitant proton pump inhibitors: which approach is better?

The GI safety profile of COX-2-selective NSAIDs still remains a matter of controversy. The VIGOR (Vioxx [rofecoxib] Gastrointestinal Outcomes Research) trial showed that rofecoxib at 50 mg/day had a significantly lower rate of serious GI complications compared with naproxen 1000 mg/day in RA patients |**17**|. However, a similar study with celecoxib, CLASS (Celecoxib Arthritis Safety Study), failed to demonstrate a significant difference in the incidence of ulcer complications between patients receiving celecoxib and those receiving diclofenac |**18**|. It has been argued that the lack of advantage of celecoxib over diclofenac was due to a large and differential dropout of susceptible patients who received diclofenac. In addition, concurrent use of low-dose aspirin may have negated the protective effect of celecoxib. A subsequent study, SUCCESS-1 (Successive Celecoxib Efficacy and Safety Studies), showed that OA patients treated with celecoxib 200–400 mg/day had a significantly lower rate of ulcer complications compared with patients treated with naproxen and diclofenac |**19**|.

Another approach for prophylaxis of NSAID-induced GI damage is concomitant use of PPIs. Several studies have shown that patients taking PPIs in addition to their NSAIDs have a significantly lower risk of developing endoscopically proven gastric and duodenal ulcers compared with those taking NSAIDs alone |**6**|. However, several issues remain unanswered. To date, there are no primary prophylaxis studies with PPIs documenting a reduction in clinically significant ulcer complications. Also, it is unlikely that PPIs will prevent lower GI complications associated with NSAID use.

Celecoxib versus diclofenac and omeprazole in reducing the risk of recurrent ulcer bleeding in patients with arthritis

Chan FKL, Hung LCT, Suen BY, *et al.* *N Engl J Med* 2002; **347**: 2104–10

BACKGROUND. Patients with a past history of peptic ulcer disease have a higher risk of recurrence and complications, particularly if they are users of NSAIDs. Against this highlighted background risk, the authors set out to compare the safety of celecoxib 200 mg twice daily versus 75 mg twice daily of diclofenac extended-release plus 20 mg of omeprazole in a 6-month, randomized, double-blind trial. They studied a total of 287 patients, 144 of whom received celecoxib and 143 diclofenac and omeprazole. All patients had a history of bleeding ulcer, with documented healing in follow-up endoscopy, and a negative test for *H. pylori* or successful eradication according to histological findings. The primary end-point was recurrent bleeding ulcer within 6 months, confirmed by endoscopy.

INTERPRETATION. In the intention-to-treat analysis, recurrent ulcer bleeding occurred in seven patients receiving celecoxib and nine receiving diclofenac plus omeprazole. The probability of recurrent bleeding during the 6-month period was 4.9% (95% CI 3.1–6.7) for patients who received celecoxib and 6.4% (95% CI 4.3–8.4) for patients who received diclofenac plus omeprazole (difference –1.5 percentage points; 95% CI for the difference –6.8 to 3.8) (Fig. 1.4).

Comment

This study shows that both celecoxib and diclofenac + PPI regimens are equally effective as a secondary prophylaxis of NSAID-induced ulcer bleeding. However, there are several interesting issues highlighted in the study. First, the annualized re-bleeding rates with both regimens were almost 10% suggestive of either a very high level of risk or inadequate protection by either of the two regimens, or both. Perhaps such patients would benefit by a combination of celecoxib and PPIs, but this regimen has not been studied. Second, the study was designed to look at only upper GI complications. The study excluded eight patients who were referred to the GI end-point adjudication committee but did not have a documented upper GI source for their bleeding. It is important to consider the possibility of NSAID-associated lower GI complications (see next paper). Third, the dyspepsia rate in the celecoxib group at 15.3% was almost twice compared with that in the diclofenac and concomitant PPI group (8.4%). This difference was not statistically significant, but the study was not powered to study dyspepsia. As dyspepsia is a frequent cause of discontinu-

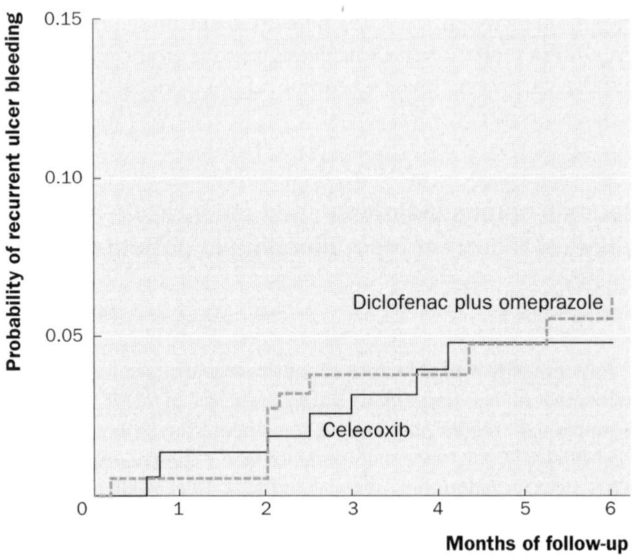

Number at risk							
Celecoxib	144	142	141	137	136	135	135
Diclofenac plus omeprazole	143	142	138	135	135	134	132

Fig. 1.4 Cumulative probability of recurrent ulcer bleeding in the group receiving celecoxib and the group receiving diclofenac plus omeprazole. The difference between groups was not significant ($P = 0.60$ by the log-rank test). Source: Chan *et al.* (2002).

ation of NSAID therapy and has a considerable impact on a patient's quality of life, concomitant PPI use should be considered seriously in such patients.

Serious lower gastrointestinal clinical events with nonselective NSAID or coxib use

Laine L, Connors LG, Reicin A, *et al. Gastroenterology* 2003; **124**: 288–92

BACKGROUND. Patients on NSAIDs are at increased risk for lower GI tract bleeding, perforations, ulcerations and symptomatic diverticular disease |3–8|. In this report, the authors performed a *post-hoc* analysis of a prospective, double-blind outcomes study of naproxen versus rofecoxib in 8076 patients. A total of 8076 RA patients 50 years or older (or 40 years or older on corticosteroid therapy) expected to require NSAIDs for 1 year or greater were randomly assigned to naproxen 500 mg twice daily or rofecoxib 50 mg daily. The rate of serious lower GI clinical events, defined as bleeding with a 2 g/dl drop in haemoglobin or hospitalization, or hospitalization for perforation, obstruction, ulceration or diverticulitis, was determined. Patients were followed for a median of 9 months (range 0.5–13 months).

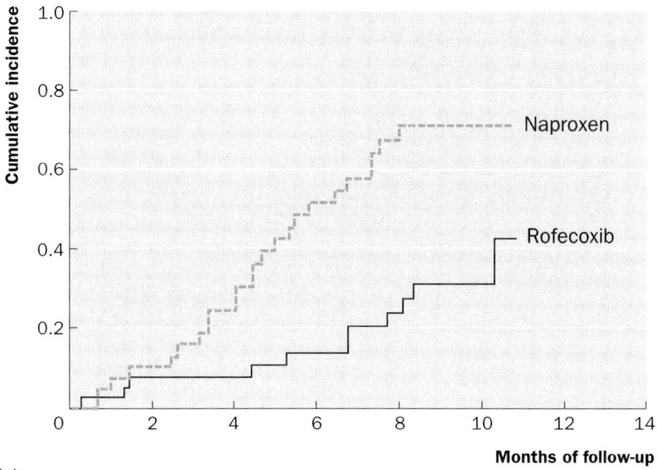

Number at risk

Rofecoxib	n = 4047	3643	3406	3180	2803	1072	533
Naproxen	n = 4029	3645	3391	3167	2793	1071	514

Fig. 1.5 Time to serious lower GI clinical events in the naproxen and rofecoxib treatment group. (Incidence expressed as rate of events per 100 patient-years.)
Source: Laine *et al.* (2003).

Interpretation. Thirty-five patients had serious lower GI events: 24 with naproxen and 11 with rofecoxib. Twenty-seven patients had serious lower GI bleeding, two had obstruction, two had diverticular perforation, three had diverticulitis without gross perforation (based on clinical plus computer tomographic evidence in each case), and one had colonic ulceration (two additional patients in the bleeding group had colonic ulcers diagnosed). Twenty-four patients were hospitalized (16 in the naproxen group, eight in the rofecoxib group). The rate of serious lower GI events per 100 patient-years was 0.41 for rofecoxib and 0.89 for naproxen. The relative risk for serious lower GI events for rofecoxib versus naproxen from the Cox model was 0.46 (95% CI 0.22–0.93; $P = 0.032$). The absolute risk difference (per 100 patient-years) was –0.48 (95% CI –0.91 to –0.05) with a number-needed-to-treat of 208.

Comment

This *post hoc* analysis of a large prospective outcomes study (VIGOR) showed that serious lower GI events occurred at an annualized incidence of 0.9% in RA patients taking the non-selective NSAID naproxen. In the same study, complicated upper GI events occurred at an annualized incidence of 1.4% with naproxen. Serious lower GI complications are common with NSAIDs and have not been well studied. Rofecoxib reduced the risk of lower GI complications by 54%. It is unlikely that concomitant PPI use would decrease lower GI complications.

Cyclo-oxyenase-2-specific inhibitors and cardiovascular complications

Today, the most important controversy surrounding the use of COX-2-specific inhibitors is the possible association of serious thrombotic complications with the use of these drugs. An unexpected finding from the VIGOR trial was a significantly increased risk of serious thromboembolic events in rofecoxib-treated patients compared with those treated with naproxen [**17**]; no increased risk was seen with celecoxib in the CLASS trial [**18**]. Some studies have suggested that a cardioprotective effect of naproxen may explain the difference in MI rate between rofecoxib and naproxen in the VIGOR trial [**20–23**]. Other studies have not found that naproxen has cardioprotective properties [**24,25**]. It is also possible that a true difference in thromboembolic event rates between the two COX-2-specific inhibitors exists. The next article is probably one of the best designed studies exploring the relationship of COX-2-specific inhibitors and AMI.

Relationship between selective cyclooxygenase-2 inhibitors and acute myocardial infarction in older adults

Solomon D, Schneeweiss S, Glynn R, *et al. Circulation* 2004; **109**: 2068–73

Background. Previous studies on the association between selective COX-2 inhibitors and AMI have come to varying conclusions. A pooled analysis of rofecoxib randomized clinical trials, including VIGOR, suggested that there may be a statistically significantly increased risk of cardiovascular events in patients taking rofecoxib compared with naproxen, but this risk was not seen when rofecoxib was compared with other NSAIDs or with placebo [6,7]. A reanalysis of the CLASS trial, which compared celecoxib with ibuprofen or diclofenac, found no increase in the risk of AMI associated with celecoxib [26]. A large observational study suggested that rofecoxib at dosages >25 mg was associated with an approximately twofold increased risk of AMI compared with celecoxib or no NSAIDs, whereas rofecoxib less than or equal to 25 mg/day was not associated with an elevated risk [25]. Solomon and colleagues conducted a matched case–control study of 54 475 patients 65 years of age or older who received their medications through two state-sponsored pharmaceutical benefits programmes in the USA. All healthcare use encounters were examined to identify hospitalizations for AMI. Each of the 10 895 cases of AMI was matched to four controls on the basis of age, gender and the month of index date. The authors constructed matched logistic regression models, including indicators for patient demographics, healthcare use, medication use and cardiovascular risk factors to assess the relative risk of AMI in patients who used rofecoxib compared with persons taking no NSAID, taking celecoxib, or taking NSAIDs.

Interpretation. Current use of rofecoxib was associated with an elevated relative risk of AMI compared with celecoxib (odds ratio [OR] 1.24; 95% CI 1.05–1.46; $P = 0.011$)

Table 1.2 Adjusted association between coxibs and AMI

	Adjusted odds ratio (95% CI)	*P*
Exposure (reference group)		
Rofecoxib (celecoxib)	1.24 (1.05–1.46)	0.011
Celecoxib (no current use)	0.93 (0.84–1.02)	0.13
Rofecoxib (no current use)	1.14 (1.00–1.31)	0.054
Celecoxib (naproxen)	0.95 (0.74–1.21)	0.7
Rofecoxib (naproxen)	1.17 (0.90–1.52)	0.2
Celecoxib (ibuprofen)	0.98 (0.76–1.26)	0.9
Rofecoxib (ibuprofen)	1.21 (0.92–1.58)	0.2
Celecoxib (other NSAID)	0.95 (0.82–1.10)	0.4
Rofecoxib (other NSAID)	1.17 (0.99–1.38)	0.073
Covariate		
Race, white	1.20 (1.12–1.29)	<0.001
No. of physician visits		
4–6	1.11 (1.05–1.18)	<0.001
7–12	1.11 (1.05–1.17)	<0.001
13+	1.09 (1.02–1.16)	0.011
Comorbid conditions		
1–2	1.25 (1.20–1.31)	<0.001
3+	1.42 (1.33–1.52)	<0.001
No. of different drugs		
6–9	1.14 (1.08–1.19)	<0.001
10+	1.18 (1.12–1.25)	<0.001
Diabetes	1.48 (1.42–1.54)	<0.001
Hypertension	1.15 (1.11–1.20)	<0.001
Previous myocardial infarction	1.56 (1.48–1.66)	<0.001
Angina	1.31 (1.25–1.38)	<0.001
Previous coronary revascularization	0.78 (0.69–0.89)	<0.001
Congestive heart failure	1.37 (1.31–1.44)	<0.001
Cerebrovascular accident	1.07 (1.01–1.27)	0.014
Use of statin	1.00 (0.94–1.04)	0.7
Use of hormone replacement therapy	0.88 (0.79–0.98)	0.02
Rheumatoid arthritis	1.16 (1.02–1.31)	0.02
Previous non-selective NSAID use	0.97 (0.90–1.04)	0.3

Conditional logistic model matched on age, gender, and month of index date. All other variables listed were adjusted for in the multivariable models. The number of AMIs in each exposure group was as follows: celecoxib 425, rofecoxib 225, ibuprofen 49, naproxen 63, other NSAID 371, and no current use 9793.
Source: Solomon *et al.* (2004).

and with no NSAID (OR 1.14; 95% CI 1.00–1.31; $P = 0.054$). The adjusted relative risk of AMI was also elevated in dose-specific comparisons: rofecoxib ≤25 mg versus celecoxib ≤200 mg (OR 1.21; 95% CI 1.01–1.44; $P = 0.036$) and rofecoxib >25 mg versus celecoxib >200 mg (OR 1.70; 95% CI 1.07–2.71; $P = 0.026$). The adjusted relative risks of AMI associated with rofecoxib use of 1–30 days (OR 1.40; 95% CI 1.12–1.75; $P = 0.005$) and 31–90 days (OR 1.38; 95% CI 1.11–1.72; $P = 0.003$) were higher than

>90 days (OR 0.96; 95% CI 0.72–1.25; $P = 0.8$) compared with celecoxib use of similar duration. Celecoxib was not associated with an increased relative risk of AMI in these comparisons (Table 1.2).

Comments

Solomon studied over 50 000 older adults in two US states with complete prescription drug coverage. The main analyses, as well as dose- and duration-specific analyses, found an elevated risk of AMI associated with rofecoxib but not with celecoxib. The risk was higher in persons taking >25 mg of rofecoxib and during the first 90 days of use, and was observed consistently in relation to several reference groups. It is important to remember that this is a retrospective, database study. There was no information on several cardiovascular risk factors, such as smoking, lipid levels, hypertension, etc. The patients were not randomized into the different treatment arms. Nevertheless, this study adds to the growing body of evidence that there may be significant differences between the COX-2-specific inhibitors and their association with AMI. Several mechanistic studies to explore the reasons for these differences are currently ongoing.

Cyclooxygenase-2 inhibitors in aspirin-sensitive asthma

Aspirin and NSAIDs sometimes cause severe bronchoconstriction, and occasionally death, in a small number of subjects with asthma. Most of these patients have the classical triad of nasal polyposis, asthma and aspirin sensitivity. This distinct clinical syndrome, called aspirin-induced asthma (AIA), is also characterized by an eosinophilic rhinosinusitis. A definitive diagnosis usually requires a provocation test with aspirin. The basic mechanism behind this response is only partially understood but seems to involve decreased formation of PGE_2, through inhibition of COX-1. PGE_2 functions as a bronchodilator and reduces the formation of cysteinyl leukotrienes that cause bronchoconstriction, inflammation and mucus production |**27**|. The remarkable susceptibility of these patients to COX-1 inhibition by NSAIDs is believed to be related to an abnormal dependency on the anti-inflammatory action of PGE_2, resulting in mast cell activation on removal of endogenous PGE_2 by NSAIDs that inhibit COX-1. The disease runs a protracted course even if COX-1 inhibitors are avoided, and the course is often severe, many patients requiring systemic corticosteroids to control their sinusitis and asthma |**27**|. The development of COX-2-selective inhibitors has been a major advance in the treatment of these patients.

Biochemical and clinical evidence that aspirin-intolerant asthmatic subjects tolerate the cyclooxygenase-2 selective analgesic drug celecoxib

Gyllfors P, Bochenek G, Overholt J, *et al. J Allergy Clin Immunol* 2003; **111**: 1116–21

BACKGROUND. In this study, Gyllfors and collaborators evaluated 33 patients with aspirin-intolerant asthma in a double-blind, randomized, crossover protocol with celecoxib and placebo. All patients had had a positive aspirin challenge test, with symptoms of intolerance and an increase in urinary leukotriene E_4 (LTE_4) within 9 months of the study, and had been clinically stable on regular medications for 3 months before the study. The subjects first underwent a double-blind, randomized, crossover, increasing dose challenge with placebo or celecoxib (10, 30 or 100 mg in suspension) on two occasions 7 days apart. Thereafter, all subjects were exposed to 400 mg of celecoxib administered during an open challenge session as two 200-mg doses 2 h apart. Lung function, clinical symptoms and urinary excretion of LTE_4 were monitored, with the latter being a sensitive biochemical marker of aspirin intolerance.

INTERPRETATION. Use of celecoxib was not associated with any significant bronchoconstrictor responses, nasal symptoms or GI symptoms, urticaria or changes in urinary LTE_4. There were no changes in lung function or extrapulmonary symptoms during the double-blind sessions. This report, with a placebo-controlled, crossover design, in stable patients, showed good tolerance to celecoxib over a 3-week period.

Comment

This study taken together with previous reports involving both celecoxib and rofecoxib, support the notion that aspirin-intolerant patients can benefit from a COX-2-selective inhibitor treatment.

Safety of selective COX-2 inhibitors in aspirin/nonsteroidal anti-inflammatory drug-intolerant patients: comparison of nimesulide, meloxicam, and rofecoxib

Bavbek S, Çelik G, Özer F, Mungan D, Misirligil Z. *J Asthma* 2004; **41:** 67–75

BACKGROUND. This study directly compared three drugs with varying amounts of COX-2 selectivity in patients with a history of aspirin/NSAID intolerance. Nimesulide, meloxicam and rofecoxib were compared by single-blind, placebo-controlled challenges. A total of 127 subjects were tested with nimesulide, 61 were challenged with meloxicam, 51 with rofecoxib and 37 with all three drugs. Placebos were given to all patients on the first day of the study. On the second day, one-quarter and three-quarters of the therapeutic doses of the active drugs (nimesulide 100 mg, meloxicam 7.5 mg or rofecoxib 25 mg) were given at 60-min intervals. A positive challenge was defined as

the occurrence of any of the following: erythema, pruritus accompanied by erythema, urticaria/angioedema, rhinorrhoea, nasal obstruction, sneezing, dyspnoea, or cough associated with a decrease of at least 20% in the forced expiratory volume (FEV_1) and hypotension.

Interpretation. Of the 127 patients challenged with nimesulide, 18 (14.3%) had a positive reaction. Meloxicam challenge produced a positive reaction in five of the 61 patients evaluated (8.1%). In contrast, only one of the 51 patients challenged with rofecoxib had a positive reaction. Only one urticaria-type reaction was observed with rofecoxib challenge in one patient who presented with anaphylaxis to aspirin/NSAIDs. All patients with asthma tolerated rofecoxib without any adverse effects. None of the patients reacted to placebo.

Comment

This study shows that among the three drugs tested, rofecoxib was least likely to provoke a positive challenge. Rofecoxib is also the most COX-1 sparing of the three drugs tested. The urticaria reaction in one subject still points out the need for caution when treating such patients. Nevertheless, the availability of COX-2-specific inhibitors finally makes it possible for the physician to be able to treat pain and inflammation effectively in these patients.

Conclusion

Serious GI complications from the use of NSAIDs remain a common and significant adverse effect. The advent of selective COX-2 inhibitors and the increasing use of PPIs are leading to a decrease in the incidence of these complications. However, a major controversy in the use of selective COX-2 inhibitors is the potential association of rofecoxib with AMI. Large outcome studies are needed to evaluate the risk–benefit ratio of these drugs in individuals at risk for serious cardiovascular complications.

What lies ahead? By the end of 2004, etoricoxib, another COX-2-selective inhibitor is expected to be approved in the USA. Several pharmaceutical companies are developing new drugs. The FDA is currently evaluating lumiracoxib, a drug developed by Novartis. Lumiracoxib has been studied in the largest clinical trial of COX-2 inhibitors designed to date. The TARGET (Therapeutic cox-189 Arthritis Research and Gastointestinal Events Trial) study is a randomized double-blinded clinical trial comparing lumiracoxib to naproxen and ibuprofen in 18 000 patients. The results of this study should be available soon, and it is expected that with its large sample size, the TARGET study will provide important information on both GI and cardiovascular complications. In the meantime, there is considerable excitement in the oncology community on the potential role of COX-2-selective inhibitors as chemoprophylactic agents and/or adjuvant drugs in the treatment of malignancies. Several definitive clinical trials are ongoing, and results from many critical studies are expected in the next 12 months.

References

1. Singh G. Treatment options for osteoarthritis. *Surg Technol Int* 2003; **11**: 285–90.
2. Singh G, Heller M, Silver D, Singleton P, Toomey P, Triadafilopoulos G. Current approach to safe osteoarthritis pharmacotherapy. *Drug Benefit Trends* 2003; **15**(Suppl E): 1–16.
3. Singh G, Ramey DR, Morfeld D, Shi H, Hatoum H, Fries JF. Gastrointestinal complications of non-steroidal anti-inflammatory drug treatment in rheumatoid arthritis: a prospective observational cohort study. *Arch Intern Med* 1996; **156**: 1530–6.
4. Singh G, Ramey DR. NSAID induced gastrointestinal complications: The ARAMIS Perspective—1997. *J Rheumatol* 1998; **25**(51): 8–16.
5. Singh G. Recent considerations in nonsteroidal anti-inflammatory drug gastropathy. *Am J Med* 1998; **105**(1B): 31–8.
6. Wolfe MM, Lichtenstein DR, Singh G. Gastrointestinal toxicity of non-steroidal anti-inflammatory drugs. *N Engl J Med* 1999; **340**: 1888–99.
7. Singh G, Triadafilopoulos G. Epidemiology of NSAID-induced GI complications. *J Rheumatol* 1999; **26**(Suppl 26): 18–24.
8. Singh G. Gastrointestinal complications of prescription and over-the-counter non-steroidal anti-inflammatory drugs: a view from the ARAMIS database. Arthritis, Rheumatism, and Aging Medical Information System. *Am J Ther* 2000; **7**(2): 115–21.
9. Singh G, Mithal A, Triadafilopoulos G. Decreasing hospitalizations due to complicated gastric and duodenal ulcers in the United States: 1988–2001. *Gastroenterology* 2004; **126**(Suppl 2): A97–8.
10. Singh G, Ramey DR, Triadafilopoulus G, Brown BW, Balise RR. GI Score: A simple self-assessment instrument to quantify the risk of serious NSAID-related complications in RA and OA. *Arthritis Rheum* 1998; **41**(Suppl 9): S75.
11. McKenna F, Weaver A, Fiechtner JJ, Bello A, Fort J. Cox-2 specific inhibitors in the management of osteoarthritis of the knee: a placebo controlled, randomized double-blind study. *J Clin Rheumatol* 2001; **7**: 151–9.
12. Geba G, Weaver AL, Polis AB, Dixon ME, Schnitzer TJ. Efficacy of rofecoxib, celecoxib, and acetaminophen in osteoarthritis of the knee: a randomized trial. *JAMA* 2002; **287**: 64–71.
13. Loll PJ, Picot D, Garavito RM. The structural basis of aspirin activity inferred from the crystal structure of inactivated prostaglandin H2 synthase. *Nat Struct Biol* 1995; **2**: 637–43.
14. Loll PJ, Picot D, Ekabo O, Garavito RM. Synthesis and use of iodinated nonsteroidal antiinflammatory drug analogs as crystallographic probes of the prostaglandin H2 synthase cyclooxygenase active site. *Biochemistry* 1996; **35**: 7330–40.
15. Catella–Lawson F, Reilly MP, Kapoor SC, Cuchiara AJ, DeMarco S, Tournier B, Vyas SN, Fitzgerald GA. Cyclooxygenase inhibitors and the antiplatelet effects of aspirin. *N Engl J Med* 2001; **345**: 1809–17.

16. Kurth T, Glynn R, Walker AM, Chan A, Buring JE, Hennekens CH, Gaziano JM. Inhibition of clinical benefits of aspirin on first myocardial infarction by nonsteroidal anti-inflammatory drugs. *Circulation* 2003; **108**: 1191–5.

17. Bombardier C, Laine L, Reicin A, Shapiro D, Burgos-Vargas R, Davis B, Day R, Ferraz MB, Hawkey CJ, Hochberg MC, Kvien TK, Schnitzer TJ; VIGOR Study Group. Comparison of upper gastrointestinal toxicity of rofecoxib and naproxen in patients with rheumatoid arthritis. VIGOR Study Group. *N Engl J Med* 2000; **343**: 1520–8.

18. Silverstein FE, Faich G, Goldstein JL, Simon LS, Pincus T, Whelton A, Makuch R, Eisen G, Agrawal NM, Stenson WF, Burr AM, Zhao WW, Kent JD, Lefkowith JB, Verburg KM, Geis GS. Gastrointestinal toxicity with celecoxib vs nonsteroidal anti-inflammatory drugs for osteoarthritis and rheumatoid arthritis: the CLASS study: A randomized controlled trial. Celecoxib Long-term Arthritis Safety Study. *JAMA* 2000; **284**: 1247–55.

19. Singh G, Fort JG, Triadafilopoulos G, Bello A. SUCCESS 1: A global osteoarthritis (OA) trial in 13,274 randomized patients: Celecoxib provides similar efficacy to diclofenac and naproxen while providing significantly improved UGI safety. *Arthritis Rheum* 2001; 44(Suppl 9): S135.

20. Konstam MA, Weir MR, Reicin A, Shapiro D, Sperling RS, Barr E, Gertz BJ. Cardiovascular thrombotic events in controlled, clinical trials of rofecoxib. *Circulation* 2001; **104**: 2280–8.

21. Rahme E, Pilote L, LeLorier J. Association between naproxen use and protection against acute myocardial infarction. *Arch Intern Med* 2002; **162**: 1111–15.

22. Solomon DH, Glynn RJ, Levin R, Avorn J. Nonsteroidal anti-inflammatory drug use and acute myocardial infarction. *Arch Intern Med* 2002; **162**: 1099–104.

23. Watson DJ, Rhodes T, Cai B, Guess HA. Lower risk of thromboembolic cardiovascular events with naproxen among patients with rheumatoid arthritis. *Arch Intern Med* 2002; **162**: 1105–10 [published erratum appears in *Arch Intern Med* 2002; **162**: 1779].

24. Schlienger RG, Jick H, Meier CR. Use of nonsteroidal anti-inflammatory drugs and the risk of first-time acute myocardial infarction. *Br J Clin Pharmacol* 2002; **254**: 327–32.

25. Ray WA, Stein CM, Hall K, Daugherty JR, Griffin MR. Non-steroidal anti-inflammatory drugs and risk of serious coronary heart disease: an observational cohort study. *Lancet* 2002; **359**: 118–23.

26. White WB, Faich G, Whelton A, Maurath C, Ridge NJ, Verburg KM, Geis GS, Lefkowith JB. Comparison of thromboembolic events in patients treated with celecoxib, a cyclooxygenase-2 specific inhibitor, versus ibuprofen or diclofenac. *Am J Cardiol* 2002; **89**: 425–30.

27. Picado C. Aspirin-induced asthma: what we know now. *Clin Pulmonary Med* 2004; **11**: 1–5.

2

Traditional disease-modifying antirheumatic drugs

KLAUS MACHOLD, DANIEL ALETAHA, JOSEF SMOLEN

Introduction

The essential pharmacological intervention in patients with rheumatoid arthritis (RA) involves disease-modifying antirheumatic drugs (DMARDs). Likewise, these have a central therapeutic role in many other rheumatological disorders, especially the seronegative arthritides. DMARDs modify the long-term outcomes of RA in terms of signs and symptoms, structural damage and functional disability. The most commonly used traditional DMARDs are methotrexate (MTX), sulphasalazine (SSZ) and antimalarials (chloroquine and hydroxychloroquine [HCQ]). In addition, leflunomide (LF), for many decades the first chemical compound specifically developed to treat RA, is a recent and potent addition to this armamentarium. Parenteral gold compounds, azathioprine, D-penicillamine, and cyclosporin A (CyA) are also less commonly used. In contrast to these 'traditional DMARDs', which are synthetic chemical compounds, the novel genetically engineered and specifically targeted compounds, which aim at interfering with specific mediators of inflammation such as tumour necrosis factor-α and interleukin-1, are produced by novel biomolecular technologies in culture systems and thus are commonly called 'biological' therapeutics.

While the modes of action of traditional DMARDs have been elucidated only in part and mostly long after recognition of their clinical usefulness, the biologicals have been specially designed to interfere with specific biological targets and processes, and have then been assessed for their efficacy. In line with the complexity of their production, the biological agents are also far more costly than the traditional DMARDs, although certain new small molecular compounds may also be expensive.

Over the years, the efficacy and safety of most traditional DMARDs have been well characterized in randomized controlled clinical trials. Subsequently, their effectiveness has been established in clinical practice, and their long-term safety profiles have been outlined. Therefore, recent studies of traditional DMARDs focus more on new regimens (including trials of novel dosing strategies or of DMARD combination therapies) and, longitudinally, on new strategies of serial DMARD applications, rather than on merely showing comparative treatment benefits. Also, certain safety issues continue to be of clinical and, therefore, also of scientific significance. LF represents an exception in some respects as it is the youngest among the traditional DMARDs, and accordingly, data on long-term benefits and safety are still of great interest.

Methotrexate

Treatment with MTX became the gold standard in RA therapy during the 1990s [**1,2**]. Despite its well documented efficacy in clinical trials, particularly in its role as a comparator drug for new agents studied, the effectiveness of its use in clinical practice has rarely been investigated. In particular, the observation of patients treated within the framework of a clinical study creates severe 'right censoring'; i.e. the later stages of treatment courses are usually omitted from documentation. This is in stark contrast to treatment in clinical practice, where therapies are continued as long as they are considered effective and well tolerated.

The methotrexate therapeutic response in rheumatoid arthritis

Ortendahl M, Holmes T, Schettler JD, Fries JF. *J Rheumatol* 2002; **29**(10): 2084–91

BACKGROUND. The authors examined 437 treatment courses in patients recruited from eight centres in the ARAMIS (Arthritis, Rheumatism, and Aging Medical Information System) database during the period 1988–96. Using the Disability Index of the Health Assessment Questionnaire (HAQ) [3], the authors note a continuous improvement through to the fourth year of disease (Fig 2.1). HAQ Disability Index values were 1.48 at baseline and improved to a minimum of 1.23 at 30 months. After this period, patients still on MTX treatment appeared to deteriorate again, to a HAQ index of 1.39 (still below baseline) after 84 months. The apparently slow rate of improvement is in contrast to the commonly noted rapid response (usually within 6 months) in clinical trials. The authors explain this finding partly by the relatively low mean peak doses of MTX (up to 11.37 mg/week in the various regional subgroups of the observation cohort) (Fig. 2.2), the late start of MTX therapy (average disease duration 16.7 years) and the maintenance of MTX despite clinical deterioration.

INTERPRETATION. MTX treatment of RA in practice differs substantially from strategies suggested by the MTX effects in clinical trials and from common perception. MTX treatment appears suboptimal by being too little, too late and too long to treatment change. The authors propose a modification of the 'sawtooth strategy', which suggests waiting for a return of disease activity to baseline: re-evaluation of MTX therapy at 3 years or when re-progression has proceeded halfway to baseline is recommended.

Comment

This is an observational long-term cohort study of the therapeutic response to MTX in RA. Of particular importance seems the notion that, even in the university centres that participated in this study, the upward titration of the MTX dose seemed to follow a very cautious approach. It took up to 30 months to reach what appeared an optimal dosage and the average peak doses were low in the eight subcohorts. This approach may have contributed to some disability, which might have been averted by a more aggressive strategy. However, the latter statement must remain speculative because the study was observational without any control population. Evidently, the main reason for this 'go low–go slow' approach was the recruitment period: in the late 1980s and early 1990s experience with MTX was still limited and the approach more cautious compared with recent years. The current approach to MTX treatment employing rapid dose escalation and doses of up to 25 and 30 mg/week is a

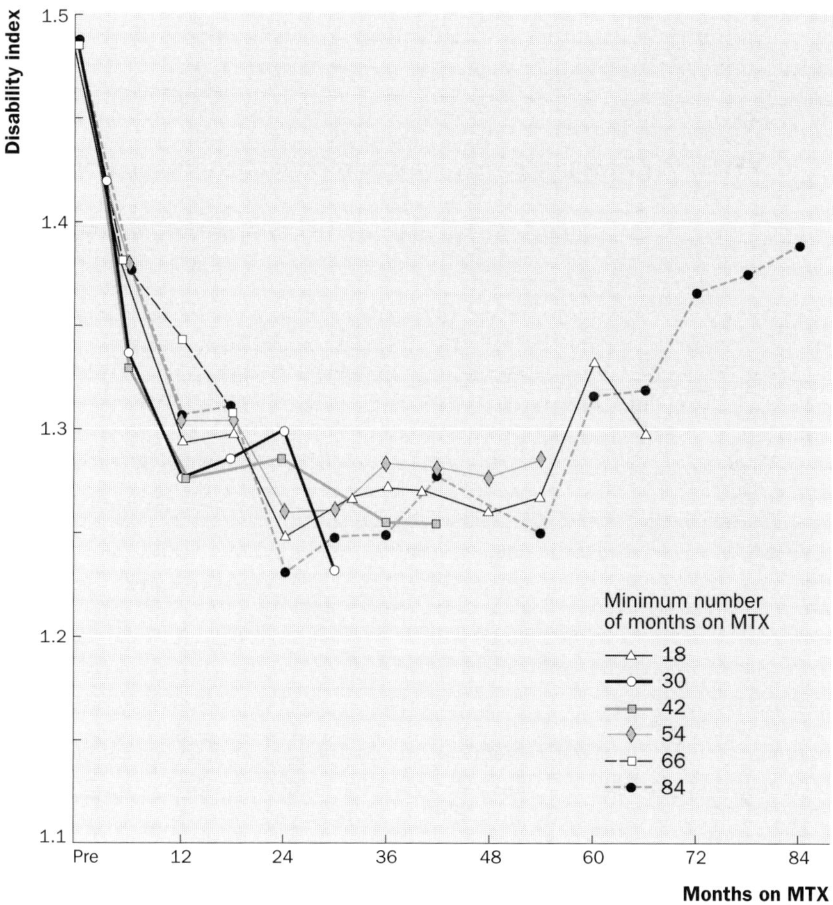

Fig. 2.1 Mean HAQ Disability Index course during MTX segments of differing lengths: retrospective analysis of overlapping groups. Source: Ortendahl *et al.* (2002).

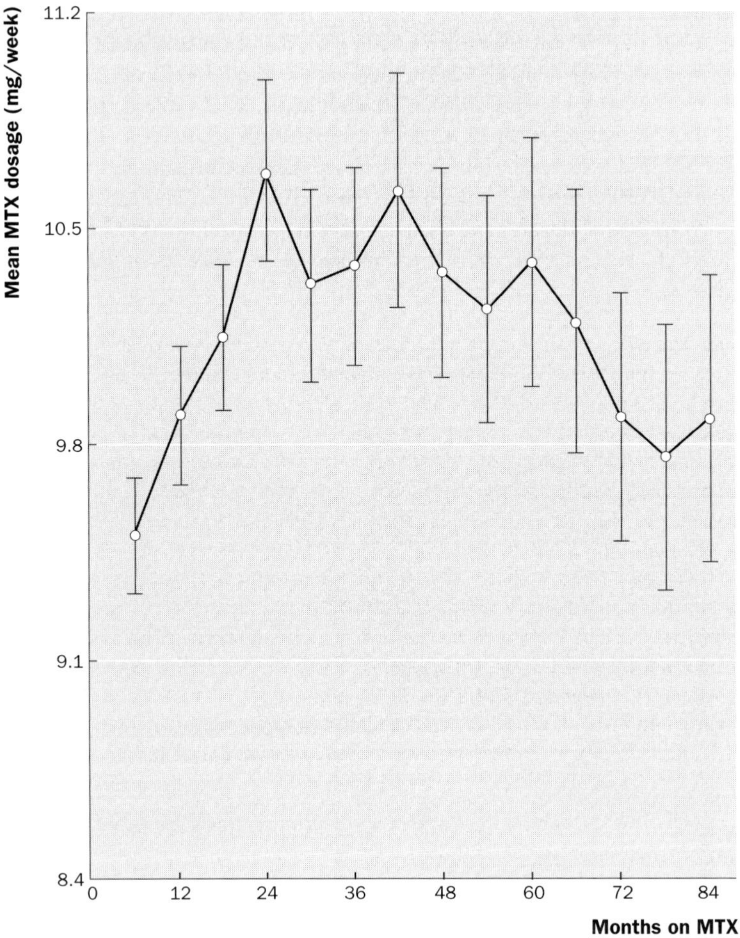

Fig. 2.2 MTX dosage plotted on elapsed months taking MTX. Source: Ortendahl *et al.* (2002).

consequence of the clinical experience of the past decade and several publications related to this experience |**1**|. Thus, it would be highly interesting to repeat the analyses for patients first treated with MTX in more recent years.

Leflunomide

LF is the first DMARD specifically developed for RA therapy in recent decades. The initial pivotal studies that led to its approval for RA treatment in 1998 proved its efficacy, which was comparable with MTX or SSZ |**4,5**|. Both studies, however, did not exceed treatment durations of 6 and 12 months, respectively. After this period, patients were offered to continue treatment in an open label extension study in order to obtain and document data on longer-term use.

The efficacy and safety of leflunomide in patients with active rheumatoid arthritis—a five-year follow-up study

Kalden JR, Schattenkirchner M, Sorensen H, *et al. Arthritis Rheum* 2003; **48**(6): 1513–20

Background. The efficacy and safety of LF beyond 2 years was investigated in a multinational, open-label extension of two phase III double-blind studies. Patients with RA who received LF (10 mg/day or 20 mg/day) in the two phase III studies and who completed 2 years of treatment were offered inclusion in the open-label extension phase and were maintained on the same dosage of LF. Patients were assessed for American College of Rheumatology (ACR) revised criteria for improvement (ACR20, 50 and 70 response rates), the Stanford HAQ scores, and C-reactive protein levels. Safety measures included monitoring of adverse events (AE) and laboratory values. A total of 214 patients (mean age 57 years, 74.8% female) were treated with LF for $>$2 years. The mean disease duration was 4.1 years (range 0.1–26.6 years), and in 44% of patients, RA was first diagnosed within 2 years of entry into the phase III studies. The mean duration of LF treatment was 4.6 years (range 2.8–5.8 years), and 32% of patients had received no previous treatment with DMARDs. ACR response rates and HAQ scores at 1 year were maintained through year 4 or until the end-point. No new types of AE were observed, and liver function was normal at baseline and at the end-point in the majority of patients.

Interpretation. The improvements in both functional ability and physician-based efficacy measures seen with LF after 1 year were maintained for more than 5 years (maximum treatment duration 5.8 years), demonstrating that the early efficacy of LF in patients with RA is sustained long term, and that the long-term safety profile of LF is no different from that observed in phase III trials.

Comment

Most clinical reports usually cover the initial study period, which rarely extends beyond 1 or 2 years, and frequently lasts even shorter, such as 6 months. This is in contrast with clinical practice in which treatments for RA are sometimes continued for much longer periods of time. Efficacy and safety in these long treated patients thus are an important issue. This report extends the findings of the published studies on the efficacy and safety of LF beyond the original 6 and 12 months. The patients who were still on LF at the end of the two mentioned phase III trials were offered to enter an extension period up to 2 years, and patients who completed the 2 years' treatment were followed for another 3 years. Thus, data on 214 patients were analysed. One hundred and sixty-three patients were still under LF therapy at the end of this study.

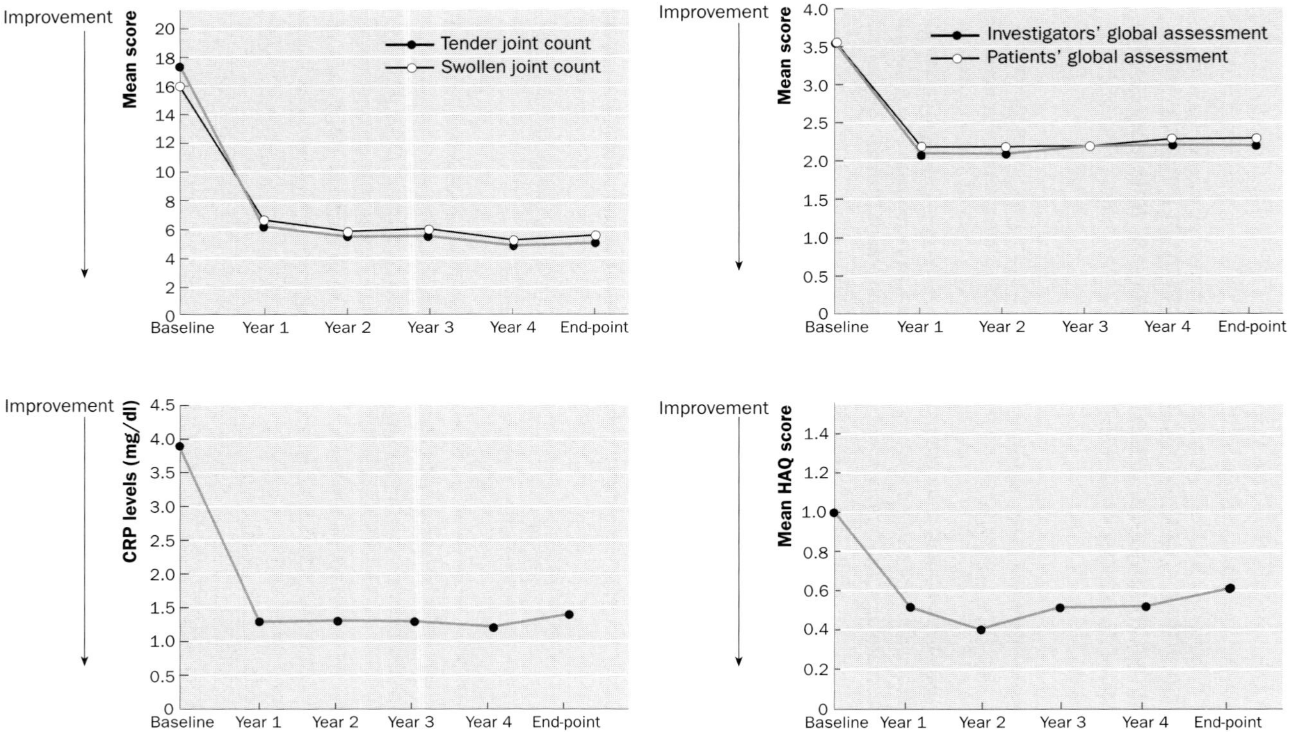

Fig. 2.3 Mean scores for tender and swollen joint counts, investigators' and patients' global assessments, C-reactive protein (CRP) levels and mean Health Assessment Questionnaire (HAQ) scores for leflunomide-treated patients. Source: Kalden *et al.* (2003).

The beneficial effects of LF appeared to be preserved within this cohort (Fig. 2.3). Only nine patients (4.2%) withdrew because of loss of efficacy. Twenty patients (9.3%) had an AE that led to discontinuation of LF therapy. Although this is a severely left censored study (only patients who already had a response, did not have adverse experiences in the preceding studies, and who opted for the extension phase entered the open label study period) the safety and, what seems more important, the sustained benefit of LF therapy has been demonstrated at least in that subgroup. As with many long-term extension studies, the limitation of the current report is the relatively low number of completers ($n = 163$) compared with the total population that entered the two trials originally (>1000).

Combination therapy

Combining DMARDs in order to reduce their lack of efficacy and/or toxicity has been investigated numerous times in past years. Whereas initial combinations (gold + HCQ, chloroquine + D-penicillamine, gold + MTX, HCQ + sulphasalazine) were shown to confer no significant benefit [6–9], combinations such as of MTX and cyclosporin [10] as well as SSZ, HCQ and MTX [11] were more efficacious than monotherapy with no increased adverse effects. These studies have led to adoption of these strategies in clinical practice and a recent report shows that these combinations may even be as efficacious as treatment with biologicals in selected patients [12]. In children with juvenile arthritis, however, data on combination therapy are scarce. The three papers discussed below, one investigating juvenile idiopathic arthritis (JIA) patients and the others adult RA, focus on efficacy of combination therapy and a possible explanation why some of these combinations are more efficient than others.

Combination therapy with methotrexate and cyclosporine A in juvenile idiopathic arthritis

Ravelli A, Moretti C, Temporini F, *et al. Clin Exp Rheumatol* 2002; **20**: 569–72

Background. The efficacy and safety of a combination therapy with MTX and CyA in patients with JIA was studied. Seventeen consecutive patients with JIA who had refractory polyarthritis despite a minimum of 6 months of MTX as a single second-line agent continued MTX with the addition of CyA (4 mg/kg per day) for 6–30 months (median 10 months). Response to therapy was assessed through the preliminary definition of improvement in JIA. At the end of the treatment, as compared with the baseline when CyA was added to MTX, eight of 17 patients (47%) met the 30% definition of improvement; among them five (29%) met the 70% definition of improvement, and two (12%) achieved complete disease control. Seven patients (41%) experienced side effects: four gastrointestinal discomfort, one liver transaminase elevation, and two an increase ≥30% in serum creatinine levels. No patient was discontinued from combination therapy due to AE.

Interpretation. In JIA patients refractory to MTX as a single second-line agent, the addition of CyA was associated with a significant clinical improvement in a sizeable proportion (close to half) of the patients. No termination of treatment due to AE was necessary.

Comment

The combination of MTX with cyclosporin has been demonstrated to confer additional clinical benefit with a reasonable safety profile in adult patients only partly responsive to MTX |**10**|. The present investigation extends these findings, albeit in an open uncontrolled study, to children with inflammatory polyarthritis. Approximately half of the patients (eight of 17) experienced improvement as defined by the criteria proposed by Giannini *et al.* |**13**|, the majority (five of eight) in this group had improvement of at least 70% of their disease activity. This comes at a relatively low 'cost' in terms of AE: no treatment had to be stopped because of side effects, although the authors do not specify the actions taken in the children with elevations of creatinine. This study thus provides additional evidence that combination therapy in children with refractory juvenile arthritis appears to bear no more risks than in adults. However, a final verdict about the best treatment modality in JIA patients with active disease despite MTX therapy is still pending.

Radiographic progression in early rheumatoid arthritis: a 12-month randomized controlled study comparing the combination of cyclosporin and methotrexate with methotrexate alone

Marchesoni A, Battafarano N, Arreghini M, *et al. Rheumatology (Oxford)* 2003; **42**(12): 1545–9

Background. The study was performed to investigate whether combination treatment with CyA and MTX in patients with early (DMARD-naïve) RA could lower the rate of radiographic progression as compared with MTX alone. Patients were randomized to receive up to 20 mg MTX i.m. or a CyA + MTX combination therapy. The radiological outcome was assessed by a blinded observer who rated radiographs using the damage score (DS) of the Sharp and van der Heijde method. Sixty-one consecutive patients with untreated RA of less than 2 years' duration were included; 30 were allocated to combination therapy, 31 to MTX monotherapy. Mean doses of the drugs were: CyA: 2.7 ± 0.3 mg/kg per day at baseline, 2.5 ± 0.6 mg/kg per day at the end; MTX: 9.9 ± 0.5 mg/week in the combination group, 10.2 ± 0.9 mg/week in monotherapy group at baseline, and 9.5 ± 1.7 in the combination group, 11.2 ± 3.4 mg/week in the monotherapy group at the end of treatment. In both groups, starting from a comparable level of damage (mean score ± SD 4.68 ± 1.24 in the combination group, 3.13 ± 0.81 in the MTX alone group), there was a significant increase in DS between baseline and 12 months (MTX/CyA 1.93 ± 0.90; MTX 7.47 ± 2.03), however, it was significantly less in the combination arm

Table 2.1 Progression of the DS and other radiographic scores

	CyA + MTX (28 patients)			MTX (30 patients)			CyA + MTX *vs* MTX
	Baseline	**Change at month 12**	***P****	**Baseline**	**Change at month 12**	***P****	***P*†**
Damage score	4.68 ± 1.24 (2.25–7.10)	1.93 ± 0.90 (0.16–3.70)	0.04	3.13 ± 0.81 (1.54–4.73)	7.47 ± 2.03 (3.49–11.44)	<0.001	0.018
Eroded joint count	0.71 ± 0.24 (0.24–1.19)	0.29 ± 0.12 (0.04–0.53)	0.03	0.77 ± 0.21 (0.35–1.18)	1.37 ± 0.40 (0.59–2.14)	0.002	0.014
Erosion score	1.11 ± 0.41 (0.30–1.92)	0.75 ± 0.33 (0.11–1.40)	0.03	1.23 ± 0.34 (0.56–1.91)	3.90 ± 1.07 (1.80–6.00)	0.001	0.008
Narrowing score	3.57 ± 1.02 (1.57–5.57)	1.18 ± 0.65 (–0.09–2.45)	NS	1.90 ± 3.21 (0.75–3.05)	3.57 ± 1.11 (1.39–5.74)	0.003	NS

Values are mean ± SEM (95% confidence limits).
**P* value for the intragroup difference between baseline and final scores.
†*P* value for the difference in the changes between the two treatment groups.
NS, not significant.
Source: Marchesoni *et al.* (2003).

($P = 0.018$). In the combination versus MTX-only groups, the proportion of ACR20, 50 and 70 responders was 53% vs 61%, 50% vs 44% and 47% vs 19%, respectively. Toxicity was rated 'acceptable' in both groups.

Interpretation. In patients with early RA, CyA + MTX combination therapy led to a significantly lower rate of 12-month radiographic progression, was effective on inflammatory articular symptoms, and was well tolerated.

Comment

The combination of MTX and CyA is long established and has been shown to confer benefit for patients who have failed MTX [10]. This is the first study to demonstrate the superior benefit of combining these drugs already during 'first-line' therapy. Despite the fact that patient numbers were small, the authors could demonstrate a significant benefit regarding an objective outcome, namely less radiographic progression in the combination group over the first year of treatment. Interestingly (and contrasting the radiological outcome), the clinical response did not differ between the two treatment modalities. Of note is the fact that retention rate (drug survival) was much higher in the MTX group (96% compared with 77% on combination treatment). This was solely related to AE. Although this difference was not significant (due to the small sample size) the latter observation should caution against premature transposition of this relatively aggressive treatment modality into clinical practice. In particular, the study was not powered to perform any risk stratification, thus the risk of side effects cannot be weighed against the benefit (decrease in risk of damage). In this respect, a larger trial seems warranted.

Combination therapy with methotrexate and hydroxychloroquine for rheumatoid arthritis increases exposure to methotrexate

Carmichael SJ, Beal J, Day RO, Tett SE. *J Rheumatol* 2002; **29**: 2077–83

Background. Combination treatment of RA with MTX and HCQ has been shown to be more potent than MTX alone. To determine a possible pharmacokinetic explanation for this observation, the bioavailability of MTX in the presence of HCQ, and vice versa, was examined. In a randomized crossover study, 10 healthy subjects, on each of five dosing occasions, received MTX alone as tablets or intravenous solution, HCQ alone as a tablet or oral solution, or a dose of MTX tablets coadministered with an HCQ tablet. The area under the concentration–time curve (AUC) was determined for each subject, on each dosing occasion, for each compound. The mean AUC for MTX was higher ($P = 0.005$) and the maximum MTX concentration (C_{max}) lower ($P = 0.025$) when MTX was coadministered with HCQ, compared with MTX administered alone. The time to reach C_{max} for MTX administration (t_{max}) was also increased during the time of coadministration with HCQ ($P = 0.072$). The AUC of HCQ showed no significant difference ($P = 0.957$) between any of the dosing occasions.

INTERPRETATION. These results may further explain the increased potency of the MTX-HCQ combination over MTX as a single agent and also the sustained effects of MTX when administered with HCQ. In addition, the reduced C_{max} of MTX observed during coadministration may explain reduction of hepatic AE. Extra vigilance for MTX adverse effects during combination therapy with HCQ is recommended, especially if renal function is known to be impaired.

Comment

This study extends the pharmacokinetic basis for the frequent observation that a combination of MTX and HCQ is superior to MTX (and HCQ) monotherapy |**14,15**| and thus strengthens the rationale for such a combination therapy. Moreover, a recent study |**16**| has shown that the MTX-HCQ combination is only marginally less effective than triple therapy with MTX, SSZ and HCQ and may be superior to the common combination of MTX and SSZ. However, in none of these trials structural damage was investigated. In this respect, the combination of MTX, SSZ and initial steroid application appears to bear more long-term benefit compared with SSZ monotherapy |**17**|.

Safety of traditional disease-modifying antirheumatic drugs

In clinical trials, the assessment of safety and efficacy is based on short-term observations at standard doses and in selected patients. However, after approval, clinicians who employ the drug will be confronted with several critical situations: (i) they might face as yet unobserved side effects, and they will therefore have to judge on association and causality; (ii) they will also usually be inexperienced in regard to follow-up examinations in patients on the respective new drug; and (iii) finally, there is the challenge of treating problematic patient groups, such as the very young or the elderly, or patients with comorbidities and co-medications, who are usually not included in clinical trials. Additionally, physicians and other caretakers will have to respond to patients' individual wishes and demands. Therefore, in the long term, it becomes increasingly important to report observations on incidences of AE, especially the type, frequency and implications of rare AE. Also, data-driven recommendations on monitoring strategies of patients receiving such drugs are important.

In this section, we will discuss three papers. Two present recent observational reports, one on AE of traditional DMARDs in RA, and the other more specifically on ocular complications related to antimalarial therapy in a large cohort of lupus patients. The third paper is particularly important as it deals with a common and critical issue in rheumatology, namely treatment of women of childbearing age with DMARDs.

Toxicity profiles of traditional disease modifying antirheumatic drugs for rheumatoid arthritis

Aletaha D, Kapral T, Smolen JS. *Ann Rheum Dis* 2003; **62**(5): 482–6

BACKGROUND. Next to inefficacy, toxicity of DMARDs limits their use in RA. Therefore, toxicity profiles and incidences in daily life are important clinical issues. Charts of 593 patients with RA (i.e. >2300 patient-years of treatment) were reviewed at two rheumatology outpatient clinics. All recorded data on toxicity and reasons for stopping treatment were collected. The key results in this report are: (i) AEs are reasons for discontinuation in 42% of treatments; (ii) 70% of AE were of subjective nature, while substantial laboratory abnormalities were seen in 9% (abnormal liver function tests in 5%; haematological abnormalities in 3%; impaired renal function in 1%); (iii) no single case of retinopathy from antimalarial drugs was found (that is, an incidence of <0.3 events/1000 patient-years), although ophthalmological examinations were abnormal 30 times per 1000 patient-years, mostly revealing keratopathy; (iv) most commonly reported symptoms were nausea, abdominal pain and rashes (Fig 2.4); (v) AE were more likely to occur with increasing number of consecutive DMARD courses; and (vi) if drugs were tolerated well during the first 4 months, AE and primarily laboratory abnormalities usually did not occur later in the treatment course.

INTERPRETATION. The first DMARD course in a patient seems to be safer than the consecutive ones. In addition, the incidence of AE seems to be similar for high and low doses of therapies, including MTX. Thus, frequency of control examinations may be reduced after the first 4 months. Data provided on types and incidences of AE are consistent with previous studies in other countries and different settings [**18**].

Comment

Many studies have been dedicated to the assessment of DMARD toxicity. This recent one presents data on observations obtained by chart review in a European outpatient setting. Its results confirm former US data from the early 1990s, and therefore constitute a validation of toxicity issues independent of the underlying cohort characteristics, ethnicity and society. The results are presented as frequency ranking of AE, where nausea, abdominal pain and rash are the most prominent ones.

The subanalyses in this paper provide additional views on toxicity, which—despite the proof of general validity of these data—should be interpreted with caution. One of these analyses suggested the notion that AE are more likely to occur with increasing number of consecutive DMARD courses; but this might have been due to prescription of 'safer' DMARDs as first drugs. Also, a similar frequency of AE is reported for low-dose and high-dose treatment groups, but this might be related to many patients who do not tolerate even low-dose therapy and therefore never reach high doses. Thus, given a gradual dose increase for most DMARDs, only a selected proportion receives high-dose treatment.

The authors also investigated whether there is any association of clinical symptoms with concurrent laboratory abnormalities, so that the latter could be predicted,

	1	2	3	4	5
All DMARDs	**Nausea (54)**	**Abd. pain (37)**	**Rash (34)**	**Urinary inf. (22)**	**Diarrhoea; infections/ fever (21)**
Methotrexate	Nausea (75)	Alopecia (40)	Abd. pain, infections/fever (39)		Urinary infection (37)
Sulphasalazine	Nausea (82)	Abd. pain (65)	Diarrhoea; rash (37)		
Antimalarial drugs	Eye symptoms (30)	Nausea (28)	Abd. pain (22)	Rash; blurred vision (17)	
Parenteral gold	Rash (120)	Pruritus (64)	Stomatitis, mucosal ulcers (46)	Infections/ fever (23)	Urinary infection (14)
Oral gold	Diarrhoea (69)	Rash (54)	Alopecia (23)	Pruritus; urinary infection; Abd. pain (15)	
D-Penicillamine	Rash; abdominal pain; nausea (37)			Respiratory (15)	
Azathioprine	Nausea (90)	Abd. pain (54)	Stomatitis, mucosal ulcers (36)	Respiratory; vomiting; vertigo (18)	
Cyclosporin A	Nausea; stomatitis; mucosal ulcers; rash; diarrhoea; urinary infection; sweat (73)				
Combinations	Nausea (119)	Infections/ fever (75)	Stomatitis, mucosal ulcers; abdominal pain (60)		

Fig. 2.4 Ranking of major symptoms in patients treated with various DMARDs. Incidence in events/1000 patient-years is given in parentheses. Source: Aletaha *et al.* (2003).

and therefore screening procedures be saved; however, no such association was found.

Such data on general safety of DMARDs provide a basis for comparison with data obtained for newer DMARDs, including the biologicals.

Adherence to ophthalmologic monitoring for antimalarial toxicity in a lupus cohort

Bernatsky S, Pineau C, Joseph L, Clarke A. *J Rheumatol* 2003; **30**(8): 1756–60

BACKGROUND. Antimalarial agents (HCQ and chloroquine) are important in the treatment of various rheumatic diseases, including systemic lupus erythematosus (SLE). Although these agents may lead to ocular complications, little is known about

adherence to policies for ophthalmological monitoring. In this study, the authors investigated adherence to the 1996 ACR guidelines (recommending yearly ophthalmological assessments), and determined the factors associated with non-adherence. This was done by chart review of the Montreal General Hospital lupus clinic cohort. In this way, 195 subjects with at least one full year of exposure to antimalarials during 1996–2001 were identified. Of the 148 patients with complete data, 47 (32%) were non-adherent (defined as missing at least one annual ophthalmology assessment). Predictors of non-adherence in adjusted logistic regression models were: cumulative damage (measured by the Systemic Lupus International Collaborating Clinics/ACR Damage Index) (odds ratio [OR] 1.2 per point in damage score; 95% confidence interval [CI] 1.0–1.5) and exposure to antimalarials ≥5 years (OR 5.2; 95% CI 2.1–13.8).

Interpretation. The results indicate incomplete adherence to ACR guidelines at the Montreal General Hospital. Because patients with higher Damage Index scores were more likely to have missed ophthalmology appointments, even after adjusting for pertinent covariates, it suggests that sicker patients may be more at risk of non-adherence. The association of non-adherence with duration of exposure to antimalarials is an important reminder that adherence to ophthalmological monitoring may decrease as risk for retinal toxicity is increasing.

Comment

This study persuades by its simplicity. The authors defined a target cohort (SLE patients with antimalarials for ≥1 year), divided the cohort into two subgroups (yearly ocular assessments versus missing ≥1 of these assessments), and finally looked at the predictors of being in the latter group using a multiple logistic regression model. Although there have been a considerable proportion of patients with missing data, the authors provide good evidence that these patients (who were excluded from the analysis) were similar to the studied ones (in respect to damage score, age, etc.). In summary, this paper is important to rheumatologists, as it emphasizes the problem of both non-compliance from the patient side, and lack of systematic follow-up by the rheumatologist. A 'record of ophthalmological examination' is now used at the Montreal General Hospital.

The detailed results on predictors of non-adherence are interesting; however, the implications of non-adherence to yearly follow-up examinations is unclear. Retinopathy is almost invariably seen in patients taking HCQ at a dose of >6.5 mg/kg per day given normal renal function |**19**|, while the role of cumulative drug toxicity in the longer term (>10 years of intake) is controversial. Therefore, it might be relevant to have evidence-based proofs of a declining monitoring compliance of these patients. The reason for the association of non-adherence with disease severity is unclear, but might be explained—as the authors do—by potentially more frequent outpatient visits of these patients. One could assume that exploration by the internist and a simple questioning of patients during such frequent visits might be a preventive means against considerable or irreversible ocular toxicity. To conclude, given the very rare incidence of irreversible retinal toxicity, and its potential prevention by dosing according to ideal body weight, antimalarials can still be considered safe DMARDs for patients with RA and especially SLE.

The use of disease modifying antirheumatic drugs in women with rheumatoid arthritis of childbearing age: a survey of practice patterns and pregnancy outcomes

Chakravarty EF, Sanchez-Yamamoto D, Bush TM. *J Rheumatol* 2003; **30**(2): 241–6

BACKGROUND. The aim of this study was to describe the practices of rheumatologists when prescribing the DMARDs MTX, LF, etanercept (ET), and infliximab (IN) to women of childbearing age with RA and the pregnancy outcomes of patients who become pregnant while taking these medications. A questionnaire was mailed to 600 members of the ACR inquiring about their perception of fetal risk, their recommendations regarding the use of birth control in women of childbearing age taking DMARD, and the pregnancy outcomes of women with DMARD exposure. One hundred and seventy-five rheumatologists (29%) returned completed surveys. Respondents were more likely to agree that pregnancy is contraindicated in women taking MTX (95%) or LF (92.7%) than for women taking ET (38.6%) or IN (46.5%). Accordingly, most required birth control for women taking MTX (95.7%) and LF (97.3%), and fewer for women taking ET (75.4%) or IN (73.4%). A total of 65 pregnancies exposed to these DMARDs were reported (MTX 38, LF 10, ET 14, IN two, MTX plus ET one). Three congenital malformations, all in the MTX group, were reported among the 52 pregnancies with known outcomes.

INTERPRETATION. Rheumatologists agree that there is a risk of teratogenicity with MTX and LF, and usually request the use of reliable methods of birth control in women taking these medications. There is no consensus about ET and IN; however, physicians still tend to discuss reliable birth control methods with their female patients. There is a risk of congenital malformations with *in utero* exposure to MTX. No malformations were reported in infants exposed to LF, ET or IN, but the number of reported pregnancy outcomes was small.

Comment

Expert opinion and surveys among a large group of professionals are useful in areas where strong evidence (e.g. clinical trials, large observational data) is missing, either because studies are unethical or too laborious and therefore unfeasible to conduct. In the case of this study, the investigators were seeking opinions and reports from fully trained and practising US rheumatologists. This synthesis of information allows a judgement of the experience basis for the opinions stated by the respondents. Sixty-five pregnancies were reported, their outcomes are shown in Table 2.2.

The question addressed in this paper is of highest clinical relevance, as a large proportion of patients with RA are women of childbearing age. MTX is the most commonly used DMARD for patients with RA and also the one with the longest history of the drugs investigated here. Therefore, the clearest evidence on safety during

Table 2.2 Number of pregnancies and reported outcomes

	Methotrexate	Leflunomide	Etanercept	Infliximab
Total number of pregnancies*	39	10	15	2
Full-term healthy deliveries, *n*	21	2	6	1
Congenital malformations (no. deliveries)†	3	0	0	0
Pre-term delivery, *n*	0	1	0	0
Elective abortions, *n*	8	2	1	0
Spontaneous abortions, *n**†	7	1	1	0
Patients still pregnant, *n*	1	2	4	0
Outcome not stated, *n*	0	2	3	1

*One pregnancy resulted in spontaneous abortion after exposure to MTX and ET at conception.
†One pregnancy (taking MTX) resulted in a spontaneous abortion; the fetus had a congenital malformation.
Source: Chakravarty *et al.* (2003).

pregnancy is available for MTX, which is also reflected by the clear consensus of the respondents that pregnancy is contraindicated in patients taking this drug (95% agreement) and that birth control is required (96%). A similar agreement exists for LF, a new DMARD with teratogenicity in animal studies and with indicated washout procedures in case of pregnancy. Like LF, the biological DMARDs have only been in use for a short time. However, for the biological agents, there is so far no evidence of teratogenicity not even in animal studies. This could be reflected by a high level of uncertainty among the respondents when asked about these drugs.

Further information will only come from new evidence, and such evidence can only develop from reports of accidental drug exposure during pregnancy. From the viewpoint of safety all women of childbearing age should be alerted about the potential danger of all new agents to their offspring, and a reliable means of contraception should be recommended.

Therapeutic strategies with traditional disease-modifying antirheumatic drugs

In recent years, the reports on the benefits of early intervention in RA have accumulated. These reports included many clinical trials of early versus delayed treatment initiation |**20**|, case–control studies |**21**|, as well as trial extension and cohort studies (see below). More recent studies have underlined a 'window of opportunity' hypothesis, which postulates a limited time frame in the beginning of the disease after which the responsiveness to treatment may decrease, and the chance for long-term remission might be lost.

Here we wish to discuss two papers looking at the long-term effects of early intervention in RA. These reports are indirectly supportive of the window of opportunity hypothesis, but underline the importance of both an early and an intensive intervention in patients with (rheumatoid) arthritis.

Five-year followup of rheumatoid arthritis patients after early treatment with disease-modifying antirheumatic drugs versus treatment according to the pyramid approach in the first year

Verstappen SM, Jacobs JW, Bijlsma JW, *et al.*; Utrecht Arthritis Cohort Study Group. *Arthritis Rheum* 2003; **48**(7): 1797–807

BACKGROUND. This study evaluates whether the clinical advantages observed after 1 year in a randomized controlled clinical trial persist after 5 years. Two hundred and thirty-eight DMARD naive early RA patients were randomized to either the pyramid group (non-steroidal anti-inflammatory drugs for at least 1 year after inclusion, giving a mean lag time of DMARD initiation of 14 ± 9 months; n = 56) or the early DMARD group (treated with a DMARD immediately after inclusion; n = 182). After 5 years, data were available for 80% of patients in both groups. 'Clinically relevant improvement' (a definition comparable with an ACR 20% response which was introduced by the authors because at the start of the study the ACR improvement criteria had not yet been established) was found more frequently in the early DMARD than in the pyramid group. However, the radiographic outcomes were not different between the treatment groups.

INTERPRETATION. The clinical results in favour of the early DMARD group, as observed after the first year, were not as evident after 5 years. This lack of distinction between immediate and delayed treatment indicates that treatment should not be reduced too early, in order to maintain the advantages obtained in the first year.

Comment

This report is an observational extension study of a randomized controlled trial in patients with early RA [**20**]. At first sight, its results do not confirm the window of opportunity hypothesis, as there was no difference in the increase of the mean radiographic damage scores between the immediate and the pyramid treatment group during the 5 years of follow-up. An editorial was dedicated to this study and its observations [**22**], in which characteristics of the original study patients and regimens are discussed as potential reasons for this discrepancy in the context of previous literature. In this editorial, it is suggested that the contrast between the treatments might have been too small, and that the study patients might have had a too low propensity for improvement, in order to achieve significant separation of the lines of disease progression between the two groups.

In fact, compared with other studies [**23**] it seems that steroids, which were used more frequently in the pyramid group in the early course of the disease might be highly important to achieve sustained reduction of disease progression [**24**]. In conclusion, although the results of the study are somewhat contrasting with previous findings, they indirectly emphasize the importance of an intensive intervention in early arthritis. Inclusion of a rapidly acting agent (such as high-dose prednisone) might be sufficient to provide some long-term benefit even if used only for a short period of time |**23**|. In addition, in patients who achieve clinically important improvement, the switch to a less aggressive DMARD (which may also be less effective) may be associated with a less favourable long-term course of disease.

Influence of disease-modifying therapy on radiographic outcome in inflammatory polyarthritis at five years: results from a large observational inception study

Bukhari MA, Wiles NJ, Lunt M, *et al. Arthritis Rheum* 2003; **48**: 46–53

BACKGROUND. The effect of early treatment with DMARDs in reducing radiographic progression over a 5-year period was assessed in 335 consecutive patients. Radiographs of the hands and feet were scored using the Larsen method, and were evaluated as a 5-year score adjusted for the first film score. Patients were stratified according to the time from symptom onset to first use of DMARDs to represent four groups (no DMARD use, <6 months, 6–12 months and >12 months). Logistic regression was used to model differences in baseline factors associated with the start of DMARDs. Negative binomial regression was used to compare Larsen score progression for each of the three treatment groups with that for patients not receiving DMARDs. Results were then adjusted for severity, based on propensity modelling. Patients who received treatment had more radiographic progression than did patients who were untreated. Coefficients (95% CI), expressed as a multiple of the Larsen score in DMARD-treated patients compared with untreated patients, were as follows: 1.6 (1.1–2.3) for <6 months, 2.4 (1.5–3.6) for 6–12 months, and 2.0 (1.4–2.8) for >12 months. Using the propensity score as a method of adjusting for baseline disease severity, the influence of treatment on outcome became attenuated as follows: 1.1 (0.8–1.7) for <6 months, 1.6 (1.0–2.6) for 6–12 months, and 1.5 (1.0–2.2) for >12 months.

INTERPRETATION. In this observational study, DMARD treatment was a marker not only of worse disease at presentation but also of the radiographic state and radiographic progression at 5 years. After adjustment for baseline disease severity, earlier therapy was shown to have a beneficial effect on outcome.

Comment

Contrary to the paper discussed before, in a cohort study like the present one, treatment groups, such as early versus delayed treated patients, cannot easily be compared because the groups are likely to be prognostically different. Bukhari and colleagues employed propensity scores for DMARD allocation (regardless of type and dosing) calculated from a pool of available baseline variables, and then assumed equal severity of disease among patients within the same propensity quintile group. The methodology of this study is discussed in a respective editorial [25]. This editorial concludes that the results have validity, although the extrapolation of baseline variables to a 5-year outcome may be insufficient to adjust for the entire course of disease and therapy in the period in between.

This study is an important piece in the early arthritis literature because it includes patients with a very small level of selection. One piece of evidence for this conclusion is the high proportion of seronegative patients (~70%) of patients at baseline (compared with ~40% in the study of Verstappen *et al.*, ~60% in the Vienna cohort [26] and 35% in the COBRA study [23]). Therefore, it might better reflect the daily life conditions, where patients with recent onset arthritis and only moderate disease activity are presenting. This advantage outweighs the methodological issues that are inherent to the analysis of inception cohorts.

Conclusion

Accumulating information about the usefulness of the 'traditional DMARDs' and their application in clinical practice has led to a number of issues that have been or need to be addressed in order to improve our knowledge. Particular concerns have been raised about toxicity of the biological agents and the associated direct and indirect costs compared with monotherapy or combination therapy with traditional DMARDs. Thus, it is still a very worthwhile undertaking for improving clinical practice to address these topics and to deepen our understanding of the subtleties of possible strategies. The papers reviewed in this article are representative of such efforts. A recent proposal for a therapeutic algorithm takes these results into account [27]. As a global summary, there are still many ways to improve care of patients treated with 'traditional DMARDs': treatment intensity may be improved, treatment timing has become a major issue, particularly the concept of early treatment, and safety of medication in various situations such as pregnancy, childhood, and its monitoring have been studied and important contributions made. Moreover, the role of traditional DMARDs will remain highly important in the age of biologicals, not only because they are often highly efficacious in clinical practice, but also because some of them, especially MTX, are invaluable for combination therapy with biological agents.

References

1. Weinblatt ME. Rheumatoid arthritis in 2003: where are we now with treatment? *Ann Rheum Dis* 2003; **62**: 94–6.

2. Cannella AC, O'Dell JR. Is there still a role for traditional disease-modifying antirheumatic drugs (DMARDs) in rheumatoid arthritis? *Curr Opin Rheumatol* 2003; **15**(3): 185–92.
3. Fries JP, Spitz P, Kraines RG, Holman HR. Measurement of patient outcome in arthritis. *Arthritis Rheum* 1980; **23**: 137–45.
4. Emery P, Breedveld FC, Lemmel EM, Kaltwasser JP, Dawes PT, Gomor B, Van Den Bosch F, Nordstrom D, Bjorneboe O, Dahl R, Horslev-Petersen K, Rodriguez De La Serna A, Molloy M, Tikly M, Oed C, Rosenburg R, Loew-Friedrich I. A comparison of the efficacy and safety of leflunomide and methotrexate for the treatment of rheumatoid arthritis. *Rheumatology* 2000; **39**(6): 655–65.
5. Smolen JS, Kalden JR, Scott DL, Rozman B, Kvien TK, Larsen A, Loew-Friedrich I, Oed C, Rosenburg R. Efficacy and safety of leflunomide compared with placebo and sulphasalazine in active rheumatoid arthritis: a double-blind, randomized, multicentre trial. *Lancet* 1999; **353**: 259–65.
6. Bunch TW, O'Duffy JD, Tompkins RB, O'Fallon WM. Controlled trial of hydroxychloroquine and d-penicillamine singly and in combination in the treatment of rheumatoid arthritis. *Arthritis Rheum* 1984; **27**: 267–76.
7. Williams HJ, Ward JR, Reading JC, Brooks RH, Clegg DO, Skosey JL, Weisman MH, Willkens RF, Singer JZ, Alarcon GS, *et al.* Comparison of auranofin, methotrexate, and the combination of both in the treatment of rheumatoid arthritis. *Arthritis Rheum* 1992; **35**: 259–69.
8. Boers M, Ramsden M. Longacting drug combinations in rheumatoid arthritis: a formal overview. *J Rheumatol* 1991; **18**: 316–24.
9. Faarvang KL, Egsmose C, Kryger P, Podenphant J, Ingeman-Nielsen M, Hansen TM. Hydroxychloroquine and sulphasalazine alone and in combination in rheumatoid arthritis: a randomised double blind trial. *Ann Rheum Dis* 1993; **52**: 711–15.
10. Tugwell P, Pincus T, Yocum D, Stein M, Gluck O, Kraag G, McKendry R, Tesser J, Baker P, Wells G. Combination therapy with cyclosporine and methotrexate in severe rheumatoid arthritis. *N Engl J Med* 1995; **333**: 137–41.
11. Mottonen T, Hannonen P, Leirisalo-Repo M, Nissila M, Kautiainen H, Korpela M, Laasonen L, Julkunen H, Luukkainen R, Vuori K, Paimela L, Blafield H, Hakala M, Ilva K, Yli-Kerttula U, Puolakka K, Jarvinen P, Hakola M, Piirainen H, Ahonen J, Palvimaki I, Forsberg S, Koota K, Friman C. Comparison of combination therapy with single-drug therapy in early rheumatoid arthritis: a randomised trial. FIN-RACo trial group. *Lancet* 1999; **353**(9164): 1568–73.
12. Bingham SJ, Buch MH, Tennant A, Emery P. The impact of escalating conventional therapy in rheumatoid arthritis patients referred for anti-tumour necrosis factor—therapy. *Rheumatology* Advance Access published December 1, 2003, 10.1093/rheumatology/keh057. 1 December 2003.
13. Giannini EH, Ruperto N, Ravelli A, Lovell DJ, Felson DT, Martini A. Preliminary definition of improvement in juvenile arthritis. *Arthritis Rheum* 1997; **40**(7): 1202–9.
14. Khraishi MM, Singh G. The role of anti-malarials in rheumatoid arthritis—the American experience. *Lupus* 1996; 5 (Suppl 1): S41–4.
15. Bensen W, Bensen W. Aim for remission or 'personal best' using combination DMARD therapy with methotrexate and hydroxychloroquine. *Clin Exp Rheumatol* 1999; **17**(6): S95–101.

16. O'Dell JR, Leff R, Paulsen G, Haire C, Mallek J, Eckhoff PJ, Fernandez A, Blakely K, Wees S, Stoner J, Hadley S, Felt J, Palmer W, Waytz P, Churchill M, Klassen L, Moore G. Treatment of rheumatoid arthritis with methotrexate and hydroxychloroquine, methotrexate and sulfasalazine, or a combination of the three medications—Results of a two-year, randomized, double-blind, placebo-controlled trial. *Arthritis Rheum* 2002; **46**(5): 1164–70.

17. Landewe RB, Boers M, Verhoeven AC, Westhovens R, van de Laar MA, Markusse HM, van Denderen JC, Westedt ML, Peeters AJ, Dijkmans BA, Jacobs P, Boonen A, van der Heijde DM, van der Linden S. COBRA combination therapy in patients with early rheumatoid arthritis: long-term structural benefits of a brief intervention. *Arthritis Rheum* 2002; **46**(2): 347–56.

18. Singh G, Fries JF, Williams CA, Zatarain E, Spitz P, Bloch DA. Toxicity profiles of disease modifying antirheumatic drugs in rheumatoid arthritis. *J Rheumatol* 1991; **18**(2): 188–94.

19. Bernstein HN. Ocular safety of hydroxychloroquine. *Ann Ophthalmol* 1991; **23**(8): 292–6.

20. Van der Heide A, Jacobs JWG, Bijlsma JWJ. The effectiveness of early treatment with 'second-line' antirheumatic drugs: a randomized, controlled trial. *Ann Intern Med* 1996; **124**: 699–707.

21. Lard LR, Visser H, Speyer I, vander Horst-Bruinsma IE, Zwinderman AH, Breedveld FC, Hazes JM. Early versus delayed treatment in patients with recent-onset rheumatoid arthritis: comparison of two cohorts who received different treatment strategies. *Am J Med* 2001; **111**(6): 446–51.

22. Boers M. Understanding the window of opportunity concept in early rheumatoid arthritis. *Arthritis Rheum* 2003; **48**(7): 1771–4.

23. Boers M, Verhoeven AC, Markusse HM, van de Laar MA, Westhovens R, van Denderen JC, van Zeben D, Dijkmans BA, Peeters AJ, Jacobs P, van den Brink HR, Schouten HJ, van der Heijde DM, Boonen A, van der Linden S. Randomised comparison of combined step-down prednisolone, methotrexate and sulphasalazine with sulphasalazine alone in early rheumatoid arthritis. *Lancet* 1997; **350**(9074): 309–18.

24. van Everdingen AA, Jacobs JW, Siewertsz Van Reesema DR, Bijlsma JW. Low-dose prednisone therapy for patients with early active rheumatoid arthritis: clinical efficacy, disease-modifying properties, and side effects: a randomized, double-blind, placebo-controlled clinical trial. *Ann Intern Med* 2002; **136**: 1–12.

25. Landewe RB. The benefits of early treatment in rheumatoid arthritis: confounding by indication, and the issue of timing. *Arthritis Rheum* 2003; **48**(1): 1–5.

26. Machold KP, Stamm TA, Eberl GJ, Nell VK, Dunky A, Uffmann M, Smolen JS. Very recent onset arthritis—clinical, laboratory, and radiological findings during the first year of disease. *J Rheumatol* 2002; **29**(11): 2278.

27. Smolen JS, Sokka T, Pincus T, Breedveld FC. A proposed treatment algorithm for rheumatoid arthritis: Aggressive therapy, methotrexate, and quantitative measures. *Clin Exp Rheumatol* 2003; **21**(5): S209–10.

3

Anticytokine therapies in rheumatic diseases: an update

NICOLÒ PIPITONE, ERNEST CHOY

Introduction

Cytokines are small proteins that serve as chemical messengers between cells. They act by binding to specific receptors expressed on the surface of the target cells, leading to the activation of different intracellular signalling pathways and ultimately to modulation of gene transcription. Cytokines are involved in numerous physiological and pathological processes, including the regulation of the immune-inflammatory response. Depending on their predominant action, cytokines can be classified as 'pro-inflammatory' or 'anti-inflammatory'. Broadly speaking, pro-inflammatory cytokines are thought to contribute to the immune-inflammatory response by activating the cells involved in such responses and by inducing the synthesis of other inflammatory mediators (Table 3.1), while anti-inflammatory cytokines suppress inflammation and promote healing. However, the role of cytokines in disease is probably more complex than that suggested by this simple classification for a number of reasons. First, the same cytokine may have a beneficial or detrimental role in different immune-mediated diseases: for example, excessive production of tumour necrosis factor α (TNF-α) is detrimental in rheumatoid arthritis (RA), while TNF-α appears to have a protective role in multiple sclerosis [**1**]. Secondly, cytokines can have a bimodal mechanism of action depending on the disease stage. For instance, TNF-α appears to be required for autoimmunity to be suppressed early in the course of systemic lupus erythematosus (SLE), whereas its presence may aid the development of lupus nephritis in established SLE. Thirdly, cytokines exert multiple functions ('pleiotropism') and can interact with other cytokines (the 'cytokine network'): this makes it difficult to dissect their specific *in vivo* effects and to predict the response to specific anticytokine therapy. Furthermore, cytokines also exert important physiological functions, and excessive blockade of a cytokine can therefore cause unwanted adverse reactions. For these reasons, extensive laboratory observations and studies in animal models are required in order to define the most appropriate therapeutic targets in different human diseases. Promising therapies must subsequently be tested in rigorous clinical trials to establish the optimal dose, timing of administration, clinical efficacy, and safety [**2**].

Table 3.1 Schematic overview of the biological effects of the principal inflammatory cytokines with particular regard to inflammatory rheumatic conditions

Inflammatory cytokines	Biological targets	Effects in inflammatory rheumatic diseases
TNF-α, IL-1	Central nervous system	Fever, fatigue, anorexia
TNF-α, IL-1	Adipocytes (enhance the release of free fatty acids and suppress lipoprotein lipase)	Weight loss, cachexia
TNF-α, IL-1	Chemokines (enhanced production)	Increase the influx of inflammatory cells from the circulation into joints
IL-8	Neutrophils (acts as chemoattractant)	Increases the influx of neutrophils into inflamed joints
TNF-α, IL-1	Cell adhesion molecules (increased synthesis and up-regulation on inflammatory cells and vascular endothelium)	Increase the influx of inflammatory cells from the circulation into joints
TNF-α, IL-1	IFN-γ and IL-12 (enhanced production)	Skew the T-cell response to the pro-inflammatory Th1 phenotype
TNF-α, IL-1	T cells (activation)	Contribute to maintenance inflammation within joints
TNF-α, IL-1	Matrix metalloproteinases (enhanced production)	Favour joint cartilage and bone damage, including periarticular osteopenia and bone erosions
TNF-α, IL-1	Angiogenic factors (enhanced production)	Favour neoangiogenesis (sprouting of new blood vessels in the inflamed synovium)
TNF-α, IL-1	Inflammatory prostaglandins (enhanced production)	Articular pain
TNF-α, IL-1	Nitrix oxide (enhanced production)	Favour joint cartilage and bone damage
TNF-α, IL-1, IL-6	Acute-phase reactants (enhanced production)	Raised acute-phase reactants

Source: Choy and Panayi (2001) |**3**|.

Role of cytokines in rheumatoid arthritis

RA is a chronic inflammatory disease characterized by a destructive arthropathy and variable extra-articular manifestations. The aetiology of RA remains elusive, but some evidence suggests a pathogenic role for $CD4^+$ T cells |**3**|. More specifically, activated $CD4^+$ T cells have been shown to stimulate B cells to produce immunoglobulins, including rheumatoid factor, and to stimulate macrophages and fibroblasts to produce inflammatory cytokines, such as TNF-α, interleukin (IL)-1 and IL-6. Most of the cytokines produced, including TNF-α and IL-1, are indeed detectable at high concentrations in the serum and synovial fluid from patients with active RA. Both TNF-α and IL-1 are able to increase the production of enzymes, such as matrix metalloproteinases, which mediate cartilage degradation and bone resorption. In addition, they also stimulate the migration of inflammatory cells from the circulation into the joints by inducing the synthesis of specific chemoattractants (chemokines) and by up-regulating cell adhesion molecules on the inflammatory cells and on the vascular endothelium. Laboratory observations and *in vivo* studies suggest that TNF-α has a dominant role in triggering the cascade of inflammatory cytokines |**4**|, while IL-1 seems to play a more important role than TNF-α in inducing cartilage and bone damage. These effects are counteracted, to some extent, by the anti-inflammatory cytokines IL-4 and IL-10. However, although both IL-4 and IL-10 are found in synovial fluid from RA patients, their amounts are insufficient to suppress inflammation.

Role of cytokines in the spondyloarthropathies, including psoriatic arthritis and ankylosing spondylitis

Psoriatic arthritis (PsA) and ankylosing spondylitis (AS) belong to the family of spondyloarthropathies, a group of diseases that share a number of genetic, pathogenic and clinical features. Recently, imaging studies have demonstrated that enthesitis (inflammation of tendon insertions) is a common and early event in the spondyloarthropathies but not in RA |**5**|. On this basis, it has been postulated that enthesitis could represent the basic lesion of the spondyloarthropathies, leading to ankylosing of the spine as well as to joint synovitis when the inflamed entheses are located in proximity to peripheral joints. However, other factors must intervene to modulate disease expression, since both PsA and AS can present with variable disease severity and with different patterns of joint involvement (for instance, some patients with AS can develop large-joint arthritis).

There is evidence that cytokines are involved both in the pathogenesis of enthesitis and in the modulation of disease severity in the spondyloarthropathies. In particular, *in situ* hybridization techniques have revealed the presence of TNF-α in inflamed entheses, the axial skeleton and peripheral joints, while IL-1 has been detected at high concentrations in the synovial fluid from affected joints. By contrast, there is evidence that patients with less severe (non-erosive) arthritis, including PsA, produce higher amounts of the anti-inflammatory cytokine IL-10 compared with those with erosive disease |**6**|. Thus, cytokines appear to be involved in the pathogenesis of both enthesitis and arthritis in the spondyloarthropathies.

Available anticytokine therapies for rheumatic diseases

There are different approaches to the suppression of inflammation, by tilting the balance between pro-inflammatory and anti-inflammatory cytokines (Fig. 3.1).

These include the neutralization of cytokines by soluble receptors or monoclonal antibodies, receptor blockade, and the activation of anti-inflammatory pathways by counter-regulatory cytokines |3|. Other potential therapeutic strategies include the

Cytokine–receptor interaction	Description	Examples
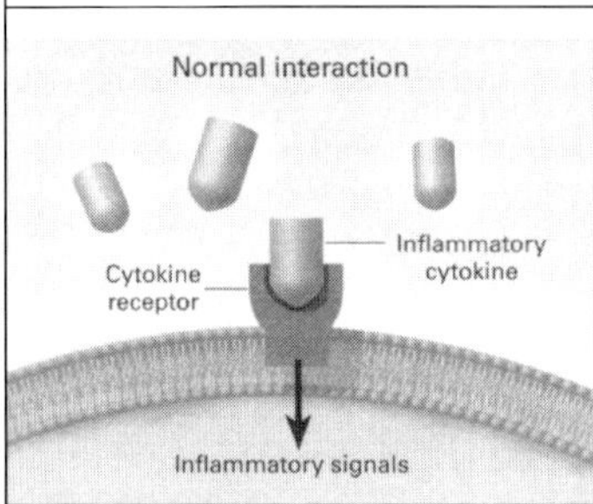	Binding of an inflammatory cytokine to its receptor leads to the production of inflammatory effector molecules	Tumor necrosis factor α, interleukin-1, and interleukin-6
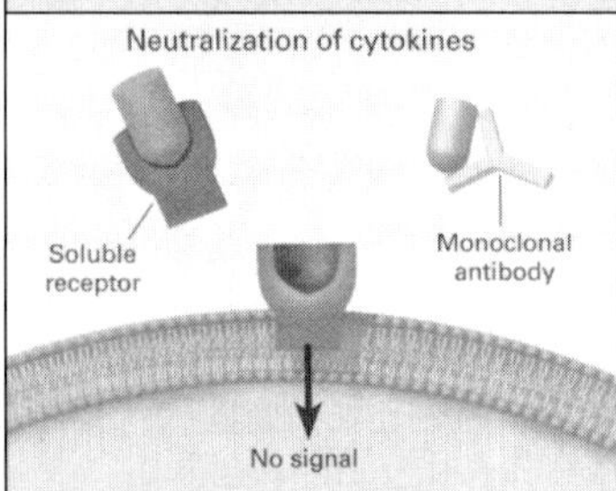	The cytokine is prevented from binding to its cell-surface receptor by soluble receptor, natural antagonists, or monoclonal antibody	Soluble tumor necrosis factor-receptor fusion proteins (etanercept), soluble interleukin-1 receptor, monoclonal antibody against tumor necrosis factor (infliximab, D2E7, nerelimomab), and monoclonal antibody against interleukin-6
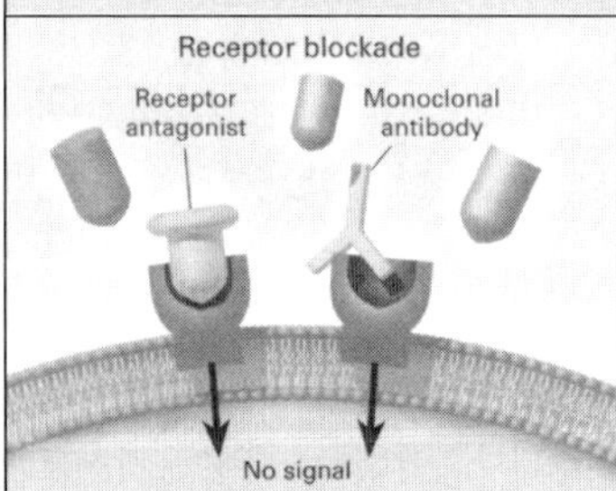	The cytokine is unable to bind its receptor because of interactions with a receptor antagonist or a monoclonal antibody against the cytokine receptor	Recombinant interleukin-1-receptor antagonist and monoclonal antibody against interleukin-6 receptor
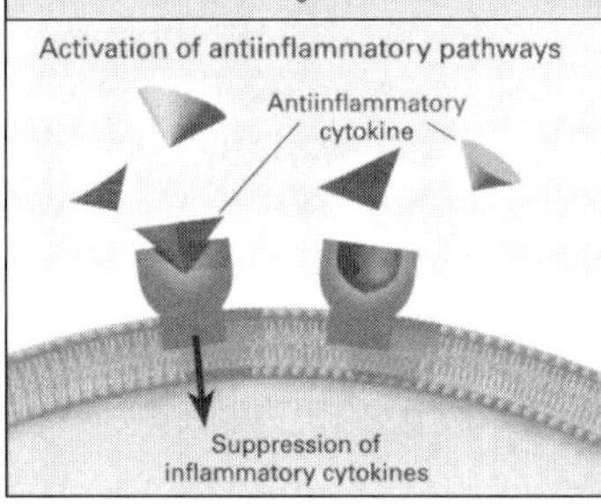	Antiinflammatory cytokines inhibit the expression of inflammatory cytokine	Interleukin-4 and interleukin-10

Fig. 3.1 Methods of blocking the activity of an inflammatory cytokine. Source: Choy and Panayi (2001) |**3**|.

use of inhibitors of cytokine intracellular signal transduction and inhibitors of the enzymes that convert cytokines from a biologically inactive to an active form.

To date, established anticytokine therapies for inflammatory rheumatic conditions are biological agents targeting TNF-α and IL-1 in view of the central role of these cytokines in driving the inflammatory response and causing joint damage. Three anti-TNF-α compounds are currently licensed for use in RA resistant to conventional disease-modifying antirheumatic drugs (DMARDs): etanercept (a recombinant human TNF-α receptor:Fc fusion protein), infliximab (a chimeric human–murine monoclonal antibody [mAb]), and adalimumab, a fully human mAb (Table 3.2) [7]. Infliximab, in combination with methotrexate (MTX), is licensed for patients with severe progressive RA, not previously treated with MTX or other DMARDs. There is only one inhibitor of IL-1 activity approved for use in DMARD-resistant RA: anakinra, a recombinant form of the human IL-1 receptor antagonist (IL-1Ra), which blocks the biological activity of IL-1 by competitively inhibiting IL-1 from binding to its receptor (Table 3.2).

Indication for anticytokine therapy in rheumatoid arthritis

RA runs a variable course but in most patients it has a poor long-term outcome, with significant disability and increased mortality. DMARDs prevent articular damage and functional deterioration; however, a sizeable proportion of patients have an incomplete clinical response, while about 10% of all RA patients are DMARD-resistant. Therefore, it is important to consider therapy with biological agents in all patients with highly active, refractory disease, not only to control the symptoms but also to improve the disease outcome. To ensure consistency across different centres, it has been agreed that severe disease activity should be properly defined using an appropriate index. To this end, in Europe the disease activity score based on a 28-joint count (DAS28) has been chosen. The DAS28 is a composite index that takes into account four variables: tender joint count, swollen joint count, erythrocyte sedimentation rate and the patient's global assessment of disease activity. In the UK, a DAS28 higher than 5.1 denotes highly active disease and is an indication for anti-TNF-α therapy if at least two DMARDs, including MTX, have been ineffective or poorly tolerated.

Using the criteria mentioned above, randomized controlled trials (RCTs) of biological agents in DMARD-resistant RA patients have clearly shown a satisfactory clinical response in at least 60% of treated subjects, with a noticeable improvement in quality of life and radiographic progression of RA also [8]. Subgroup analysis of the ATTRACT (Anti TNF Trial in Rheumatoid Arthritis with Concomitant Therapy) trial suggested the benefit was greatest in patients with disease for less than 3 years [9]. There are no head-to-head studies comparing the different biological agents, but TNF-α blockers appear to have similar efficacy overall.

Table 3.2 Biological agents used in rheumatic conditions

Agent	Specificity	Structure	Mode of action	Half-life	Administration
Infliximab (Remicade®, Centocor, Malvern, PA, USA)	Soluble and membrane-bound TNF-α	Chimeric monoclonal antibody with a murine antigen-binding domain linked to the Fc of human IgG1	Binds soluble and membrane-bound TNF-α with a lytic effect on cells expressing TNF-α	8–9 days	3–10 mg/kg intravenously every 8 weeks together with methotrexate
Etanercept (Enbrel®, Immunex Co., Seattle, WA, USA)	Soluble and membrane-bound TNF-α	Dimer of the extracellular domain of the p75 TNF-α receptor and of the Fc of human IgG1	Binds soluble and membrane-bound TNF-α (non-lytic)	4 days	25 mg subcutaneously twice weekly
Adalimumab (Humira®, Abbott Immunology, Abbott Park, IN, USA)	Soluble and membrane-bound TNF-α	Anti-TNF-α monoclonal antibody indistinguishable from human IgG1	Binds soluble and membrane-bound TNF-α, probably with a lytic effect on cells expressing TNF-α	11–12 days	40 mg subcutaneously every second week
Anakinra® (Amgen, Thousand Oaks, CA, USA)	Soluble and membrane-bound IL-1	Human IL-1 receptor antagonist	Acts as a competitive inhibitor of IL-1 binding to its receptor	4–6 hours	100 mg subcutaneously daily

Long-term safety and efficacy of biological therapies in rheumatoid arthritis

Infliximab and etanercept have been used for the treatment of refractory RA for nearly a decade, with encouraging results. However, the issue has arisen whether the clinical benefit conferred by anti-TNF-α inhibitors (with or without concomitant MTX therapy) and by the more recent IL-1Ra can be sustained, and whether toxicity will emerge in the longer term. So far, a number of serious adverse reactions during anti-TNF-α therapy have been reported. These include (1) reactivation of tuberculosis (TB), (2) the development and/or worsening of heart failure and demyelinating disorders, and (3) increased susceptibility to infection and worsening of pre-existing infections [10]. An updated list of adverse events is available on the website of the Food and Drug Administration (www.fda.gov).

The longer-term safety profile of the IL-1Ra anakinra is less well established, but available data suggest that reactions at injection sites occur in approximately 70% of treated patients, only a small minority of patients developing serious infections [11]. Here we discuss a number of recent studies that have addressed the issues of the longer-term efficacy and safety (separately or in combination) of biological agents in active RA.

Etanercept added to background methotrexate therapy in patients with rheumatoid arthritis: continued observations

Kremer JM, Weinblatt ME, Bankhurst AD, *et al.* *Arthritis Rheum* 2003; **48**: 1493–9

BACKGROUND. MTX is considered the DMARD of choice for RA because of its superior long-term effectiveness and favourable safety profile. However, a significant number of patients do not achieve an adequate clinical response even at a full therapeutic dose. It has been shown previously that therapy with infliximab or etanercept added to background MTX is more effective than therapy with MTX alone, but questions remain regarding whether the benefit can be sustained and whether toxicity will emerge. In a previous 6-month RCT in patients with active RA despite MTX therapy, etanercept added to MTX was significantly superior to MTX alone in terms of clinical efficacy, and was also well tolerated. To address the question of longer-term efficacy and safety, 79 of the 89 patients enrolled in the original blinded study were recruited in an open-label extension of the study of 3 years' duration.

INTERPRETATION. At the 3-year assessment, 77% of the 57 patients available for evaluation met the American College of Rheumatology (ACR) 20 criteria, 47% met the ACR50 criteria, and 23% met the ACR70 criteria (Fig. 3.2). Thirty out of 36 patients on corticosteroids (83%) were able to decrease their dosages of corticosteroids and 20 (56%) were able to discontinue corticosteroid therapy. The dosage of MTX was decreased in 41 of 66 patients (62%) and MTX therapy was discontinued in 19 patients (29%).

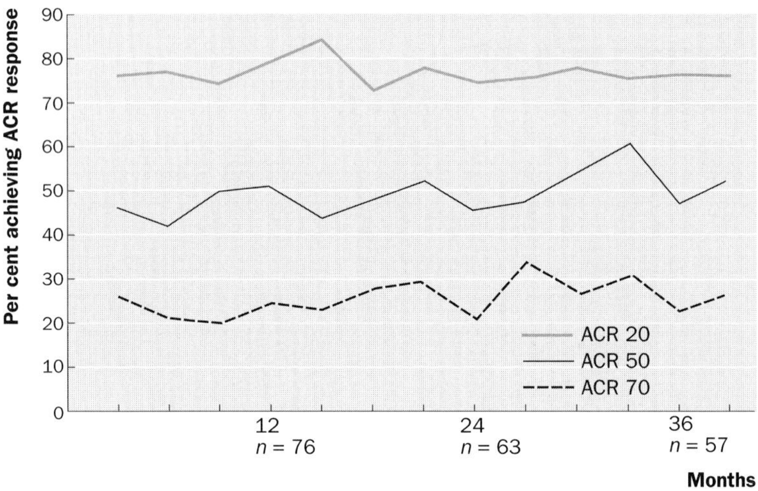

Fig. 3.2 American College of Rheumatology 20% improvement (ACR20), ACR50, and ACR70 rates over time. Patients were not always available for evaluation. Source: Kremer *et al.* (2003).

Comment

This observational continuation study shows that the addition of etanercept to background MTX provides sustained clinical benefit over 3 years. The clinical amelioration is clearly reflected by the high ACR response rates as well as by the trends to dosage reduction or discontinuation of MTX and corticosteroids. Regrettably, no X-rays were taken to ascertain whether this clinical benefit was paralleled by a delay in the radiographic progression of the disease. No increase in the rate of adverse events was observed. However, because of the limited number of patients recruited, it is difficult to make any conclusive statement about long-term safety, which is best evaluated by post-marketing surveillance.

Sustained improvement over two years in physical function, structural damage, and signs and symptoms among patients with rheumatoid arthritis treated with infliximab and methotrexate

Maini RN, Breedveld FC, Kalden JR, *et al. Arthritis Rheum* 2004; **50**: 1051–65

Background. For the proportion of RA patients who fail to respond to DMARDs and continue to manifest disease activity and structural damage, together with diminished quality of life, treatment with infliximab has been found to be effective and safe over a

1-year period. The ATTRACT trial was designed to evaluate the prolonged efficacy of infliximab plus MTX. This paper describes the sustained benefit in physical function as assessed by using the Health Assessment Questionnaire and the improvements in signs and symptoms over a 2-year period. Due to the improvements apparent at the end of the 1-year, placebo-controlled phase of the study, the second year was an open-label follow-up since, given the extent of improvements with infliximab treatment, it was considered unethical to allow patients to be treated with placebo.

Interpretation. This was a multinational, placebo-controlled, 1-year study, with a 2-year open follow-up, during which 428 patients with active RA were treated with infusions of 3 mg/kg or 10 mg/kg infliximab or placebo, in addition to MTX at the same dose as patients had been receiving prior to study entry. In one group, patients received either 3 mg/kg or 10 mg/kg infusions every 4 weeks; in the other group, patients received the infliximab infusions every 8 weeks with placebo infusions at the interim 4-week visits. The Health Assessment Questionnaire was administered every 4 weeks. The primary analysis was the mean change in the Health Assessment Questionnaire over the two-year period. Reduced disability was associated with a positive mean response. In addition, quality of life (SF-36), structural damage to hands and feet (total radiographic scores), clinical response (ACR20), and safety (adverse events and lab evaluations) were assessed. Of 259 patients who entered the second year of treatment, 216 continued to receive infliximab plus MTX for 102 weeks; 94 experienced a gap in therapy of >8 weeks. At 102 weeks, despite the gap in therapy for almost half the patients, the infliximab plus MTX regimens resulted in significantly greater improvement in Health Assessment Questionnaire scores ($P \leq 0.006$) and SF-36 Physical Component Summary scores ($P \leq 0.011$) compared with the MTX-only group; the Mental Component Summary score remained stable. Median changes in the total radiographic score were 0.50 for patients who received the infliximab plus MTX regimen compared with 4.25 for patients on the MTX-only regimen. Forty per cent to 48% of patients in the infliximab plus MTX groups achieved an ACR20 response at week 102 compared with 16% for the MTX-only group. Serious adverse event profiles were similar in the infliximab plus MTX and MTX-only groups.

Comment

In patients who failed to achieve a sufficient response to MTX alone, the combination of infliximab plus MTX was effective and well tolerated over a two-year period. There were clinically meaningful and statistically significant improvements in physical function and quality of life, along with inhibition of progressive joint damage and improved signs and symptoms of RA.

Treatment of rheumatoid arthritis with tumor necrosis factor inhibitors may predispose to significant increase in tuberculosis risk: a multicenter active-surveillance report

Gomez-Reino JJ, Carmona L, Valverde VR, Mola EM, Montero MD. *Arthritis Rheum* 2003; **48**: 2122–7

Background. Recent evidence based on spontaneous reporting has shown an association of anti-TNF-α agents with reactivation of TB. This study aimed to determine

the long-term safety of two such agents, infliximab and etanercept, in rheumatic diseases based on a Spanish surveillance system following the commercialization of the drugs. To this end, the safety data collected in a database launched in February 2000 by the Spanish Society of Rheumatology were analysed. For the estimation of TB risk, the annual incidence rate in patients treated with these agents was compared with the background rate and with the rate in a cohort of patients with arthritis assembled before the era of anti-TNF-α treatment.

Interpretation. Seventy-one participating centres in Spain sent data on 1578 treatments with infliximab (86%) or etanercept (14%) in 1540 arthritic patients. Seventeen cases of culture-confirmed TB were found in patients (15 RA, 2 PsA) treated with infliximab. The estimated incidence of TB associated with infliximab in arthritic patients was 1893 per 100 000 in 2000 and 1113 per 100 000 in 2001. These findings represent a significantly increased risk compared with the background rate in the overall population, assumed to amount to 21 cases per 100 000 based on the official report for 2000. Prophylaxis against TB was not implemented in 13 patients, and it is unclear whether the remaining five patients received it. TB protein derivative skin testing was negative in four patients (who also had normal chest X-rays), and was not done in nine patients; there are no data on the remaining patients. Sixty-five per cent of the study patients developed extrapulmonary TB, with disseminated or hepatosplenic disease in 35% of cases and involvement of the central nervous system in 29% of cases. Two patients (12%) died of TB, compared with an average mortality rate of less than 5% in the general population in the USA in 2000. However, in the first 5 months of 2002, after official guidelines had been established for TB prevention in patients treated with biologicals, only one new TB case was registered (in January).

Comment

This study confirms previous observations that therapy with infliximab is associated with an increased risk of developing active TB. The study did not evaluate the incidence of TB while on adalimumab therapy, but other sources indicate that the TB risk associated with adalimumab (18 cases among 2334 treated patients in pre-marketing studies) falls somewhere between those of the two older anti-TNF-α agents. It is noteworthy that no new cases of TB were recorded in Spanish patients treated with biological agents after February 2002, following the establishment of official guidelines for TB prevention. These guidelines require that any patients with risk factors for developing active TB (exposure to active TB, previous inadequately treated TB, and positive PPD test) scheduled to undergo anti-TNF-α therapy should receive isoniazid (5 mg/kg/day up to 300 mg/daily) prophylaxis for 9 months. The optimal timing of TB prophylaxis remains to be established, but a minimum of 1 month of isoniazid treatment prior to anti-TNF-α therapy seems to be prudent. The Spanish guidelines are in good agreement with data from the American Thoracic Society, which have demonstrated that a 9-month course of isoniazid treatment decreases the rate of developing TB by at least 70%.

It is unclear whether all patients receiving biological agents were actually registered in the database; this information would be required in order to ascertain how reliable the reported high TB incidence rates are. Still, the data of this study are in keeping with previous results showing an increased risk of active TB while on infliximab therapy, and constitute a valuable source of information not only on the incidence of TB but also on the effectiveness of TB prophylaxis in a large number of rheumatic patients treated with biological agents.

Case reports of heart failure after therapy with a tumor necrosis factor antagonist

Kwon HJ, Cote TR, Cuffe MS, Kramer JM, Braun MM. *Ann Intern Med* 2003; **138**: 807–11

BACKGROUND. More than a decade ago, patients with advanced heart failure were shown to have increased serum levels of TNF-α, which correlated with the severity of the disease. On this basis, treatment of such patients with TNF-α inhibitors was proposed. However, a phase II trial of infliximab versus placebo in 150 patients with heart failure was stopped early because it showed excessive mortality (7 deaths versus 0) and hospitalization rates in the infliximab group. Subsequently, there have been various articles linking anti-TNF-α therapy to cardiac failure. In this case series study, Kwon *et al.* have reviewed adverse events of heart failure after TNF-α antagonists reported to the US Food and Drug Administration's Med Watch programme up to February 2002.

INTERPRETATION. After TNF-α antagonist therapy, 38 patients developed new-onset heart failure and nine patients experienced heart failure exacerbation. The mean time from onset of anti-TNF-α therapy to the diagnosis of heart failure was approximately 4 months. Of the 38 patients with new-onset heart failure, 19 (50%) had no identifiable risk factors. Ten patients younger than 50 years developed new-onset heart failure after receiving TNF antagonists; again, no risk factors were identified in this subset of patients. After TNF antagonist therapy was discontinued and heart failure therapy was started in these ten patients, three had complete resolution of heart failure, six improved and one died.

Comment

This case series provides evidence that, in a proportion of patients, TNF-α antagonists may induce new-onset heart failure or exacerbate a pre-existing disease. The prevalence of heart failure in patients receiving TNF-α therapy appears to be low, although the actual prevalence may be higher because reporting to Med Watch is voluntary. Heart failure is common (more than 5%) in subjects aged 60–69 years, while RA patients have an increased risk of cardiovascular complications. Thus, it may be argued that the link between TNF-α therapy and cardiac failure remains tenuous. However, the occurrence of heart failure in young patients and the resolution or improvement of this condition after withdrawal of TNF-α therapy suggest a causal connection. Clinicians should be aware of this potential complication and be vigilant when patients on TNF-α inhibitors develop symptoms and/or signs of cardiac failure.

Long-term safety and maintenance of clinical improvement following treatment with anakinra (recombinant human interleukin-1 receptor antagonist) in patients with rheumatoid arthritis: extension phase of a randomized, double-blind, placebo-controlled trial

Nuki G, Bresnihan B, Bear MB, McCabe D. *Arthritis Rheum* 2002; **46**: 2838–46

BACKGROUND. The efficacy and safety of anakinra have been demonstrated previously in the short term in a 24-week RCT in 472 patients with active RA. The aim of this 52-week, double-blind, parallel-group extension phase of the trial was to establish the longer-term efficacy and safety of therapy with anakinra.

INTERPRETATION. Of the 345 patients, 309 of those enrolled initially continued in a 52-week double-blind extension phase of the study. Patients received subcutaneous injections of anakinra (30, 75 or 150 mg) once daily. Two hundred and eighteen patients completed the extension phase. Ninety-one patients withdrew prematurely, 46 because of adverse events and 26 due to lack of efficacy. Among patients receiving anakinra who entered the extension phase, the level of improvement was maintained for 48 weeks. At week 48, the ACR20 response was 46%, while ACR50 and ACR70 responses were demonstrated in 18 and 3% of patients, respectively, who continued taking anakinra (all dose groups) and in 20 and 1% of patients, respectively, who were originally receiving placebo and were then randomized to all doses of anakinra. There was a significant improvement in acute-phase reactants in the patients switched from placebo to anakinra; similarly, the tender and swollen joint count significantly improved in the patients switched from placebo to anakinra (except for those treated with 30 mg daily) and remained stable in the patients continuing to receive anakinra (Table 3.3). However, there was a small but significant decline in functional capacity, as evaluated by the Health Assessment Questionnaire. The results of the radiographic assessments, published in a separate study, showed that anakinra reduced the progression of articular damage. Anakinra was well tolerated; the only side effect was judged to be treatment-related injection-site reactions.

Comment

This study demonstrates that the clinical benefit of treatment with anakinra in active RA patients was maintained for up to 48 weeks. The ACR response rates observed appeared to be somehow lower than those reported in most clinical trials with anti-TNF-α therapy. This study was not ideally suited to the evaluation of treatment safety, but the results of a study that aimed specifically to investigate the longer-term safety of therapy with anakinra are reported below.

Table 3.3 Changes in ACR component outcome measures during the second 6 months of treatment with anakinra during extension study*

Outcome measure	Placebo to anakinra				Anakinra to anakinra			
	All doses (*n* = 76)	**30 mg (*n* = 30)**	**75 mg (*n* = 24)**	**150 mg (*n* = 22)**	**All doses (*n* = 233)**	**30 mg (*n* = 81)**	**75 mg (*n* = 79)**	**150 mg (*n* = 73)**
No. of swollen joints	–4.1 ± 1.1†	–3.2 ± 2.1	–5.0 ± 2.1‡	–4.4 ± 1.2§	–0.9 ± 0.5	–0.3 ± 0.9	–1.5 ± 0.9	–0.9 ± 1.1
No. of tender joints	–5.6 ± 1.3†	–5.2 ± 2.6	–6.1 ± 1.9§	–5.5 ± 1.8‡	–0.2 ± 0.9	–0.3 ± 1.2	–1.2 ± 1.8	+1.0 ± 1.6
Patient global assessment	–0.3 ± 0.1‡	–0.2 ± 0.2	–0.3 ± 0.1‡	–0.3 ± 0.2	+0.1 ± 0.1	+0.1 ± 0.1	0.0 ± 0.1	+0.2 ± 0.1‡
Investigator assessment	–0.3 ± 0.1‡	–0.4 ± 0.2	–0.3 ± 0.1	–0.2 ± 0.2	0.0 ± 0.1	0.0 ± 0.1	0.0 ± 0.1	0.1 ± 0.1
Pain assessment	–0.09 ± 0.03§	–0.08 ± 0.04	–0.07 ± 0.05	–0.12 ± 0.07	+0.03 ± 0.02	+0.04 ± 0.03	–0.01 ± 0.03	+0.07 ± 0.03‡
Health Assessment Questionnaire	–0.26 ± 0.05†	–0.33 ± 0.1§	–0.11 ± 0.1	–0.35 ± 0.1§	+0.06 ± 0.03‡	+0.08 ± 0.05	–0.01 ± 0.04	+0.1 ± 0.05‡
C–reactive protein level, mg/dl	–1.0 ± 0.3§	–1.2 ± 0.5‡	–0.8 ± 0.5	–1.1 ± 0.6	+0.02 ± 0.2	–0.02 ± 0.3	–0.07 ± 0.3	–0.01 ± 0.3
Erythrocyte sedimentation rate, mm/h	–11.9 ± 2.2†	–11.9 ± 3.4§	–15.0 ± 3.4†	–8.2 ± 4.9	–1.7 ± 1.4	–1.3 ± 2.3	–3.2 ± 2.0	–0.5 ± 2.9

ACR, American College of Rheumatology. *Values are the mean ± SEM. †$P < 0.001$ by paired *t*-test. ‡$P < 0.05$ by paired *t*-test. §$P < 0.005$ by paired *t*-test.
Source: Nuki *et al.* (2002).

Anakinra, a recombinant human interleukin-1 receptor antagonist (r-metHuIL-1ra), in patients with rheumatoid arthritis: a large, international, multicenter, placebo-controlled trial

Fleischmann RM, Schechtman J, Bennett R, *et al. Arthritis Rheum* 2002; **48**: 927–34

BACKGROUND. This study aimed to evaluate the safety of anakinra in a large population of patients with RA representative of those seen in community practices.

INTERPRETATION. A total of 1414 patients were randomly assigned to treatment with 100 mg of anakinra (n = 1116) or placebo (n = 283), administered daily subcutaneously (15 patients were randomized but did not receive any study drug). Background medications included DMARDs, corticosteroids and non-steroidal anti-inflammatory drugs (NSAIDs), alone or in combination. The study was designed to exclude as few patients as possible, but patients with malignancies, infections or serious uncontrolled medical conditions and pregnant and breast-feeding women were not included. Safety was evaluated by recording adverse events, discontinuation from the study due to adverse events, and death. Baseline demographics, disease characteristics and concomitant medications were similar in the anakinra and placebo groups. The study group included patients with numerous co-morbid conditions and a wide range of RA disease activity. Serious adverse events were observed at similar rates in the anakinra group and the placebo group (7.7 and 7.8%, respectively). Serious infectious episodes were observed more frequently in the anakinra group (2.1 versus 0.4% in the placebo group). The rate of withdrawal due to adverse events was 13.4% in the anakinra group and 9.2% in the placebo group. Reactions at injection sites were more common in the anakinra (72.6%) than in the placebo group (32.9%).

Comment

This study is well suited to the identification of adverse reactions due to anakinra for two reasons: first, because of the large number of patients enrolled, and secondly because the study population was representative of community patients, including those with co-morbidities and those using multiple concomitant therapies. The results demonstrate that anakinra is safe and well tolerated in a diverse population of patients with RA. The frequency of serious infection was slightly higher in the anakinra group; however, no infection was attributed to opportunistic micro-organisms or resulted in death.

Treatment of DMARD-resistant RA with the new monoclonal antibody adalimumab and MTX

As we mentioned above in this chapter, patients treated with the chimeric mAb infliximab may develop an immune reaction to its murine component, resulting in decreased clinical efficacy and a heightened risk of adverse events. More recently, a fully humanized anti-TNF-α mAb, adalimumab, has been developed and successfully used as monotherapy or together with MTX in numerous trials to treat recalcitrant RA. Strictly speaking, adalimumab need not be co-prescribed with MTX as it lacks a murine component. However, since there is some evidence that the combination of MTX and anti-TNF-α therapy is synergistic, trials have been conducted to investigate the effectiveness of combined therapy with adalimumab and MTX. We report here the results of a recent study.

Adalimumab, a fully human anti-tumor necrosis factor alpha monoclonal antibody, for the treatment of rheumatoid arthritis in patients taking concomitant methotrexate: the ARMADA trial

Weinblatt ME, Keystone EC, Furst DE, *et al. Arthritis Rheum* 2003; **48**: 35–45

BACKGROUND. The ARMADA (Anti-TNF Research study program of the Monoclonal antibody Adalimumab [D2E7] in rheumatoid Arthritis] trial was designed to establish the efficacy and safety profile of adalimumab therapy added to MTX.

INTERPRETATION. In this 24-week RCT, 271 patients with active RA were randomly assigned to receive injections of adalimumab (20, 40 or 80 mg subcutaneously) or placebo every other week while continuing to take MTX at a stable dosage (mean dosage, 16.7 mg/week). At the study end, an ACR20 response was achieved by a significantly greater proportion of patients in the 20-, 40- and 80-mg adalimumab plus MTX groups (47.8, 67.2 and 65.8%, respectively) than in the placebo plus MTX group (14.5%) ($P < 0.001$) (Fig. 3.3). ACR50 response rates with the 20-, 40- and 80-mg adalimumab dosages (31.9, 55.2 and 42.5%, respectively) were also significantly greater than that with placebo (8.1%) ($P < 0.01$) (Fig. 3.3). The 40- and 80-mg doses of adalimumab were associated with statistically higher ACR70 response rates (26.9 and 19.2%, respectively) than that with placebo (4.8%) ($P < 0.001$ and $P = 0.020$) (Fig. 3.3). Responses were rapid, the greatest proportion of adalimumab-treated patients achieving an ACR20 response at week 1. In addition, there was an improvement in quality of life and a significant decrease in the levels of acute-phase reactants in the adalimumab group. Comparable numbers of adalimumab-treated and placebo-treated patients reported adverse events, although injection-site reactions were recorded more frequently in the adalimumab group (15.3%) than in the placebo group (3.2%).

Comment

This trial demonstrates that the addition of adalimumab to background MTX in patients with active RA provided significant, rapid and sustained improvement in disease activity over 24 weeks compared with MTX plus placebo. The optimal clinical response was observed with 40 mg, which is now the standard dosage for adalimumab therapy. A clear limitation of this trial is the lack of other active arms,

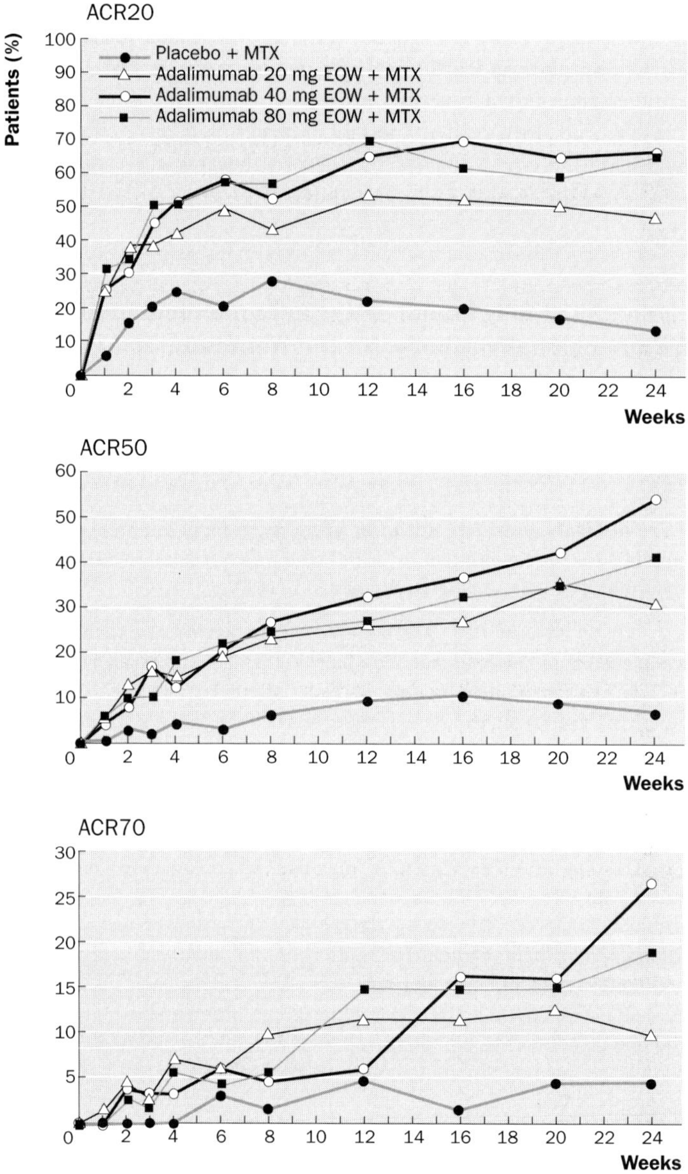

Fig. 3.3 Percentages of rheumatoid arthritis patients who met the American College of Rheumatology criteria for 20%, 50% and 70% improvement (ACR20, ACR50 and ACR70, respectively) during treatment with methotrexate (MTX) plus either placebo or adalimumab at a dosage of either 20 mg, 40 mg, or 80 mg administered subcutaneously every other week (EOW). Source: Weinblatt *et al.* (2003).

i.e. adalimumab alone and MTX alone. An RCT involving these additional arms is needed to clarify whether combined adalimumab/MTX therapy is indeed clinically superior to either agent alone.

Predicting the response to TNF-α blockade in RA: lessons from a study on the polymorphism of the TNF-α gene

Although TNF-α antagonists have been a major breakthrough in the management of RA, approximately 20% of patients respond inadequately to therapy with these drugs. Since anti-TNF-α treatment is expensive and has significant side effects, it is important to be able to predict which patients can benefit from this treatment. As the regulatory region of the TNF-α gene is polymorphic and certain alleles, such as –308A, are associated with high TNF-α production, theoretically genotyping may predict the response to TNF inhibitors. The following study investigated the relationship between the polymorphism at position –308 and the clinical response to infliximab in 59 RA patients treated over a 22-week period.

Polymorphism at position –308 of the tumor necrosis factor alpha gene influences outcome of infliximab therapy in rheumatoid arthritis

Mugnier B, Balandraud N, Darque A, Roudier C, Roudier J, Reviron D. *Arthritis Rheum* 2003; **48**: 1849–52

BACKGROUND. This study was set up to test whether the G→A polymorphism at position –308 in the promoter of the TNF-α gene influences the response to infliximab therapy in patients with RA.

INTERPRETATION. Fifty-nine RA patients were genotyped by the polymerase chain reaction and were subdivided into two groups: those with the A/A or A/G genotype and those with the G/G genotype. Clinical responses to infliximab treatment were compared between groups after 22 weeks, using the DAS28. The average improvement in the DAS28 score was 1.24 in the A/A and A/G patients and 2.29 in the G/G patients ($P = 0.029$).

Comment

These data suggest that patients with the TNF-α –308G/G genotype are better infliximab responders than are patients with the A/A or A/G genotype. This could be due to the fact that in A/A and A/G patients the TNF-α blockade is overwhelmed by the high production of TNF-α associated with these genotypes; however, this interpretation should be confirmed by showing that higher doses of TNF-α antagonists lead to better responses in A/A and A/G patients.

TNF-α inhibitors for psoriatic arthritis

PsA has traditionally been considered mostly a benign disease, but this assumption has been challenged. The current perception is that PsA can run a quite variable course, ranging from mild enthesitis to severe, destructive peripheral arthritis. In addition, a minority (about 5%) of patients develop inflammatory disease of the axial skeleton (psoriatic pelvispondylitis), which is notoriously resistant to treatment with conventional DMARDs. Recently, etanercept therapy has been demonstrated to be effective in PsA patients with recalcitrant peripheral synovitis and to have a beneficial effect on psoriatic skin lesions. Indeed, recent randomized control trials of infliximab and etanercept confirmed that these agents are effective treatment both for the skin disease as well as for the arthritis [12]. Here, we report an open study of infliximab treatment for psoriatic arthritis that shows similar encouraging results.

Open-label study of infliximab treatment for psoriatic arthritis: clinical and magnetic resonance imaging measurements of reduction of inflammation

Antoni C, Dechant C, Hanns-Martin Lorenz PD, *et al. Arthritis Rheum* 2002; **47**: 506–12

BACKGROUND. The purpose of this study was to evaluate infliximab efficacy and safety in disease-modifying antirheumatic drug-unresponsive PsA.

INTERPRETATION. In this 54-week, open-label study, ten patients with PsA received intravenous infliximab at a dose of 5 mg/kg at weeks 0, 2 and 6; the dose was individualized after week 10. Patients continued their current therapy (stable dose) until week 10. Assessments were performed at weeks 2, 6, 10 and 54. Magnetic resonance imaging (MRI) detection of gadolinium-DTPA was used to measure joint inflammation at weeks 0 and 10. All patients achieved an ACR20 response by week 2. Eight patients achieved an ACR70 response at week 10, which was sustained in six patients after week 54. MRI revealed an 82.5% mean reduction in gadolinium-DTPA uptake from baseline. The skin involvement was quantified by the psoriasis area and severity index (PASI), a measure of overall psoriasis severity and extension: a reduction of PASI score by 71 $\pm$ 17% was observed. No serious adverse events were recorded.

Comment

In this open trial, infliximab therapy significantly ameliorated arthritis and psoriasis in all ten PsA patients evaluated. The clinical benefit was very substantial; eight patients achieved an ACR70 response, which was sustained in six patients. The clinical improvement was paralleled by a major decrease in inflammation, as measured by MRI.

This trial confirms the efficacy of TNF-α blockade in PsA and is in agreement with the results of a previous RCT with etanercept. In addition, it demonstrates that MRI can be useful for monitoring the response to therapy with biological agents. The study has a number of limitations, including the lack of a placebo arm and the small number of patients enrolled. In addition, no patients with pelvispondylitis were included, which does not permit the extrapolation of the favourable response observed to this subset of patients. Nevertheless, the excellent clinical response, together with the concomitant reduction of joint inflammation on MRI, provides further evidence for the usefulness of TNF-α inhibitors in refractory PsA.

Treatment of ankylosing spondylitis with TNF-α inhibitors

AS is a chronic inflammatory disease that predominantly affects the axial skeleton. It is characterized by widespread inflammation and subsequent variable ossification of the entheses (insertions of tendons, ligaments and capsule into bone), mainly in the region of the spine and sacroiliac joints. Clinically, AS causes pain and stiffness of the spine, with progressive loss of spinal movements.

The treatment of AS is based on NSAIDs associated with physiotherapy. DMARDs are not effective for axial disease, although they can be beneficial when peripheral arthritis is present.

There is now mounting evidence from clinical studies, including RCTs, that TNF-α blockade is efficacious in patients with AS. More specifically, TNF-α inhibitors have been shown to (1) induce significant clinical amelioration, (2) suppress inflammation measured by MRI, and (3) counteract disease-related bone density loss. In patients with AS and concomitant Crohn's disease, infliximab has been shown to be effective for treating both conditions |**13**|. Hitherto, in Crohn's disease, etanercept seems ineffective whilst the effect of adalimumab is currently being tested. Here we present the results of recent studies that have investigated these issues.

Six-month results of a double blind, placebo-controlled trial of etanercept treatment in patients with active ankylosing spondylitis

Brandt J, Kharicuzov A, Listing J, *et al. Arthritis Rheum* 2003; **48**: 1667–75

BACKGROUND. There is increasing evidence that TNF-α is centrally involved in the pathogenesis of ankylosing spondylitis (AS) and other spondylarthritides. This study was designed to investigate the efficacy of anti-TNF-α therapy with etanercept, a 75-kDa receptor fusion protein, in active AS. This multicentre trial had two phases: an initial placebo-controlled period of 6 weeks' duration and an observational phase lasting 24 weeks.

INTERPRETATION. Thirty patients with active AS in spite of NSAID therapy were randomized to receive etanercept 25 mg subcutaneously twice weekly (n = 14) or placebo

($n = 16$) for 6 weeks; all patients received etanercept in the subsequent observational phase, lasting 24 weeks. DMARDs and steroids were withdrawn prior to the study. The primary outcome measure was a 50% improvement in the Bath AS Disease Activity Index (BASDAI), an index of disease activity that evaluates fatigue, pain and stiffness. Ancillary outcome measures included the Bath AS Functional Index (BASFI), which evaluates the impact of disability on different activities of daily living, the Bath AS Metrology Index (an index of spinal mobility), pain level on a numeric rating scale, quality of life (using the Short Form 36), and C-reactive protein levels. Fifty-seven per cent of the etanercept-treated patients but only 6% of patients receiving placebo ($P = 0.004$) had a 50% improvement in the BASDAI at week 6 (Fig. 3.4); when the placebo-treated patients switched to etanercept, 56% improved. Similarly, the other outcome variables improved significantly with etanercept but not with placebo at week 6. Disease relapses occurred on average 6 weeks after cessation of etanercept therapy. No severe adverse events were observed.

Comment

This study, in line with previous trials, confirms that etanercept is very effective in decreasing pain and improving function in the majority of patients with active AS resistant to NSAIDs. After cessation of therapy, almost all patients experienced a relapse within a few weeks. Thus, it seems probable that etanercept should be administered continuously in most AS patients to achieve permanent inhibition of the inflammatory process.

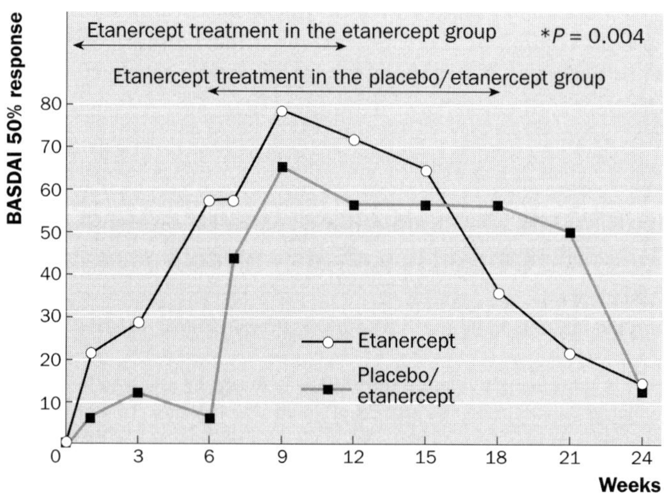

Fig. 3.4 Percentage of patients achieving at least 50% improvement in Bath Ankylosing Spondylitis Disease Activity Index. Source: Brandt *et al.* (2003).

Magnetic resonance imaging examinations of the spine in patients with ankylosing spondylitis, before and after successful therapy with infliximab: evaluation of a new scoring system

Braun J, Baraliakos X, Golder W, *et al. Arthritis Rheum* 2003; **48**: 1126–36

BACKGROUND. A fundamental question that remains to be answered is whether biological agents have truly disease-modifying properties in AS, i.e. whether they are able to suppress spinal inflammation effectively and to prevent the progressive ossification of the axial skeleton. Theoretically, the disease-modifying effect of anti-TNF-α therapy in AS could be assessed by evaluating its capacity to delay or halt radiographic disease progression. However, given the low sensitivity to change of X-ray lesions, 1 or 2 years may be required to capture significant differences. An alternative approach is to measure spinal inflammation by MRI, which is more sensitive than conventional radiography. The use of MRI to monitor the degree and extent of spinal inflammation has long been hampered by the lack of a validated method. Braun *et al.* demonstrate in the following study that inflammatory spinal lesions due to AS can be quantified by an activity and chronicity index based on MRI. This method can be useful in monitoring the response to biological agents in AS.

INTERPRETATION. Twenty patients with AS were examined at baseline and after 3 months. Nine patients received infusions of infliximab (5 mg/kg body weight) at weeks 0, 2 and 6, and eleven patients received placebo. Three MRI sequences and two scoring systems were used. Chronic lesions were evaluated by T_1-weighted turbo spin-echo (TSE) sequences and were assigned a chronicity score ranging from 0 to 6 (0 = no lesions, 6 = vertebral fusion) (Table 3.4). Active lesions were evaluated either by repetition of T_1-weighted TSE sequences after infusion of gadolinium-DTPA or by short-inversion recovery (STIR) sequences, and were assigned an activity score ranging from 0 to 6 (0 = normal, 6 = major [>50%] erosion with bone marrow oedema) (Table 3.4). Active spinal lesions were detected in 75% of the patients; the frequency as determined by STIR was equal in the two groups. The active lesion score, determined by gadolinium-DTPA, improved by 40% in the infliximab group compared with 6% in the placebo group (see the example in Fig. 3.5), while the active lesion score, determined by STIR, improved by 60% in the infliximab group but deteriorated by 21% in the placebo group. The chronic lesion score, determined by T_1, improved by 7% in the infliximab group but worsened by 35% in the placebo group. The acute MRI changes correlated with clinical improvement, as assessed by the BASDAI.

Comment

This novel MRI scoring system performed well in assessing acute inflammation by using STIR and post-gadolinium-DTPA sequences. The clinical improvement in patients with active AS treated with infliximab correlated with a significant regression of spinal inflammation according to the MRI activity scores. Thus, this study supports the use of MRI in monitoring the response to biological agents in AS and suggests that TNF-α inhibitors have disease-modifying properties in this condition.

Table 3.4 Scoring system using MRI to evaluate spinal lesions for acute and chronic changes in patients with AS

Activity score
0 = Normal, no lesions
1 = Minor bone marrow oedema/enhancement ≤25%
2 = Moderate bone marrow oedema/enhancement ≤50%
3 = Major bone marrow oedema/enhancement >50%
4 = Minor erosion (≤25%), with bone marrow oedema/enhancement
5 = Moderate erosion (>25% but ≤50%), with bone marrow oedema/enhancement
6 = Major erosion (>50%), with bone marrow oedema/enhancement

Chronicity score
0 = Normal, no lesions
1 = Minor sclerosis/suspicion of relevant changes
2 = Sclerosis/vertebral squaring/possible syndesmophyte
3 = 1–2 syndesmophytes/small erosions
4 = >2 syndesmophytes/spondylodiscitis/severe erosions
5 = Vertebral bridging
6 = Vertebral fusion

MRI, magnetic resonance imaging; AS, ankylosing spondylitis.
For scoring purposes, a vertebral unit (VU) was defined as the region between two virtual lines through the middle of each vertebra. For the activity score, enhancement and bone marrow oedema are graded as mild if covering ≤25% of a VU (grade 1), moderate if covering >25% but ≤50% of a VU (grade 2), and severe if covering >50% of a VU (grade 3). If, in addition to the signs of any acute inflammation, erosions are present, these are graded as minor if eroding ≤25% of a VU (grade 4), intermediate if eroding >25% but ≤50% of a VU (grade 5), and major if eroding >50% of a VU (grade 6). For the chronicity score, T1 sequences were used to assign a score ranging from 0 to 6, according to the presence and visibility of sclerosis, erosions, small and large syndesmophytes, and partial or complete ankylosis. Almost the complete spine was examined (from the middle of the second cervical vertebra to the middle of the first sacral vertebra), comprising 23 VUs. Thus, the maximum possible MRI score for both activity and chronicity was 138 (6 × 23).
Source: Braun *et al.* (2003).

Increase in bone mineral density of patients with spondyloarthropathy treated with anti-tumour necrosis factor

Allali F, Breban M, Porcher R, Maillefert J F, Dougados M, Roux C. *Ann Rheum Dis* 2003; **62**: 347–9

BACKGROUND. Patients with AS have an increased prevalence of osteoporosis (18.7–62% according to some reports) and a five-fold risk of developing pathological vertebral fractures (mainly in the spine) compared with age- and gender-matched controls. The pathogenesis of AS-associated osteoporosis is not fully elucidated, but excessive synthesis of inflammatory mediators, including TNF-α, and decreased mobility of the patient both probably play a role. The optimal treatment of osteoporosis secondary to AS remains to be established. In particular, at present there are no data addressing the value of bisphosphonates |14|. TNF-α has been shown to be an important

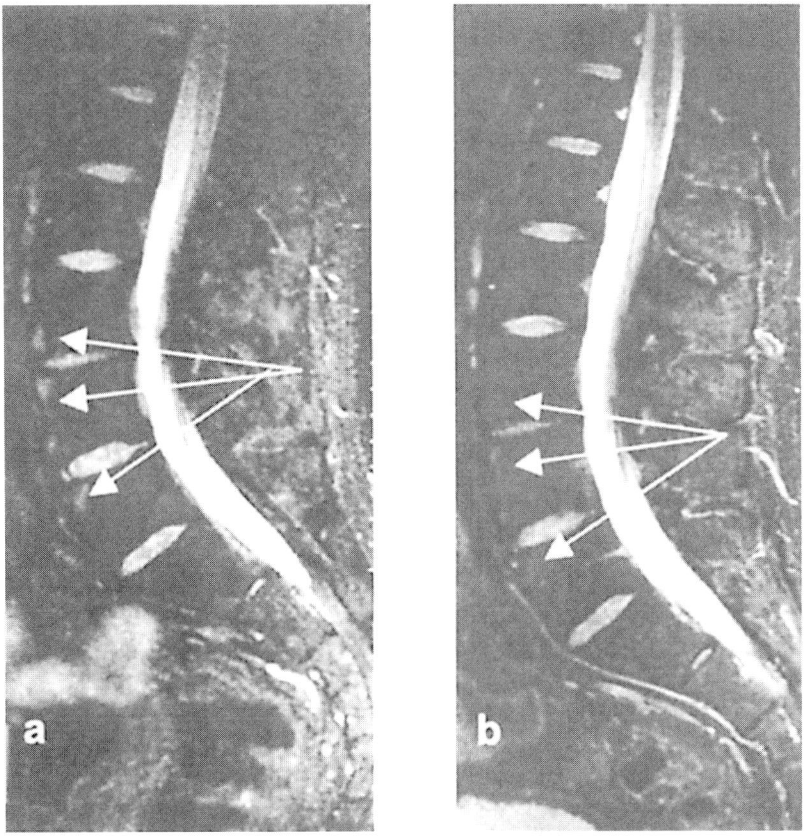

Fig. 3.5 Spondylitis anterior (L2, L3, L4) after application of Gd-DTPA, before (a) and after (b) 12 weeks of therapy with infliximab. The hyperintensity of the anterior edges of the vertebra is no longer detectable after therapy with infliximab. Source: Braun *et al.* (2003).

pathogenic factor in the spondyloarthropathies, including AS, and to mediate bone resorption in different conditions. Therefore, it may be hypothesized that TNF-α blockade may increase bone mineral density (BMD) in AS. The following study investigated this issue in a group of 29 patients with spondyloarthropathy, including 17 patients with inflammatory spinal pain as the leading symptom.

Interpretation. Twenty-nine patients (six women; 23 men) aged 22–68 years, with active spondyloarthropathy refractory to standard therapies, were treated with infliximab 5 mg/kg (n = 25) and 3 mg/kg (n = 4) at weeks 0, 2, 6 and then received either no infusion (n = 3) or an additional infusion of infliximab every other month (n = 6). The remainder received one infusion only in case of a relapse. Lumbar and femoral BMDs were measured by dual-energy X-ray absorptiometry at baseline and 6 months later. Serum osteocalcin (a marker of bone formation) and urinary deoxypyridinoline (a marker of bone resorption) were measured in 19 patients at weeks 0, 2 and 24 and in 13 patients at all visits. Over 6 months, BMD increased by 3.6% in the spine and by 2.2% in the total hip. There was also an increase in osteocalcin between baseline and week 6, but no change in urinary deoxypyridinoline was observed. There was no change in biochemical markers between the baseline and final visits. There was a trend for a correlation between the decrease at 6 months in erythrocyte sedimentation rate and BMD change in the lumbar spine ($r = -0.35$, $P = 0.06$).

Comment

These data suggest that anti-TNF-α therapy can lead to an increase in BMD in patients with spondyloarthropathy, including those with predominant axial disease. The increase in BMD seems genuine and not due to progression of ossification at the spine, since radiographic changes such as syndesmophytes and facet joint ankylosis do not vary significantly over 6 months. The mechanisms by which infliximab therapy results in increased BMD are not entirely clear. The increase in osteocalcin levels in the absence of changes in urinary deoxypyridinoline excretion suggests an uncoupling effect on bone turnover, with augmented bone formation but stable resorption. Further studies are warranted to clarify the mechanisms by which anti-TNF-α therapy interferes with bone metabolism.

Conclusion

Biological agents represent one of the major advances in the treatment of numerous inflammatory disorders, including refractory RA, PsA and AS. However, the introduction of these agents has raised a number of issues that ought to be considered in order to achieve optimal patient management. First, not all patients respond adequately to these agents, and one of today's challenges is therefore to try to identify those patients that can respond better to biological treatment without developing side effects. A second issue is whether the favourable efficacy and safety profile observed in most treated patients is maintained over time. The experience accrued so far suggests that this is indeed the case, but it will be important to monitor patients for the uncommon adverse events that usually emerge in the long term, such as lymphoma and other malignancies. Thirdly, all patients receiving biological agents should be monitored appropriately to document the effect of therapy on pain, articular disease, function, quality of life and radiographic disease progression. Fourthly, combination therapy with conventional DMARDs and possibly other agents should be further actively investigated to obtain the maximum clinical benefit. Finally, it is important that the use of biological agents be entrusted to physicians who have specific expertise in both the diseases treated and in the agents employed. This will ensure that optimal treatment schedules are developed in order to achieve long-term efficacy and safety.

References

1. Robinson WH, Genovese MC, Moreland LW. Demyelinating and neurologic events reported in association with tumor necrosis factor alpha antagonism: by what mechanisms could tumor necrosis factor alpha antagonists improve rheumatoid arthritis but exacerbate multiple sclerosis? *Arthritis Rheum* 2001; **44**: 1977–83.
2. Kollias G, Kontoyiannis D. Role of TNF/TNFR in autoimmunity: specific TNF receptor blockade may be advantageous to anti-TNF treatments. *Cytokine Growth Factor Rev* 2002; **13**: 315–21.
3. Choy EH, Panayi GS. Cytokine pathways and joint inflammation in rheumatoid arthritis. *N Engl J Med* 2001; **344**: 907–16.
4. Andreakos ET, Foxwell BM, Brennan FM, Maini RN, Feldmann M. Cytokines and anti-cytokine biologicals in autoimmunity: present and future. *Cytokine Growth Factor Rev* 2002; **13**: 299–313.
5. McGonagle D, Conaghan PG, Emery P. Psoriatic arthritis: a unified concept twenty years on. [Review]. *Arthritis Rheum* 1999; **42**: 1080–6. [Published erratum appears in *Arthritis Rheum* 1999; **42**: 1997].
6. Huizinga TW, Keijsers V, Yanni G, Hall M, Ramage W, Lanchbury J, Pitzalis C, Drossaers-Bakker WK, Westendorp RG, Breedveld FC, Panayi G, Verweij CL. Are differences in interleukin 10 production associated with joint damage? *Rheumatology* 2000; **39**: 1180–8.
7. Criscione LG, St Clair EW. Tumor necrosis factor-alpha antagonists for the treatment of rheumatic diseases. *Curr Opin Rheumatol* 2002; **14**: 204–11.
8. Kroot EJ, van de Putte LB, van Riel PL. Management of therapy-resistant rheumatoid arthritis. *Baillières Best Pract Res Clin Rheumatol* 1999; **13**: 737–52.
9. Breedveld FC, Emery P, Keystone E, Patel K, Furst DE, Kalden JR, St Clair EW, Weisman M, Smolen J. Lipsky PE, Maini RN, Infliximab in active early rheumatoid arthritis. *Ann Rheum Dis* 2004; **63**(2): 149–55.
10. Pressman LS. Use of biologics for rheumatoid arthritis tempered by concerns over safety, cost. *JAMA* 2003; **289**: 3229–30.
11. Jiang Y, Genant HK, Watt I, Cobby M, Bresnihan B, Aitchison R, McCabe D. A multicenter, double-blind, dose-ranging, randomized, placebo-controlled study of recombinant human interleukin-1 receptor antagonist in patients with rheumatoid arthritis: radiologic progression and correlation of Genant and Larsen scores. *Arthritis Rheum* 2000; **43**: 1001–9.
12. Kavanaugh A, Krueger G, De Vlam K, Birbara C, Beutler A, Guzzo C, Zhou B, DeWoody K, Antoni C. Infliximab improves arthritis and psoriasis in patients with active polyarticular psoriatic arthritis: results of the IMPACT 2 trial. *Ann Rheum Dis* 2004; **63**(Suppl I): Abstr. No. SAT0050.
13. Braun J, Kellner H, Deodhar A, Inman R, Han CL, DeWoody K, Williamson P, Bala M, van der Heijde D. Infliximab improves quality of life in patients with ankylosing spondylitis: results of a randomized, placebo-controlled trial (ASSERT). *Ann Rheum Dis* 2004; **63**(Suppl I): Abstr. No. SAT0049.
14. Bessant R, Keat A. How should clinicians manage osteoporosis in ankylosing spondylitis? *J Rheumatol* 2002; **29**: 1511–19.

4

Cardiovascular disease in rheumatoid arthritis

NAVEED SATTAR

Introduction

There are abundant data to indicate an excess cardiovascular morbidity and mortality in patients with rheumatoid arthritis (RA) |**1**| but the responsible mechanisms remain unclear. It is evident that traditional coronary heart disease (CHD) risk factors do not explain the excess risk for CHD in this population. For example, in relevant studies that have measured cholesterol, blood pressure or smoking, the risk for CHD in patients with RA is often only minimally attenuated following adjustment for such factors |**2**|.

More recent research has focused on the potential for systemic inflammation to accelerate CHD risk in RA. Indeed, several groups of researchers from differing disciplines have proposed systemic inflammation as the likely major determinant of the accelerated CHD risk in RA |**1,3**|. Consequently, dampening systemic inflammation may be a major means by which to lower CHD risk in RA. Of course, numerous RA-specific factors may contribute but it increasingly appears as if the relative contribution of systemic inflammation is dominant in accelerating CHD risk in RA.

Patients with RA tend to have lower cholesterol concentrations than those in the general population—but again this can be linked back to the inflammatory response. Nevertheless, such findings indicate that the role of conventional modalities to lessen CHD risk in RA, for example statins, requires further investigation. Independent of their lipid-lowering actions, the statins class of drugs may offer particular benefit to RA patients by virtue of their anti-inflammatory effects |**4,5**|. However, formal clinical studies are required to test this hypothesis. It is likely that CHD risk is not being widely addressed in RA patients.

The papers chosen herein elaborate on the above observations. First, there is a strong prospective study supportive of an elevated CHD risk in women with RA (Solomon *et al.* 2003). Thereafter, a recent excellent review on the topic is presented with suggestions on to how to manage CHD risk in RA (Kitas and Erb 2003). This is followed by a paper (Wong *et al.* 2003) consistent with a series of similar papers demonstrating independent and consistent relationships between measures of blood vessel stiffness—a surrogate for CHD risk—and systemic inflammatory parameters in RA. Next, data from Leung *et al.* (2003) demonstrating potent anti-inflammatory effects of statins in the collagen-induced arthritis mouse model are presented. A replication of such findings in humans would be very exciting and such work is likely to emerge in the near future. To end, there is a recent review/hypothesis published by Sattar *et al.* (2003) in Glasgow that seeks to summarize the available evidence in the literature linking numerous metabolic aberrations back to the systemic inflammatory response in RA.

In summary, there is an emerging concept that systemic inflammation may be the major driver of accelerated CHD in RA. Future studies should hopefully confirm this notion by examining the metabolic effects of dampening inflammation and, in addition, determine whether conventional CHD preventative therapies are able to reduce CHD risk in the context of ongoing high-grade inflammation.

Cardiovascular morbidity and mortality in women diagnosed with rheumatoid arthritis

Solomon DH, Karlson EW, Rimm EB, *et al.* *Circulation* 2003; **107**: 1303–7

Background. There are numerous studies suggestive of excess CHD risk in patients with RA. Solomon *et al.* had the opportunity to test this question in the large prospective Nurses' Health Study.

Interpretation. Incidence rates of myocardial infarction and stroke in subjects with and without RA among the 114 342 women participating in the Nurses' Health Study who were free of cardiovascular disease and RA at baseline in 1976 were compared. Multivariate pooled logistic regression was used to adjust for potential cardiovascular risk factors. Five hundred and twenty-seven incident cases of RA and 3622 myocardial infarctions and strokes were confirmed during 2.4 million person-years of follow-up. The adjusted relative risk of myocardial infarction in women with RA compared with those without was 2.0 (95% confidence interval [CI] 1.23–3.29). For stroke, the adjusted relative risk was 1.48 (95% CI 0.70–3.12). Women who had RA for at least 10 years had a risk for myocardial infarction of 3.10 (95% CI 1.64–5.87).

Comment

This study by Solomon *et al.* is important for several reasons. First, it is one of the very few that has recruited a community-based cohort rather than a referral population of more severely ill patients. It also prospectively collected information on CHD outcomes rather than retrospectively and similarly controlled for important potential confounders such as body mass index, blood pressure, diabetes and smoking. The authors were also very careful in checking the validity of end-point data with careful record acquisition. The study therefore has several strengths over previously published data. The authors were able to confirm a significant increased CHD risk; about double that of women without RA. The data were also in keeping with the notion that conventional CHD risk factors do not explain this excess risk, as the relative risk was hardly attenuated with adjustment for such factors (age adjusted risk 2.07 [1.28–3.24] versus multivariable risk 2.00 [1.23–3.29]). Interestingly, an excess risk for stroke was not confirmed in this study but the study may have been underpowered to answer this question. The authors suggested that inflammation may be the culprit for excess CHD risk but the one limitation in their study was the absence of C-reactive protein (CRP) or other acute phase reactant measurements to test this hypothesis directly. Nevertheless, this important study adds considerable weight to the RA-accelerated CHD risk proposal.

Tackling ischaemic heart disease in rheumatoid arthritis

Kitas GD, Erb N. *Rheumatology* 2003; **42**: 607–13

BACKGROUND. RA is the commonest form of chronic inflammatory arthritis. It causes significant disability and the efforts of the scientific community have concentrated on controlling symptoms, decelerating joint damage and improving function. However, it has been known for 50 years that RA is also associated with increased mortality. For severe RA, this compares with that of major killers such as triple-vessel CHD and some lymphomas. Despite advances in treatment, the mortality of RA does not appear to have changed over the last three decades. Its control, therefore, merits at least as much attention as the reduction of disability. An obvious target is reduction of cardiovascular mortality, which accounts for almost half of all deaths in RA. This article describes the nature and significance of the problem, discusses the evidence for the involvement of atherosclerotic CHD, outlines the role of classical and some novel cardiovascular risk factors, introduces potential lines for intervention, and provides a literature base for the interested reader.

INTERPRETATION. Kitas and Erb have put together a very useful overview of the risk factors for CHD in RA. They make the point that increased CHD in RA is likely to be multifactorial in nature but allude also to the strong link to inflammation. They draw a nice parallel between RA and diabetes as populations at risk for CHD. Excess CHD risk is of similar magnitude in both pathologies and both are independent risk factors for CHD. Moreover, the prevalence of the two conditions is not dissimilar particularly in women aged 45–75+.

Comment

Not only does this article provide comprehensive references for the interested reader, it is also well balanced. In particular, in discussing systemic inflammation as a major cause of CHD in RA, Kitas and Erb are correct in pointing out that despite evidence supporting the reduction in CHD with anti-inflammatory therapies, caution should still remain in view of other evidence linking anti-tumour necrosis factors with worsening heart failure. Clearly, future careful studies examining vascular effects of tumour necrosis factor blockers in RA are required. The other useful aspect of this article is in its comparison of RA and diabetes as causes of excess CHD risk. In this respect, it is noteworthy that while CHD risk reduction is a major priority in patients with diabetes worldwide and that many such patients are on lipid-lowering agents |**6**|, the same is certainly not true for patients with RA.

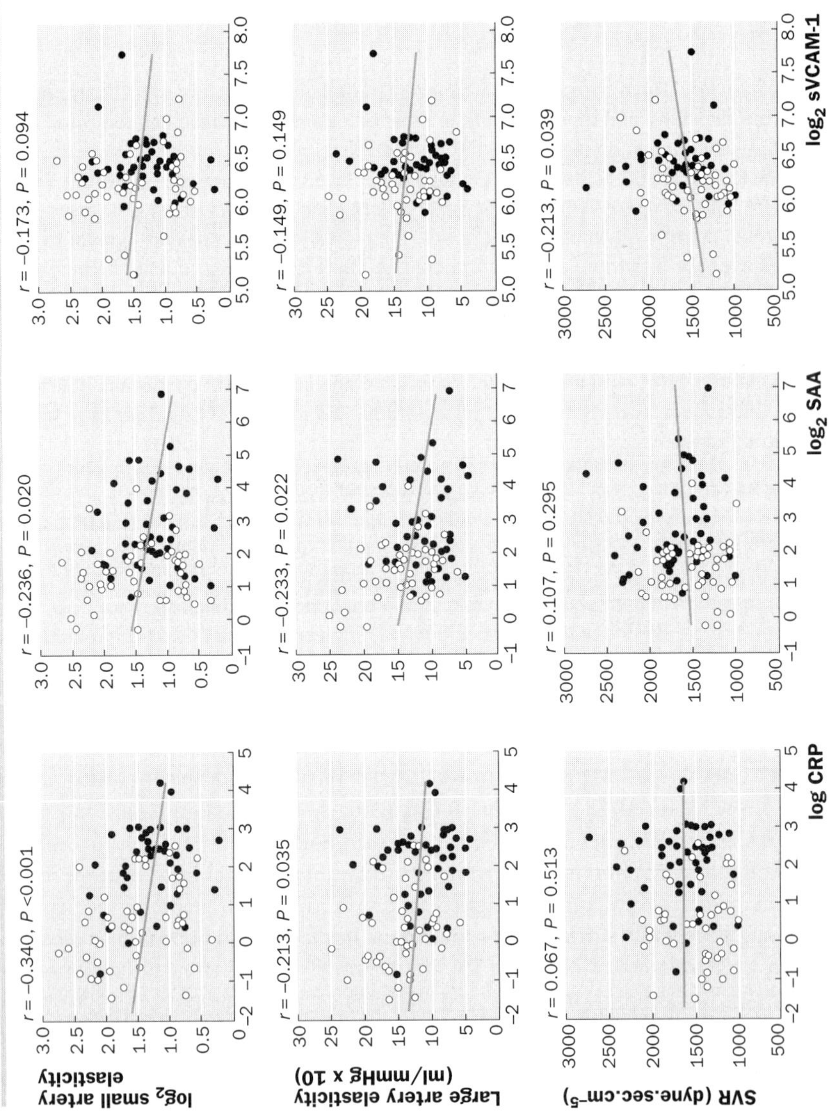
log2 small artery elasticity
Large artery elasticity (ml/mmHg x 10)
SVR (dyne.sec.cm−5)
r = −0.340, P <0.001
r = −0.236, P = 0.020
r = −0.173, P = 0.094
r = −0.213, P = 0.035
r = −0.233, P = 0.022
r = −0.149, P = 0.149
r = 0.067, P = 0.513
r = 0.107, P = 0.295
r = −0.213, P = 0.039
log CRP
log2 SAA
log2 sVCAM-1

Reduced arterial elasticity in rheumatoid arthritis and the relationship to vascular disease risk factors and inflammation

Wong M, Toh L, Wilson A, *et al.* *Arthritis Rheum* 2003; **48**: 81–9

BACKGROUND. Blood vessel stiffness has emerged as a potential surrogate marker of CHD risk [7]. RA is associated with increased rates of cardiovascular disease but data on blood vessel stiffness have until recently been lacking.

INTERPRETATION. Wong *et al.* used the technique of pulse wave analysis (PWA) to examine arterial elasticity/stiffness in 43 RA patients together with 43 controls. They observed impaired elasticity (increased stiffness) in RA patients in both small and large vessels. However, conventional risk factors were not related to impaired vessel elasticity in RA patients. Rather, measures of inflammation predicted impaired elasticity (Fig. 4.1).

Comment

The concept of endothelial dysfunction has long been established as a potential intermediate marker for subsequent CHD. A recent panel of non-invasive measures to determine endothelial function has been developed in the CHD arena [**7**]. Among these is the technique of PWA and there is now evidence that impairment in PWA predicts CHD events independent of conventional risk factors. Thus, the finding of enhanced arterial stiffness in RA patients is in keeping with their elevated risk for CHD. The further observation that markers of inflammation rather than conventional CHD risk markers were predictive of arterial stiffness, albeit only modestly, further underscores the role of systemic inflammation in accelerating CHD risk in RA. Whether techniques such as PWA will find clinical utility in determining which patients with RA (or indeed with other pathologies or in primary prevention) necessitate interventions to lessen CHD risk remains uncertain at this present time.

Fig. 4.1 Correlations between small artery elasticity, large artery elasticity and systemic vascular resistance (SVR) and markers of inflammation in patients with rheumatoid arthritis (solid circles) and control subjects (open circles). Coefficients and *P* values refer to partial correlations, adjusted for age and sex. CRP, C-reactive protein (high sensitivity); SAA, serum amyloid A; sVCAM-1, soluble vascular cell adhesion molecule 1.
Source: Wong *et al.* (2003).

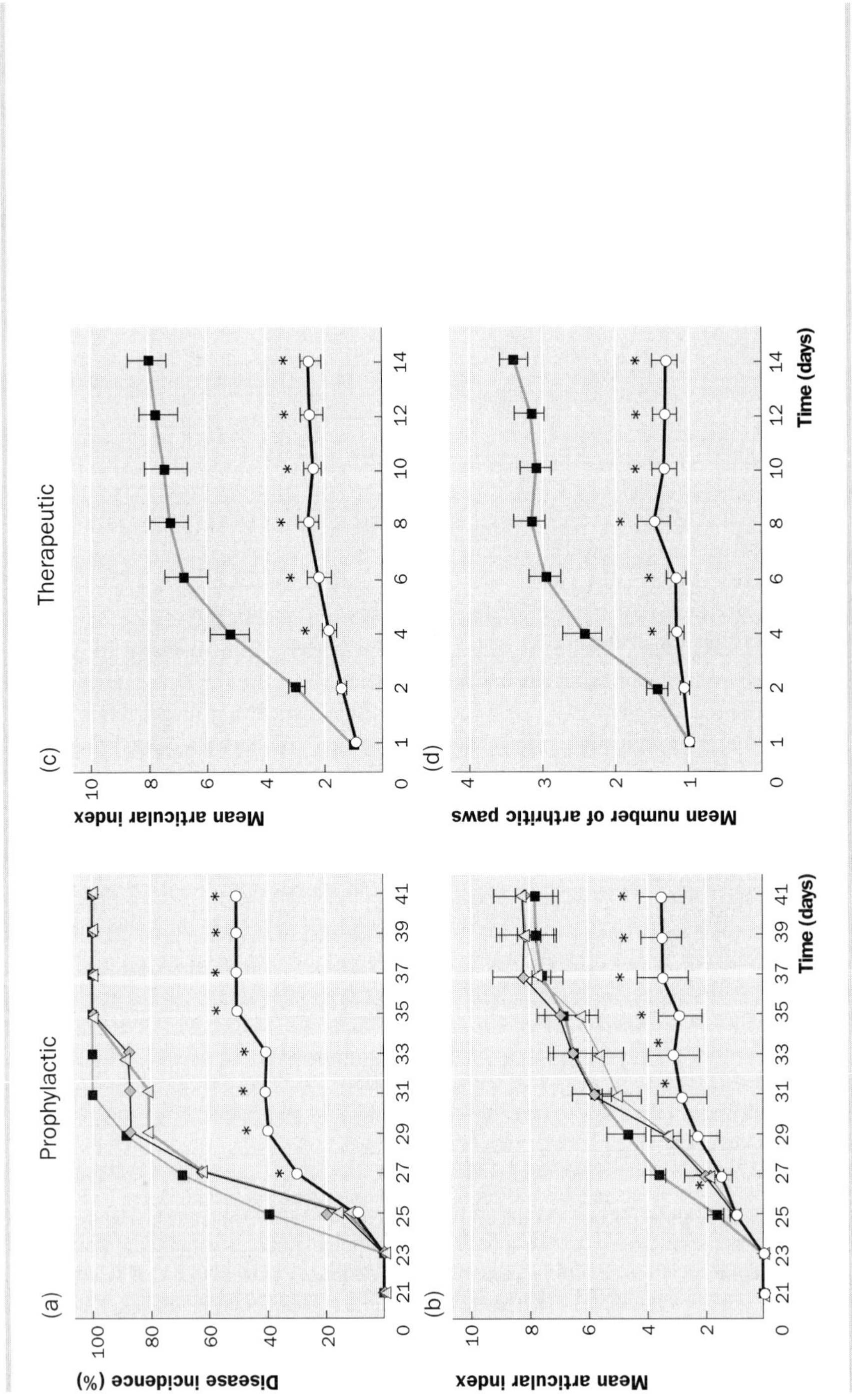
Prophylactic
Therapeutic
(a)
Disease incidence (%)
(b)
Mean articular index
Time (days)
(c)
Mean articular index
(d)
Mean number of arthritic paws
Time (days)

A novel anti-inflammatory role for simvastatin in inflammatory arthritis

Leung BP, Sattar N, Crilly A, *et al. J Immunol* 2003; **170**: 1524–30

BACKGROUND. There is abundant evidence from CHD studies and *in vitro* and *ex vivo* observations suggesting statins possess anti-inflammatory effects |5|. This study tested for the first time whether such effects could attenuate the development of arthritis in the collagen-induced mouse model. The study was designed as a proof of concept study to test the therapeutic potential of statin-sensitive pathways in inflammatory arthritis.

INTERPRETATION. We explored the activities of simvastatin, a lipophilic statin, in a T-helper 1-driven model of murine inflammatory arthritis. We noted that simvastatin markedly inhibited not only developing, but also clinically evident, collagen-induced arthritis (Fig. 4.2) in doses that were unable significantly to alter cholesterol concentrations *in vivo*. *Ex vivo* analysis demonstrated significant suppression of collagen-specific T-helper 1 humoral and cellular immune responses. Moreover, simvastatin reduced anti-CD3/anti-CD28 proliferation and interferon-γ release from mononuclear cells derived from peripheral blood and synovial fluid. Proinflammatory cytokine production *in vitro* by T cell contact-activated macrophages was suppressed by simvastatin, suggesting that such observations may have direct clinical relevance.

Comment

These data clearly illustrate the therapeutic potential of statin-sensitive pathways in inflammatory arthritis. The study was important as it provided the best available evidence to indicate statins may well proffer clinically relevant anti-inflammatory effects in RA. The major caveat, however, was that the dose given to the mice was far in excess of that used in humans for cardioprotection—due to the ability of mice to rapidly upregulate their HMG-COA reductase—and thus direct extrapolation to the human situation must be tempered. Nevertheless, the results of this study made the case for a clinical trial in humans more compelling.

Fig. 4.2 Effects of simvastatin on developing (prophylactic) and clinically evident (therapeutic) CIA. DBA/1 mice were immunized with CII and an i.p. challenge injection was given at day 21. (a) and (b) Prophylactic protocol: mice were treated daily from days 21 to 40 with increasing doses of simvastatin starting from 10 mg/kg (◆ *n* = 10), 20 mg/kg (▲ *n* = 8), 40 mg/kg (○ *n* = 10), or PBS (■ *n* = 10). The appearance of arthritis was monitored daily and presented as disease incidence or mean articular index (calculated only from arthritic mice). Simvastatin administered at 40 mg/kg significantly lowered incidence and severity of arthritis (*P <0.05 by Mann–Whitney *U* test). There was no statistically significant difference between the 10 mg/kg, 20 mg/kg and PBS groups. (c) and (d) Therapeutic protocol: mice were treated 1 day postonset of clinically evident articular disease for a total of 14 days either with simvastatin 40 mg/kg (○ *n* = 13) or PBS (■ *n* = 14). Significant suppression of disease activity (*P <0.05) was observed in simvastatin-treated mice as indicated by mean articular index and mean number of arthritic paws. Data are expressed as mean ± SEM. Source: Leung *et al.* (2003).

Explaining how 'high-grade' systemic inflammation accelerates vascular risk in rheumatoid arthritis

Sattar N, McCarey DW, Capell H, McInnes IB. *Circulation* 2003; **108**: 2957–63

BACKGROUND. There is intense interest in mechanisms whereby low-grade inflammation could interact with conventional and novel vascular risk factors to promote the atheromatous lesion. Patients with RA, who manifest by definition persistent high levels of inflammation, are at greater risk of developing cardiovascular disease. Mechanisms mediating this enhanced risk are ill-defined.

INTERPRETATION. Based on available evidence, the authors argued that the systemic inflammatory response in RA is critical to accelerated atherogenesis operating via accentuation of established and novel risk factor pathways (Figs. 4.3 and 4.4). By implication, long-term suppression of the systemic inflammatory response in RA should be effective in reducing CHD risk. Early epidemiological observational and clinical studies are commensurate with this hypothesis |**1,3**|. By contrast, risk factor modulation using conventional agents, such as statins, may provide unpredictable clinical benefit in the context of uncontrolled systemic inflammatory parameters. Unravelling such complex relationships in which exaggerated inflammation–risk factor interactions are prevalent may elicit novel insights to effector mechanisms in vascular disease generally.

Comment

The above paper, we believe, is important for several reasons. First, it provides a comprehensive literature base on the links between inflammation and CHD risk pathways (as reviewed in Table 4.1). Second, the article re-examines older data on novel CHD risk pathways such as insulin action and demonstrates how the apparent 'paradoxical' effects of steroids in improving insulin sensitivity in RA strongly implicates the inflammatory response in mediating insulin resistance in RA |**8,9**|. Third, the article draws some interesting pathogenic parallels to other diseases associated with both systemic inflammation and accelerated atherogenesis, e.g. lung cancer |**10,11**|. Fourth, it predicts that risk factor modulation using conventional agents, such as statins, may provide unpredictable clinical benefit in the context of uncontrolled systemic inflammatory parameters. Finally, although some points expressed in the article require confirmation, it brings together many previously apparent 'disparate' pieces of information in a logical framework amenable to future interrogation. If we are correct, then one of the best means to reduce CHD risk in RA is by long-term suppression of the systemic inflammatory response in RA.

Table 4.1 Risk factor perturbances in RA, their association with the inflammatory response in cross-sectional studies, and documented improvements upon inflammatory suppression

CHD risk factors	Strength of evidence for abnormality of risk factor in RA	Strength of evidence linking metabolic perturbances to inflammatory response in RA	Evidence for improvement in risk factor upon inflammatory suppression*
Obesity/insulin resistance			
Body fat redistribution	+	ND	Steroids and SSZ paradoxically enhance insulin sensitivity in RA
Hyperinsulinaemia	+	+	
Insulin resistance	++	+	
Dyslipidaemia			
Free fatty acids	+	+	Anti-inflammatory treatment increases HDL-cholesterol but data on other lipid mediators generally lacking
Triglyceride	+/0	+	
↓ HDL-cholesterol	++	++	
↓ HDL_2	++	+	
Small, dense LDL	+	+	
Lipoprotein (a)	++	+	
Endothelial dysfunction			
sICAM-1	++	+	sICAM declines with SSZ. FMD improves with anti-tumour necrosis factor-α therapy
vWF	+	+	
Microalbuminuria	+	+	
Impaired vasoreactivity	++	+	
Arterial stiffness	++	+	
Oxidative stress			
MDA	+	+	Not examined but ibuprofen ↑ antioxidant levels in cancer subjects
↓ Vitamin antioxidants	+	+	
Haemostatic alterations			
Fibrinogen	++	++	Limited data
PAI-1	+	0	
Blood pressure	+	ND	No data
Homocysteine pathway			
↓ Vitamin B6	++	+	Steroids reduced homocysteine levels in RA
Homocysteine	++	+	

Majority of data stem from small, uncontrolled studies. 0, lack of, or conflicting evidence; +, moderate supporting evidence; ++, consistent evidence; ND, no data; SSZ, sulphasalazine; MDA, malondialdehyde; vWF, von Willebrand factor; FMD, flow-mediated dilation; LDL, low-density lipoprotein; HDL, high-density lipoprotein; sICAM, soluble intercellular adhesion molecule. Modified from Sattar *et al.* (2003).

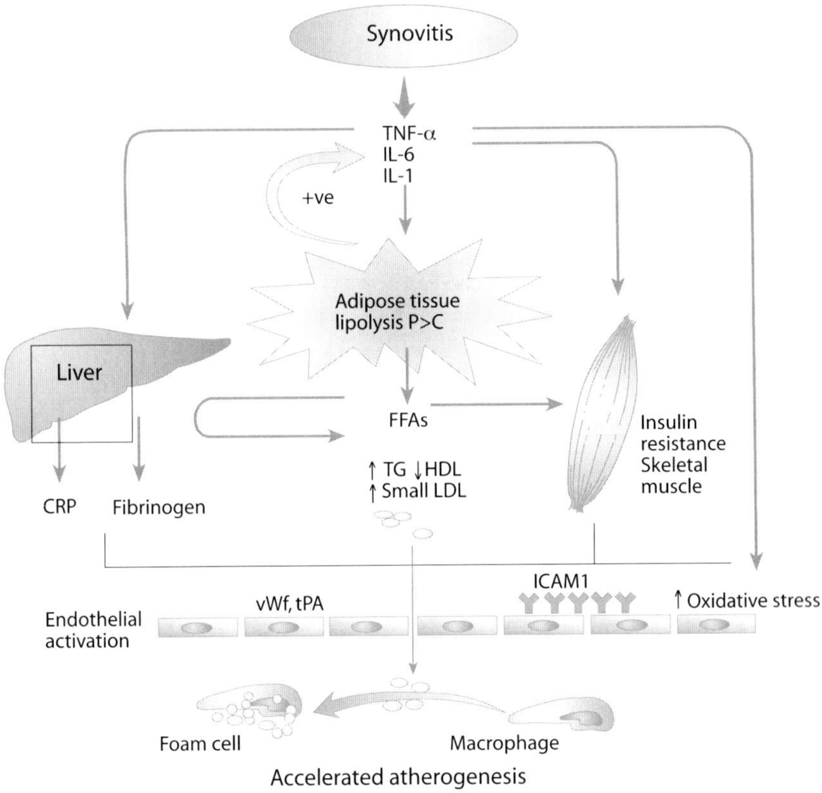

Fig. 4.3 In RA, the primary site of inflammation is the synovial tissue from which cytokines can be released into the systemic circulation. These circulating cytokines alter the function of distant tissues including adipose, skeletal muscle, liver and vascular endothelium, to generate a spectrum of proatherogenic changes that include insulin resistance, a characteristic dyslipidaemia, pro-oxidative effects, and endothelial dysfunction and damage. Source: Sattar *et al.* (2003).

Conclusion

The topic of CHD in RA appears to be of increasing interest to clinical and academic rheumatologists and the wider vascular research community in general—this interest has in part been stimulated by the accumulating evidence for low-grade inflammation as a major contributor to atherogenesis |**4**|. It has been fuelled also by the finding that many conventional vasculo-protective modalities such as statins |**5**| and angiotensin-converting enzyme inhibitors proffer anti-inflammatory actions. It

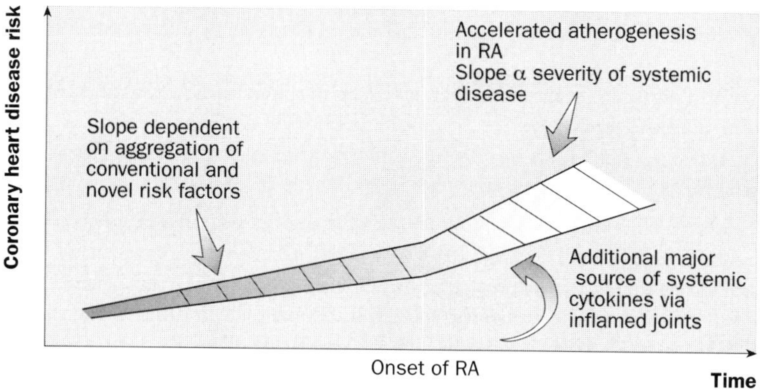

Fig. 4.4 Prior to onset of RA, classical risk factors predict risk of an event. However, following onset of disease, the severity of the systemic inflammation secondary to RA joint disease is critical in the acceleration of atherogenesis and thus risk factors influenced by systemic inflammation will predict risk of future events. Source: Sattar *et al.* (2003).

is likely that we will soon discover whether statins offer clinically apparent anti-inflammatory effects in RA, and whether they simultaneously lessen CHD risk either by their lipid-lowering or anti-inflammatory actions, or a combination of both. The thrust of recent research has clearly identified systemic inflammation as the likely major driver for accelerated CHD in RA. Future intervention studies examining risk factor pathways and novel surrogate markers of CHD upon inflammatory suppression should confirm this notion. They should also hopefully lead in turn to more formalized measures to identify, treat and lessen the burden of vascular disease in RA.

References

1. Van Doornum S, McColl G, Wicks IP. Accelerated atherosclerosis: an extraarticular feature of rheumatoid arthritis? *Arthritis Rheum* 2002; **46**: 862–73.
2. del Rincon ID, Williams K, Stern MP, Freeman GL, Escalante A. High incidence of cardiovascular events in a rheumatoid arthritis cohort not explained by traditional cardiac risk factors. *Arthritis Rheum* 2001; **44**: 2737–45.

3. Choi HK, Hernan MA, Seeger JD, Robins JM, Wolfe F. Methotrexate and mortality in patients with rheumatoid arthritis: a prospective study. *Lancet* 2002; **359**: 1173–7.
4. Libby P, Ridker PM, Maseri A. Inflammation and atherosclerosis. *Circulation* 2002; **105**: 1135–43.
5. Palinski W, Tsimikas S. Immunomodulatory effects of statins: mechanisms and potential impact on arteriosclerosis. *J Am Soc Nephrol* 2002; **13**: 1673–81.
6. Haffner SM. Statin therapy for the treatment of diabetic dyslipidemia. *Diabetes Metab Res Rev* 2003; **19**: 280–7.
7. Oliver JJ, Webb DJ. Non-invasive assessment of arterial stiffness and risk of atherosclerotic events. *Arterioscler Thromb Vasc Biol* 2003; **23**: 554–66.
8. Paolisso G, Valentini G, Giugliano D, Marazzo G, Tirri R, Gallo M, Tirri G, Varricchio M, D'Onofrio F. Evidence for peripheral impaired glucose handling in patients with connective tissue diseases. *Metabolism* 1991; **40**: 902–7.
9. Hallgren R, Berne C. Glucose intolerance in patients with chronic inflammatory diseases is normalized by glucocorticoids. *Acta Med Scand* 1983; **213**: 351–5.
10. Yoshikawa T, Noguchi Y, Doi C, Makino T, Nomura K. Insulin resistance in patients with cancer: relationships with tumor site, tumor stage, body-weight loss, acute–phase response, and energy expenditure. *Nutrition* 2001; **17**: 590–3.
11. De Vita F, Orditura M, Infusino S, Auriemma A, Catalano G. Increased serum levels of tumor necrosis factor-alpha are correlated to soluble intercellular adhesion molecule-1 concentrations in non-small cell lung cancer patients. *Int J Mol Med* 1998; **1**: 605–8.

5

Anti-CCP2: a marker with a high diagnostic potential for the detection of (early) rheumatoid arthritis

ANIL VASISHTA, WALTHER van VENROOIJ

Introduction

Rheumatoid arthritis (RA) is a common, systemic autoimmune disease affecting 0.5–1% of the population. It is characterized by chronic inflammation of the synovium, which commonly leads to progressive joint destruction and in most cases to disability and reduction of quality of life. With the availability of more sophisticated and effective therapies (reviewed by Smolen and Steiner [1]) and with increasing evidence that the first few months of disease represent a unique therapeutic opportunity and that such early therapeutic intervention is crucial in preventing irreversible joint damage [2–4], it is widely accepted that early and accurate diagnosis of RA is critical in disease management. Although widely employed, the 1987 American College of Rheumatology (ACR) criteria [5] are not very well suited for the diagnosis of early RA [6–8] as they rely heavily on the presence of clinical symptoms of RA, and these are often absent in early RA. In light of the above, the ideal serological marker for RA would have to be not only specific and sensitive, but also present very early in the disease. Within the last 2 years a number of publications have reported that the anti-CCP (cyclic citrullinated peptide) test may become the marker of choice for early RA as it appears to be highly specific and sensitive for the disease. In this review we discuss the evidence supporting the utility of anti-CCP in early RA.

Antibodies in rheumatoid arthritis

Throughout the last decades several autoantibody systems have been described that are associated with RA. The best known RA-associated antibody system has been the rheumatoid factor (RF), an antibody directed to the Fc part of IgG molecules. While this antibody can be detected in up to 80% of RA patients, it is also present in several

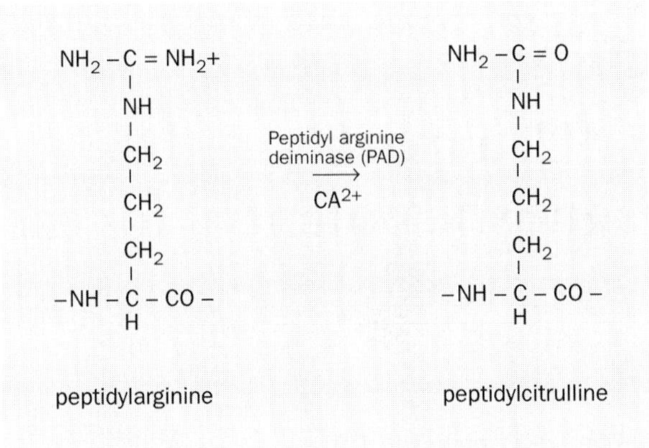

Fig. 5.1 Citrullination (deimination) of peptidylarginine to peptidylcitrulline by peptidylarginine deiminase enzyme. Source: Vossenaar *et al.* (2003) |**21**|.

other diseases and healthy controls (especially in the elderly: 10–30%), thus limiting its specificity for RA.

Several other RA-associated antibody systems have also been described, such as anticalpastatin, anti-RA33, anti-GPI, anticollagen type II, anti-BiP (p68) and anti-neutrophil cytoplasmic antibodies (reviewed in |**9–11**|). However, due to a lack of sensitivity and/or specificity most of these systems have never made it as routine serological tests for RA.

In terms of specificity, the so-called anticitrullinated protein antibodies including antiperinuclear factor (APF), antikeratin antibodies, antifilaggrin antibodies, anti-Sa and the anti-CCP antibodies are highly associated with RA |**12–19**|.

Citrullination is a process whereby the non-standard amino acid citrulline is generated by post-translational modification of arginine residues in proteins by the enzyme peptidylarginine deiminase |**20,21**| (Fig. 5.1). Using a citrulline-containing peptide derived from filaggrin sequences, as the antigenic source on a solid phase, antibodies were detected in up to 48% of RA sera with a very high specificity (up to 98%) |**16**|.

To increase the low sensitivity of these linear citrulline-containing peptides, modifications were carried out to enable the peptide to adopt a more stringent structure in which the citrulline moiety is optimally exposed for antibody binding |**22**|. With a single CCP, antibodies could be detected in about 68% of RA sera with a very high specificity (98%) |**22**|. This filaggrin-derived cyclic peptide was used as the antigenic substrate in the CCP1 test.

Although the sensitivity of the CCP1 assay was higher than that of the classical APF and antikeratin antibody assays and most antifilaggrin antibody assays, it was not as high as that of the RF test (reviewed by van Boekel *et al.* |**9**|). In an effort to improve this low sensitivity, a dedicated library of citrulline-containing peptides was screened for additional antigenic peptides. This work succeeded in identifying unique peptides that are present in the current CCP2 enzyme-linked immunosorbent assay test.

As discussed above an ideal serological marker for a given disease is only useful to the clinician when the desired antibodies are not only present in the majority of patients but are also highly specific for the disease. Furthermore, the antibodies should preferably be present very early in the disease and able to predict disease outcome. Recent data from several laboratories indicate that the CCP2 system meets all these requirements in RA.

Anti-CCP sensitivity and specificity

A good serological marker for RA should be highly specific for the disease and be able to distinguish RA from other diseases that mimic RA. From the original studies of Schellekens *et al.* [22], in which anti-CCP was measured in cohorts of patients with RA, other rheumatic diseases, infectious diseases and in healthy controls, it was concluded that anti-CCP antibodies (anti-CCP1 in this case) were indeed very specific for RA. These results were subsequently confirmed by Bizzaro *et al.* [23], Palosuo *et al.* [24] and several other investigators (reviewed by van Boekel *et al.* [9]). Newer recent studies have also confirmed this specificity with the second-generation CCP2 test.

In a large multicentre trial comprising 1189 sera, 78% of RA patients, 15% of healthy controls and 50% of disease controls tested positive for IgM-RF, while 79% of RA patients, none of the healthy controls and only 5% of the disease controls were positive for anti-CCP2 [25]. In another large cohort study anti-CCP2 was positive in 82% of (chronic) RA patients, 1% of healthy controls and 2% of disease controls; as compared with 80%, 1% and 12%, respectively, for IgM-RF [26]. CCP2 thus has a comparable sensitivity but a much higher specificity for RA than RF. In a recent study of 264 patients the diagnostic potential of RF and CCP2 for RA were directly compared. When the cut-off was defined in such a way that a specificity for RA of 98.5% was maintained, the sensitivity of RF was only 12.8%, compared with 73.7% for CCP2 [27]. A summary of the results from these cohorts, supplemented with data from other (some not yet published) studies is given in Tables 5.1 and 5.2.

In addition to diagnosing RA there are reports that anti-CCP may distinguish true RA from other diseases that mimic early RA. Patients with early systemic lupus erythematosus (SLE) for instance, can often be misdiagnosed as having RA, because they can be RF positive and present with erosive polyarthritis [33]. Mediwake *et al.* [34] reported that anti-CCP status can be used to distinguish RA from erosive SLE. In this study employing a large cohort of SLE patients, 10 of whom had erosive disease, the antibody findings were as follows: six were RF positive (60%), six were anti-RA-33 positive (60%), whereas only two were anti-CCP1 positive (20%). Of the non-erosive patients the positivity rates were 18% for RF positive, 6% for RA-33 and only 0.5% for CCP1 [34].

Patients with chronic hepatitis C virus (HCV) infection often display extrahepatic manifestations among which arthropathy is common, affecting up to as many as

Table 5.1 Sensitivity and specificity of the anti-CCP2 and IgM-RF antibody systems (combined results of CCP2 cohorts [**25,26,29**]

	CCP2			IgM-RF		
	n	pos	(%)	*n*	pos	(%)
RA	1117	865	(77)	1119	827	(74)
Healthy individuals	431	1	(0)	335	38	(11)
Osteoarthritis	81	7	(9)	79	14	(18)
Juvenile RA*	21	6	(29)	21	8	(38)
Various connective tissue diseases†	814	44	(5)	573	217	(38)
Various inflammatory diseases‡	225	2	(1)	160	14	(9)
Various arthropathies§	297	13	(4)	72	5	(7)
Various viral infections¶	188	2	(1)	171	43	(25)
Various bacterial infections**	147	2	(1)	179	21	(12)
Various parasitic infections††	93	2	(2)	99	22	(22)
Total non-RA	2297	79	(3)	1689	382	(23)
Specificity			97%			77%

*Including adult JRA patients, described in [**28,29**].
†Including systemic lupus erythematosus, mixed connective tissue disease, scleroderma, Sjögren's syndrome, CREST syndrome, polymyositis/dermatomyositis.
‡Including Crohn's disease, colitis ulcerosa, polymyalgia rheumatica, vasculitis, Wegener's granulomatosis, sarcoidosis, autoimmune thyroiditis.
§Reactive arthritis, gout, psoriatic arthritis, fibromyalgia, Reiter's syndrome, inflammatory polyarthritis, ankylosing spondylitis.
¶Including Epstein–Barr, hepatitis C, parvovirus B19, rubella, viraemia.
**Including inflammatory endocarditis, *Legionella, Lyme borrelia, Yersinia, Salmonella*, tuberculosis, *Streptococcus pyogenis*.
††Including malaria, *Mycoplasma, Toxoplasma*, Chaga's disease, *Schistosoma, Leishmania*.
Source: Vossenaar and van Venrooij [**28**].

20% of HCV-infected individuals. As many HCV-infected patients are RF positive, especially those that display mixed cryoglobulinaemia (MC), RF cannot be used to discriminate HCV-related arthritis from RA [**35,36**]. In a group of 50 randomly selected HCV patients, none was positive for anti-CCP2 (44% were positive for RF) and of 29 HCV patients with MC only two tested positive for anti-CCP (76% were RF positive) [**37**]. Similar data were obtained in a study by Bombardieri *et al.* [**38**]. In this study anti-CCP was detected in 77% of patients with RA (RF in 90%) but in none of the patients with HCV, while RF was present in 15% of the HCV patients. In the subset of HCV patients that presented with joint involvement, RF was even positive in 37.5%.

In summary, due to its high specificity, the use of anti-CCP testing offers a reliable diagnostic tool for RA.

Anti-CCP is present early in disease

When a random population attending a rheumatology clinic is tested for anti-CCP, about 2–5% of the patients test positive but do not suffer from RA (our unpublished

Table 5.2 Summary of recent diagnostic CCP2 studies

Study	Ref.	RA/controls	Sensitivity %	Specificity %	Outcome/remarks
van Venrooij*	[26]	390/904	82	98	Specificity: CCP >RF; sensitivity: CCP = RF
Vasishta*	[25]	682/1189	79	97	CCP also useful for early RA
Pinheiro	[30]	150/NM	80	98	Good sensitivity of CCP in established RA
Lee	[29]	103/146	66	90	CCP false positivity in JRA perhaps because of childhood onset RA
Suzuki	[31]	549/528	88	89	Discriminative ability of CCP >RF
Dubucquoi	[32]	140/131	65	96	Cohort with various stages of RA (sensitivity in established RA: 77%)
de Rycke	[27]	118/146	75	97	At 98.5% specificity, the sensitivity of RF was 12.8% compared with 73.7 for CCP2

NM, not mentioned. *Some overlap in cohorts.
Source: Zendman *et al.* (in press) [39].

observations). A similar phenomenon can be observed when the population of an early arthritis clinic is tested. Two recent studies have provided clear evidence that such supposedly 'false' positives might in fact be in the early phase of developing RA. Rantapää-Dahlqvist *et al.* [40] analysed blood samples from 83 blood donors who subsequently developed RA. Anti-CCP2 positivity was detected in 25% of the subjects 1.5–9 years before onset of disease symptoms and, not surprisingly, in the last 1.5 years before first presentation to the clinician this increased to 52%. For IgM-RF, IgG-RF and IgA-RF the corresponding figures were 15 and 30%, 12 and 27%, and 29 and 39%, respectively. More than 70% of the patients were anti-CCP2 positive at their first visit to the clinic. These workers concluded that anti-CCP2 antibody was superior to RF in its ability to predict the development of RA. In a similar type of study Nielen *et al.* [41] measured anti-CCP1 and IgM-RF levels in serial blood donations from 72 donors that subsequently developed RA. In this cohort 27% of RF-negative and 46% of RF-positive RA patients were positive for anti-CCP1, 4.8 and 5.5 years before the onset of complaints, respectively. Thus, anti-CCP detected more positive subjects and longer before the start of the complaints compared with IgM-RF.

Other recent studies also point to a similar conclusion. For example, Jansen *et al.* [42] tried to discriminate RA from undifferentiated polyarthritis at presentation. They reported that the combined presence of IgM-RF and anti-CCP1 was able to predict those patients with early arthritis who subsequently developed RA at a sensitivity of 55.4% and a specificity close to 97% |**42**|. A similar study using the CCP2 test was performed by van Gaalen *et al.* |**43**|. This group followed 318 patients of a cohort of 936 attending an early arthritis clinic, who could not be diagnosed as having RA at first presentation and were thus classified as undifferentiated arthritis (UA). After 3 years of follow-up 40% of the UA patients were clinically classified as RA. Of the UA patients that were negative for anti-CCP2 at baseline, 25% developed RA within 3 years. By contrast, of the UA patients with a positive anti-CCP2 test at baseline, 93% developed RA (odds ratio [OR] 38). A very recent study of Vittecoq *et al.* |**44**| studying 314 early arthritis patients confirmed these results. At 1 year follow-up 90% of the patients that were CCP positive at baseline were classified as established RA patients |**44**|.

The conclusion from these studies is that anti-CCP antibodies are present early in disease, and that their presence can accurately predict the likely development of RA.

Anti-CCP may predict erosive disease

It has been known for some time that APF antibodies are able to predict joint erosion in (early) RA patients. Typically, APF-positive patients exhibit higher radiological damage scores than APF-negative patients, and in some studies the performance of APF was reported to be superior to that of IgM-RF |**42**|. Given the relationship between APF and CCP, it might be expected that anti-CCP antibodies may also be able to predict erosive disease. Several studies have been published to support this.

Kroot *et al.* |**45**| were the first to study the predictive value of anti-CCP1 in patients with recent onset RA. They reported that patients positive for the anti-CCP1 antibody developed significantly more severe radiological damage after 6 years of follow-up than CCP1-negative patients. However, in multiple regression analysis the additional predictive value of this antibody in this cohort of patients was rather moderate |**45**|. This may be attributable in part to the relatively low sensitivity of the CCP1 test.

In another interesting study Visser *et al.* |**8**| performed a standardized diagnostic evaluation on 524 newly referred patients with early arthritis. Their objective was to develop a clinical model for the prediction, at first visit, of three forms of arthritis outcomes, namely, self-limiting, persistent erosive and persistent non-erosive. Seven potential diagnostic determinants, including IgM-RF and CCP1, were entered in a logistic regression analysis and arthritis outcome was recorded at 2 years' follow-up. The discriminative ability of the model and various parameters was expressed as a receiver operating characteristic (ROC) area under the curve (AUC). The ROC/AUC of the new model was 0.84 for discrimination between self-limiting and persistent arthritis, and 0.91 for discrimination between persistent non-erosive and persistent erosive arthritis. By contrast the discriminative ability of the 1987 ACR criteria for RA was significantly lower with ROC/AUC values of 0.78 and 0.79, respectively. Furthermore in their prediction model, of the seven criteria studied, anti-CCP1 had the highest odds ratios |**8**|.

Vencovský *et al.* also confirmed that anti-CCP1 antibodies were able to predict erosive and progressive disease |**46**|. They reported that the combined presence of anti-CCP1 and IgM-RF provided the most accurate prediction. In another report Meyer *et al.* followed 191 patients with recent onset RA prospectively for 5 years |**47**|. Their results showed that the likelihood of a total Sharp score increase after 5 years was significantly greater among patients with anti-CCP1 antibodies (67%; OR 2.5) than patients with RF (OR 0.7). They concluded that antibodies to citrullinated proteins/peptides are good predictors of radiographic joint damage. Similar results with the anti-CCP1 test were obtained by Bas *et al.* |**48**|, and Saraux *et al.* |**49**| (Table 5.3).

Although the above studies employed the CCP1 test, similar findings have also been published for the more sensitive CCP2 test. Forslind *et al.* |**52**| measured anti-CCP2 at baseline in 379 patients and assessed radiological joint damage and disease progression after a 2 years follow-up. They observed that the presence of anti-CCP2 was associated with significantly higher Larsen scores both at baseline and at end-point compared with RF, C-reactive protein, erythrocyte sedimentation rate and other parameters |**52**|. Similarly Kastbom *et al.* |**53**| followed 242 patients with recent onset RA for 3 years. Their results showed that, although both anti-CCP2 antibody and RF had similar diagnostic sensitivities in early RA, CCP2 was superior as a predictor of the disease course over 3 years. Interestingly, they also found that anti-CCP antibody positivity remained essentially unchanged 3 years after diagnosis and initiation of therapy |**53**|.

Can anti-CCP be used in predicting which individuals may develop rheumatoid arthritis?

All the studies mentioned above suggest that the presence of anti-CCP antibodies may indicate the likelihood of developing (erosive) disease, although in not all individuals. However, this raises the interesting point as to how can we be sure that (erosive) RA is developing in a CCP-positive individual who has no obvious clinical complaints.

The answer to this question is the Holy Grail in RA and without doubt needs further study. There is, however, some light in the darkness. For example, it is possible that the anti-CCP titre might give an indication that erosive disease is likely to develop. Our own, as yet incomplete and unpublished, data seem to indicate that higher titres of anti-CCP (>5 times cut-off) correlate somewhat stronger with erosive disease than lower titres. It is thus possible that anti-CCP titre measurements in carefully controlled follow-up studies may be helpful in monitoring outcome/development.

In the original study of Rantapää-Dahlqvist *et al.* |**40**| the OR for anti-CCP2 to predict future development of RA was about 25, a significantly high number when compared with the OR of about 2 for both RF and shared epitope positivity (SE). The latter is typically associated with more aggressive disease and poor prognosis. Similarly van Gaalen *et al.* reported OR values of 38 for CCP2, 1.7 for RF and about 2 for SE |**43**|. Given the fact that RA is a multifactorial disease the presence of two or more of these parameters in an individual patient may drastically increase the likelihood of

Table 5.3 Features of predictive and prognostic CCP studies

Study	Ref.	Test	Cohort	Outcome/remarks
Predictive				
Nielen	|**41**|	CCP1*	79 RA (pre-patient)	CCP detectable >14 years before clinical manifestation
Rantapää	|**40**|	CCP2	83 RA (pre-patient)	CCP detectable >10 years before clinical manifestation; 70% CCP+ first clinical presentation
van Gaalen	|**43**|	CCP2	936 early arthritis	75% of undifferentiated arthritis patients that were CCP+ at baseline fulfil ACR criteria for RA after 1-year follow-up (93% after 3 years)
Vittecoq	|**44**|	CCP2	314 early arthritis	90% of early arthritis patients that were CCP+ at baseline were classified RA at the end of 1 year follow-up
Prognostic				
Visser	|**8**|	CCP1*	524 early arthritis	Prediction model for RA development including CCP far better than without CCP (both for persistence and erosiveness of arthritis)
Kroot	|**45**|	CCP1*	273 early RA	CCP+ at baseline (66%) is a predictor for development of significantly more severe radiological damage after 6 years
van Jaarsveld	|**50**|	CCP1*	249 early RA	CCP+ at baseline (52%) has prognostic value in addition to RF in predicting joint damage, but mainly for mild disease
Jansen	|**51**|	CCP1*	282 early RA	CCP+ at baseline (32%) correlates significantly with radiographic progression at 2 years follow-up (especially in RF-negative group; OR 21)
Meyer	|**47**|	CCP1	145 early RA	CCP+ at baseline (57%) is a good predictor for development of radiographic joint damage after 5 years (OR 2.5)
Vencovský	|**46**|	CCP1	104 early RA	CCP+ at baseline (42%) is a prognostic marker for erosive disease in early RA patients at 2 years follow-up
Bas	|**48**|	CCP1	27 early arthritis	CCP+ at baseline (30%) associates with RA disease severity at 8 years follow-up
Saraux	|**49**|	CCP1	243 early RA	CCP+ at baseline (47% at 93% specificity) is a predictor for erosive disease (43% CCP+) versus non-erosive (16% CCP+) after 2–4 years follow-up
Forslind	|**52**|	CCP2	379 early RA	CCP+ at baseline (55%) predicts radiological damage (OR 3.6) and progression (OR 2.9) at 2 years follow-up
Kastbom	|**53**|	CCP2	242 early RA	CCP+ at baseline (64%) predicts disease activity at 3 years follow-up

*'In house' CCP1 test, following the procedures described by Schellekens *et al.* |**22**|.
Source: Zendman *et al.* (in press) |**39**|.

their developing RA. This hypothesis was tested by Berglin *et al.* [54] who, using the patient material from the Rantapää-Dahlqvist *et al.* study [40], found that the combination of RF and SE gave an OR of about 40, while the combination of SE and anti-CCP2, for predicting the future development of RA, was about 67. It is therefore likely that a combination of serological and genetic factors may be able to predict accurately the development of (erosive) RA in an individual. Arguably a future genetic and serological 'RA passport' could be of considerable value in the therapeutic management of the disease, especially in individuals at high risk. There is already an increased understanding of the evolution of pre-clinical autoimmunity in other autoimmune diseases, such as SLE and type 1 diabetes mellitus [55].

Conclusion

From several recent publications the anti-CCP2 system has been shown to be a highly specific and sensitive test in the diagnosis of RA. Without doubt CCP antibodies are present very early in the disease and an increasing number of studies indicate that elevated titres of these antibodies may predict the development of erosive disease. In the near future, a combination of serological (CCP2, RF) and genetic (SE) factors may be used as powerful tools in the decision process to identify which individuals without obvious clinical symptoms may develop erosive disease and would therefore benefit from aggressive therapy.

References

1. Smolen JS, Steiner G. Therapeutic strategies for rheumatoid arthritis. *Nat Rev Drug Discov* 2003; 2: 473–88.
2. Bukhari MA, Wiles NJ, Lunt M, Harrison BJ, Scott DG, Symmons DP, Silman AJ. Influence of disease-modifying therapy on radiographic outcome in inflammatory polyarthritis at five years: results from a large observational inception study. *Arthritis Rheum* 2003; **48**: 46–53.
3. Landewe RB. The benefits of early treatment in rheumatoid arthritis: confounding by indication, and the issue of timing. *Arthritis Rheum* 2003; **48**: 1–5.
4. Lard LR, Visser H, Speyer I, van der Horst-Bruinsma IE, Zwinderman AH, Breedveld FC, Hazes JM. Early versus delayed treatment in patients with recent-onset rheumatoid arthritis: comparison of two cohorts who received different treatment strategies. *Am J Med* 2001; **111**: 446–51.
5. Arnett FC, Edworthy SM, Bloch DA, McShane DJ, Fries JF, Cooper NS, Healey LA, Kaplan SR, Liang MH, Luthra HS. The American Rheumatism Association 1987 revised criteria for the classification of rheumatoid arthritis. *Arthritis Rheum* 1988; **31**: 315–24.

6. Kaarela K, Kauppi MJ, Lehtinen KE. The value of the ACR 1987 criteria in very early rheumatoid arthritis. *Scand J Rheumatol* 1995; **24**: 279–81.
7. Saraux A, Berthelot JM, Chales G, Le Henaff C, Thorel JB, Hoang S, Valls I, Devauchelle V, Martin A, Baron D, Pennec Y, Botton E, Mary JY, Le Goff P, Youinou P. Ability of the American College of Rheumatology 1987 criteria to predict rheumatoid arthritis in patients with early arthritis and classification of these patients two years later. *Arthritis Rheum* 2001; **44**: 2485–91.
8. Visser H, Le Cessie S, Vos K, Breedveld FC, Hazes JM. How to diagnose rheumatoid arthritis early? A prediction model for persistent (erosive) arthritis. *Arthritis Rheum* 2002; **46**: 357–65.
9. van Boekel MA, Vossenaar ER, van den Hoogen FH, van Venrooij WJ. Autoantibody systems in rheumatoid arthritis: specificity, sensitivity and diagnostic value. *Arthritis Res* 2002; **4**: 87–93.
10. Steiner G, Smolen J. Autoantibodies in rheumatoid arthritis and their clinical significance. *Arthritis Res* 2002; **4** (Suppl 2): S1–5.
11. Marcelletti JF, Nakamura RM. Assessment of serological markers associated with rheumatoid arthritis: diagnostic autoantibodies and conventional disease activity markers. *Clinical and Applied Immunology Reviews* 2003; **4**: 109–23.
12. Nienhuis RLF, Mandema EA. A new serum factor in patients with rheumatoid arthritis. The antiperinuclear factor. *Ann Rheum Dis* 1964; **23**: 302–5.
13. Young BJ, Mallya RK, Leslie RD, Clark CJ, Hamblin TJ. Anti-keratin antibodies in rheumatoid arthritis. *Br Med J* 1979; **2**: 97–9.
14. Hoet RM, Boerbooms AM, Arends M, Ruiter DJ, van Venrooij WJ. Antiperinuclear factor, a marker autoantibody for rheumatoid arthritis: colocalisation of the perinuclear factor and profilaggrin. *Ann Rheum Dis* 1991; **50**: 611–18.
15. Sebbag M, Simon M, Vincent C, Masson-Bessière C, Girbal E, Durieux JJ, Serre G. The antiperinuclear factor and the so-called antikeratin antibodies are the same rheumatoid arthritis-specific autoantibodies. *J Clin Invest* 1995; **95**: 2672–9.
16. Schellekens GA, de Jong BA, van den Hoogen FH, van de Putte LB, van Venrooij WJ. Citrulline is an essential constituent of antigenic determinants recognized by rheumatoid arthritis-specific autoantibodies. *J Clin Invest* 1998; **101**: 273–81.
17. Girbal-Neuhauser E, Durieux JJ, Arnaud M, Dalbon P, Sebbag M, Vincent C, Simon M, Senshu T, Masson-Bessière C, Jolivet R, Jolivet M, Serre G. The epitopes targeted by the rheumatoid arthritis-associated antifilaggrin autoantibodies are posttranslationally generated on various sites of (pro)filaggrin by deimination of arginine residues. *J Immunol* 1999; **162**: 585–94.
18. Menard HA, Lapointe E, Rochdi MD, Zhou ZJ. Insights into rheumatoid arthritis derived from the Sa immune system. *Arthritis Res* 2000; **2**: 429–32.
19. Vossenaar ER, Despres N, Lapointe E, van der Heijden A, Lora M, Senshu T, van Venrooij WJ, Menard HA. Rheumatoid arthritis specific anti-Sa antibodies target citrullinated vimentin. *Arthritis Res Ther* 2004; **6**: R142–50.
20. Vossenaar ER, Radstake TR, van der Heijden A, van Mansum WAM, Dieteren C, de Rooij DJ, Barrera P, Zendman AJW, van Venrooij WJ. Expression and activity of citrullinating PAD enzymes in monocytes and macrophages. *Ann Rheum Dis* 2004; **63**: 373–81.
21. Vossenaar ER, Zendman AJW, van Venrooij WJ, Pruijn G. PAD, a growing family of citrullinating enzymes: genes, features and involvement in disease. *BioEssays* 2003; **25**: 1106–18.

22. Schellekens GA, Visser H, de Jong BA, van den Hoogen FH, Hazes JM, Breedveld FC, van Venrooij WJ. The diagnostic properties of rheumatoid arthritis antibodies recognizing a cyclic citrullinated peptide. *Arthritis Rheum* 2000; **43**: 155–63.

23. Bizzaro N, Mazzanti G, Tonutti E, Villalta D, Tozzoli R. Diagnostic accuracy of the anti-citrulline antibody assay for rheumatoid arthritis. *Clin Chem* 2001; **47**: 1089–93.

24. Palosuo T, Tilvis R, Strandberg T, Aho K. Filaggrin related antibodies among the aged. *Ann Rheum Dis* 2003; **62**: 261–3.

25. Vasishta A. Diagnosing early-onset rheumatoid arthritis: the role of anti-CCP antibodies. *Am Clin Lab* 2002; **21**: 34–6.

26. van Venrooij WJ, Hazes JM, Visser H. Anticitrullinated protein/peptide antibody and its role in the diagnosis and prognosis of early rheumatoid arthritis. *Neth J Med* 2002; **60**: 383–8.

27. de Rycke L, Peene I, Hoffman IEA, Kruithof E, Union A, Meheus L, Lebeer K, Vincent C, Mielants H, Boullart L, Serre G, Veys E, de Keyser F. Rheumatoid factor and anti-citrullinated protein antibodies in rheumatoid arthritis: diagnostic value, associations with radiological progression rate, and extra-articular manufestations. *Ann Rheum Dis*, in press.

28. Vossenaar ER, van Venrooij WJ. Anti-CCP antibodies, a specific marker for (early) rheumatoid arthritis. *Clin Applied Immunol Rev* 2004; **4**: 239–62.

29. Lee DM, Schur PH. Clinical utility of the anti-CCP assay in patients with rheumatic diseases. *Ann Rheum Dis* 2003; **62**: 870–4.

30. Pinheiro GC, Scheinberg MA, Aparecida-da Silva M, Maciel S. Anti-cyclic citrullinated peptide antibodies in advanced rheumatoid arthritis. *Ann Intern Med* 2003; **139**: 234–5.

31. Suzuki K, Sawada T, Murakami A, Matsui T, Tohma S, Nakazono K, Takemura M, Takasaki Y, Mimori T, Yamamoto K. High diagnostic performance of ELISA detection of antibodies to citrullinated antigens in rheumatoid arthritis. *Scand J Rheumatol* 2003; **32**: 197–204.

32. Dubucquoi S, Solau-Gervais E, Lefranc D, Marguerie L, Sibilia J, Goetz J, Dutoit V, Fauchais A, Hachulla E, Flipo R, Prin L. Evaluation of anti-citrullinated filaggrin antibodies as hallmarks for the diagnosis of rheumatic diseases. *Ann Rheum Dis* 2004; **63**: 415–19.

33. Isenberg DA, Horsfall AC. Systemic lupus erythematosus in adults. In: Madisson PJ, Isenberg DA, Woo P, Glass DN, eds. *Oxford Textbook of Rheumatology*, 2nd edn. Oxford: Oxford University Press, 1998; 5.7.1: 1145–80.

34. Mediwake R, Isenberg DA, Schellekens GA, van Venrooij WJ. Use of anti-citrullinated peptide and anti-RA33 antibodies in distinguishing erosive arthritis in patients with systemic lupus erythematosus and rheumatoid arthritis. *Ann Rheum Dis* 2001; **60**: 67–8.

35. Olivieri I, Palazzi C, Padula A. Hepatitis C virus and arthritis. *Rheum Dis Clin North Am* 2003; **29**: 111–22.

36. Leone N, Pellicano R, Ariata M, Maiocco I, Modena V, Marietti G, Rizzetto M, Ponzetto A. Mixed cryoglobulinaemia and chronic hepatitis C virus infection: the rheumatic manifestations. *J Med Virol* 2002; **66**: 200–3.

37. Wener MH, Hutchinson K, Monshima C, Gretch DR. Absence of antibodies to cyclic citrullinated peptides in sera of patients with hepatitis C virus infection and cryoglobulinaemia. *Arthritis Rheum*, in press.

38. Bombardieri M, Alessandri C, Labbadia G, Iannuccelli C, Carlucci F, Riccieri V, Paoletti V, Valesini G. Role of anti-cyclic citrullinated peptide antibodies in discriminating patients with rheumatoid arthritis from patients with chronic hepatitis C infection-associated polyarticular involvement. *Arthritis Res Ther* 2004; **6**: R137–41.

39. Zendman AJW, Vossenaar ER, van Venrooij WJ. Autoantibodies to citrullinated (poly) peptides: a key diagnostic and prognostic marker for rheumatoid arthritis. *Autoimmunity*, in press.

40. Rantapää-Dahlqvist S, de Jong BA, Berglin E, Hallmans G, Wadell G, Stenlund H, Sundin U, van Venrooij WJ. Antibodies against citrullinated peptide and IgA rheumatoid factor predict the development of rheumatoid arthritis. *Arthritis Rheum* 2003; **48**: 2741–9.

41. Nielen MMJ, van Schaardenburg D, Reesink HWR, van de Stadt RJ, van der Horst-Bruinsma IE, de Koning MHM, Habibuw MR, Vandenbroucke JP, Dijkmans BA. Specific autoantibodies precede the symptoms of rheumatoid arthritis: a study of serial measurements in blood donors. *Arthritis Rheum* 2003; **50**: 380–6.

42. Jansen AL, van der Horst-Bruinsma IE, van Schaardenburg D, van de Stadt RJ, de Koning MHM, Dijkmans BA. Rheumatoid factor and antibodies to cyclic citrullinated peptide differentiate rheumatoid arthritis from undifferentiated polyarthritis in patients with early arthritis. *J Rheumatol* 2002; **29**: 2074–6.

43. van Gaalen FA, Linn-Rasker SP, van Venrooij WJ, de Jong BA, Breedveld FC, Verweij CL, Toes REM, Huizinga TW. In undifferentiated arthritis, autoantibodies to cyclic citrullinated peptides (CCP) predict progression to rheumatoid arthritis: a prospective cohort study. *Arthritis Rheum* 2004; **50**: 709–15.

44. Vittecoq O, Incaurgarat B, Jouen-Beades F, Legoedec J, Letourneur O, Rolland D, Gervasi G, Menard JF, Gayet A, Fardellone P, Daragon A, Jolivet M, Le Loet X, Tron F. Autoantibodies recognizing citrullinated rat filaggrin in an ELISA using citrullinated and non-citrullinated recombinant proteins as antigens are highly diagnostic for rheumatoid arthritis. *Clin Exp Immunol* 2004; **135**: 173–80.

45. Kroot EJ, de Jong BA, van Leeuwen MA, Swinkels H, van den Hoogen FH, van't Hof MA, van de Putte LB, van Rijswijk MH, van Venrooij WJ, van Riel PL. The prognostic value of anti-cyclic citrullinated peptide antibody in patients with recent-onset rheumatoid arthritis. *Arthritis Rheum* 2000; **43**: 1831–5.

46. Vencovský J, Machacek S, Sedova L, Kafkova J, Gatterova J, Pesakova V, Ruzockova S. Autoantibodies can be prognostic markers of an erosive disease in early rheumatoid arthritis. *Ann Rheum Dis* 2003; **62**: 427–30.

47. Meyer O, Labarre C, Dougados M, Goupille P, Cantagrel A, Dubois A, Nicaise-Roland P, Sibilia J, Combe B. Anticitrullinated protein/peptide antibody assays in early rheumatoid arthritis for predicting five year radiographic damage. *Ann Rheum Dis* 2003; **62**: 120–6.

48. Bas S, Genevay S, Meyer O, Gabay C. Anti-cyclic citrullinated peptide antibodies, IgM and IgA rheumatoid factors in the diagnosis and prognosis of rheumatoid arthritis. *Rheumatology (Oxford)* 2003; **42**: 677–80.

49. Saraux A, Berthelot JM, Devauchelle V, Bendaoud B, Chales G, Thorel JB, Hoang S, Jousse S, Baron D, Le Goff P, Youinou P. Value of antibodies to citrulline-containing peptides for diagnosing early rheumatoid arthritis. *J Rheumatol* 2003; **30**: 2535–9.

50. van Jaarsveld CH, ter Borg EJ, Jacobs JW, Schellekens GA, Gmelig-Meyling FH, van Booma-Frankfort C, de Jong BA, van Venrooij WJ, Bijlsma JW. The prognostic value of the antiperinuclear factor, anti-citrullinated peptide antibodies and rheumatoid factor in early rheumatoid arthritis. *Clin Exp Rheumatol* 1999; **17**: 689–97.

51. Jansen LM, van Schaardenburg D, van der Horst-Bruinsma IE, van de Stadt RJ, de Koning MHM, Dijkmans BA. The predictive value of anti-cyclic citrullinated peptide antibodies in early arthritis. *J Rheumatol* 2003; **30**: 1691–5.

52. Forslind K, Ahlmén M, Eberhardt K, Hafström I, Svensson B. Prediction of radiological outcome in early RA in clinical practice: role of antibodies to citrullinated peptides (anti-CCP). *Ann Rheum Dis*, in press.

53. Kastbom A, Strandberg G, Lindroos A, Skogh T. Anti-CCP antibody test predicts the disease course during three years in early rheumatoid arthritis (the TIRA project). *Ann Rheum Dis*, in press.

54. Berglin E, Padyukov L, Hallmans G, van Venrooij WJ, Klareskog L, Rantapää-Dahlqvist S. Presence of the shared epitope genes increase the predictive value of antibodies against cyclic citrullinated peptide (CCP) for rheumatoid arthritis. *Arthritis Rheum* 2003; **48**(Suppl 9): S678 (Abstract).

55. Majka DS, Holers VM. Can we accurately predict the development of rheumatoid arthritis in the preclinical phase. *Arthritis Rheum* 2003; **48**: 2701–5.

Part II

Seronegative arthropathies

6

Seronegative arthropathies

IAIN McINNES

Introduction

Considerable advances have been made in treatment across the range of inflammatory arthropathies, in particular those derived from the therapeutic utility of pro-inflammatory mediators detected in synovium. Studies focused initially on rheumatoid arthritis (RA) have now been extended to encompass the seronegative arthropathies, including psoriatic arthritis (PsA) and ankylosing spondylitis (AS). This short review will focus upon the latter conditions and will especially highlight articles published in 2003 that elucidate clinical progress and novel therapeutics. These treatment advances are remarkable in that they provide opportunity in an area of rheumatology for which existing therapies have been particularly limited, and for which there has been only a small evidence base of randomized controlled trials upon which to formulate clinical decisions. In particular, the introduction of tumour necrosis factor (TNF)-α inhibiting agents provides not only clinical utility but also challenges current treatment paradigms and health economic models.

Papers have been selected that define the extent and significance of the clinical problem in prospective cohorts in PsA. It is now apparent that a substantial proportion of patients with PsA progress and exhibit structural decline, assessed by radiographic means. The factors that predict and mediate such decline remain unclear. Genetic evaluation represents one approach to this question. PsA resembles a polygenic disorder. Although known to be associated with HLA-Cw*0602, two recent studies in Iceland and Canada now provide evidence for an additional non-major histocompatibility complex (MHC) locus on chromosome 16q that links to PsA. This locus is shared with other autoimmune diatheses. The clinical relevance of the latter will be of considerable interest. Thereafter a paper is discussed that exemplifies the use of infliximab in treating resistant PsA. These data presage the publication of larger controlled trials in the use of infliximab in PsA, but are persuasive when considered in context of previous studies |**1**| showing the benefits of etanercept in PsA. Alternate approaches to targeting PsA arise from the recognition of the key role played by T lymphocytes prompting the use of a lymphocyte depletion strategy.

In AS the key advance in 2003 has been the publication of randomized clinical trials that demonstrate the efficacy of TNF blocking agents. I have focused therefore upon these studies but provide also two papers that describe the use of magnetic resonance imaging (MRI) and of immunological analysis *ex vivo* to gain further insight into the action of biologics in AS and in turn offer pathogenetic insight to the disease. The selection in this chapter will inevitably omit papers of importance and potential relevance to practice. For this I apologise but plead only space limitation in defence—nevertheless I trust that papers selected are of interest.

Progression of peripheral joint disease in psoriatic arthritis: a 5-yr prospective study

McHugh NJ, Balachrishnan C, Jones SM. *Rheumatology* 2003; **42**: 778–83

BACKGROUND. PsA has an estimated incidence of approximately 6.5/100 000. The prevalence of the disease is disparate across populations, with marked differences reported dependent upon the community or specialist care environment. With the advent of novel therapeutics, it is increasingly important to derive predictive factors for clinical patterns of disease most associated with functional disability. Only a few studies have adopted a prospective study design to determine the progression of PsA. Recent data have challenged the performance over time of the original classification criteria of Moll and Wright [2]. In particular the asymmetric articular distribution of PsA in comparison with RA was not sustained when models adjusted for the number of peripheral joints involved [3]. McHugh and colleagues have re-evaluated a cohort of patients originally studied in cross-section to determine outcomes over a median follow-up of 65 months.

INTERPRETATION. One hundred patients consecutively recruited into a cross-sectional cohort were included in this prospective study. Nine patients had died at median age 70 (five of cardiovascular disease), and four declined, or were lost to, follow-up. Of 87 patients analysed at median 65 months, there were significant increases in the number of joints involved and in Health Assessment Questionnaire scores at follow-up. Thirty-seven of 51 polyarticular patients had progressed the number of peripheral joints involved at a rate of 0.42 peripheral joints per year. Only 13 patients were available that had presented at outset within 1 year of disease onset—this group showed higher rates of progression. Distribution of disease across the cohort showed progression of polyarticular involvement but also emphasized that the frequency of distal interphalangeal (hand) and interphalangeal (feet) involvement provided distinction from RA disease distribution. Three patients became seropositive for rheumatoid factor. Fifty-seven per cent of patients had elevated plasma viscosity at baseline and initial plasma viscosity correlated with rate of progression of joint damage. Forty of 75 radiographs showed erosion at baseline and this increased to 51 of 75 at follow-up.

Comment

This study re-emphasizes that PsA is a progressive disease and that disease categorization may not be consistent over time. Polyarthritis is the predominant clinical phenotype in practice. This is commensurate with the observations of Marsal *et al.* who identified only two patterns of disease over time namely peripheral versus axial disease [4]. Isolated distal interphalangeal disease was rare but its presence with other joint involvement served as a useful distinguishing feature from RA. The rates of disease progression are similar to those reported by Gladman *et al.* [5]. Importantly, very few patients were in remission at 5 years, which again was similar to the reported rates in Toronto [5]. Plasma viscosity was, as expected, a predictor of progression. However, it is notable that almost half of patients did not have elevated plasma viscosity at baseline emphasizing the limitations of acute phase response in practice for a proportion of patients who may yet progress. Given the recent interest in early aggressive intervention in inflammatory arthritis, it will be imperative to derive information about initial progression. Although a subset of baseline patients in this cohort presented within 12 months of disease onset and appeared to progress more rapidly, the numbers are too small to inform properly as to early versus established disease progression rates. For this, inception subsets from early synovitis cohorts are necessary.

A prospective, clinical and radiological study of early psoriatic arthritis: an early synovitis clinic experience

Kane D, Stafford L, Bresnihan B, FitzGerald O. *Rheumatology* 2003; **42**: 1460–8

Background. Only two previous studies have addressed the outcome of PsA using an early inception cohort design in which only disease of short duration is admitted. The increasing emphasis on early and aggressive intervention using immunosuppressive agents in inflammatory arthritis, particularly RA, gives priority to evaluating the nature and rate of early disease progression in PsA. Moreover early inception cohorts lend the possibility of identifying predictive factors that in due course may prove of clinical utility.

Interpretation. One hundred and twenty-nine of 1018 patients recruited via an early synovitis clinic were diagnosed with PsA of mean disease duration 9 months (mean age 41 years). A majority of patients had polyarticular disease at outset. Importantly as synovitis was required for clinic referral, no patients with isolated spinal disease were included. Enthesopathy was present in 38% at presentation and 39% had distal interphalangeal involvement. One hundred and nineteen patients had psoriasis at presentation of mean age of onset 30 years. Baseline disease activity parameters included a visual analogue score of 4.8 cm (possible range 1–10), Health Assessment Questionnaire 0.71, Ritchie index 5.6, swollen joint count 6.9, erythrocyte sedimentation rate 24, serum amyloid A protein 145 mg/l and C-reactive protein 28 mg/l. One hundred and nineteen patients were reassessed at 1 year of whom 70 were taking a disease-modifying antirheumatic drug (DMARD). At 2 years 97 patients were reassessed, of whom 54 were on a DMARD. DMARD use included sulphasalazine (SASP), methotrexate (MTX), and more rarely cyclosporin (CyA) and combination MTX/CyA, MTX/SASP and MTX/azathioprine. Although improvements in inflammation and functional measures were observed up to 2 years, only 31 patients were in remission. Moreover, only 11 patients were in DMARD-free remission at 2 years. Radiographic progression was evaluable in

86 patients with median follow-up of 24 months. Forty-seven per cent of patients had erosive disease measured at follow-up—mean Sharp erosion score was 3 and Sharp narrowing score was 3.2.

Comment

This study provides important information as to the early progression of PsA and provides a powerful incentive to intervene early in patients presenting with synovitis and psoriasis. The study is the largest yet provided but is comparable with previously reported early cohorts. A proportion of PsA patients clearly exhibit significant disease activity and erosive changes even at baseline and the majority will exhibit disease progression, and require a DMARD despite which a subset will continue to exhibit functional and structural decline. This group have previously observed that psoriasis is itself a poor prognostic factor in a general spondyloarthropathy cohort |**6**| suggesting that PsA represents a particularly 'at-risk' group within the seronegative spectrum. Further prospective follow-up is ongoing to test this hypothesis. The rate of radiological erosive progression was significant but modest. It may be important to consider the distinctive anatomical localization of inflammatory disease in PsA compared with RA (for which the scoring systems were developed). As such ultrasound or MRI-based evaluation that is capable of including non-articular sites including entheses may be useful in determining progression and improving sensitivity to change after an intervention.

The foregoing papers, together with extensive datasets describing established PsA disease particularly from the Toronto cohort, clearly define the need for predictive and diagnostic indices in PsA. Extensive pathogenetic investigations are now ongoing with the aim of identifying such indices. PsA arises from a combination of genetic and environmental interactions resulting in aberrant host immune function. Genetic factors have until now focused upon immune response related genes primarily in the MHC. Two studies in 2003 re-examined genetic risk in PsA and were remarkable in identifying a locus outside the MHC that is associated with PsA.

A susceptibility gene for psoriatic arthritis maps to chromosome 16q: evidence for imprinting

Karason A, Gudjonsson JE, Upmanyu R, *et al. Am J Hum Genet* 2003; **72**: 125–31

BACKGROUND. Psoriasis is a polygenic disease for which several loci have now been described. That PsA has a genetic component to pathogenesis is indicated by segregation within families and high concordance rates in monozygotic twins (approximately 30–70%). Epidemiological analysis suggests more PsA patients have affected fathers than affected mothers. Commensurate with a proposed immune-mediated aetiology, genetic associations for psoriasis have been described at HLA-Cw*0602 with lesser associations noted with HLA-B13, HLA-B17 and HLA-B57.

PsA has a less pronounced association with HLA-Cw*0602 that is most evident in early onset patients. Iceland has a comprehensive genealogical database that facilitates genetic analyses that can identify extended family groups within study populations. This analysis created families that contained PsA patients separated by up to seven meioses (six meioses separate second cousins).

Interpretation. Of 906 patients with chronic plaque psoriasis, 178 were identified with PsA. Using the genealogical database, 100 of these patients were in turn connected to 39 families. Patients were genotyped using 1000 microsatellite markers with an average density of 3 cM and thereafter a multipoint, affected-only, allele sharing linkage analysis was performed. Further detailed mapping was performed in promising loci to characterize candidate loci. The strongest linkage was found at marker D16S3038 on chromosome 16q (LOD score 2.17). This is close to a marker previously linked to psoriasis. Linkage analysis using only paternal transmissions to affected individuals gave a LOD score of 4.19 at marker D16S267, close to the marker linked in the entire cohort. In contrast, no similar LOD score was observed when maternal transmission was investigated. The authors note that this locus is close to the *NOD2* gene (MIM605956) that has been linked to other autoimmune diseases, particularly Crohn's disease.

CARD15: a pleiotropic autoimmune gene that confers susceptibility to psoriatic arthritis

Rahman P, Bartlett S, Siannis F, *et al. Am J Hum Genet* 2003; **73**: 677–81

Background. This study was conducted in PsA patients in a Newfoundland population that exhibits relative genetic isolation, reminiscent of Hutterites or Amish communities. The investigators noted that the locus of maximum LOD score in the foregoing study was within 20 Mb of the *CARD15* gene (MIM605956) that has been associated with Crohn's disease. Epidemiological studies have suggested an increased incidence of psoriasis and PsA in patients with Crohn's disease. Three common independent sequence mutations are described in the *CARD15* gene that may be demonstrated by polymerase chain reaction amplification of genomic DNA collected from patients and population healthy volunteer controls. By this means possible overrepresentation of *CARD15* mutations in PsA patients may be examined.

Interpretation. One hundred and eighty-seven patients with PsA were compared with 136 healthy controls from the same Newfoundland population. In all, 53 of 187 (28%) PsA patients had a variant at the *CARD15* gene compared with 16 of 136 (12%) controls (odds ratio 2.97). The prevalence of *CARD15* mutation was similar in the entire PsA population as in familial PsA (at least one first degree relative involved). Allele frequencies were compared at each site: R702W (PsA 10.4% vs control 3.3%), leu1007fsinsC (3.2% vs 2.6 %) and G908R (1.6% vs 0.4%). One hundred and seventy-six patients were also genotyped at HLACw*0602. No relationship was noted between *CARD15* mutations and the presence of HLACw*0602.

Comment

PsA arises from a complex series of interactions between environmental agents acting upon a genetically predisposed host. It is suspected but not proven that many of these genetic loci will identify molecules of importance in host defence. The availability of technology for large population gene sequencing of marker sets mapping the human genome, and in this case rather unique clinical cohorts for evaluation, provides great potential for identification of candidate genes that offer pathogenetic insight. These studies identify for the first time a non-MHC gene of potential importance in susceptibility to PsA. The study in the Icelandic population identified a locus on chromosome 16q that was close to the *NOD2/CARD15* gene that has been associated with Crohn's disease and with Blau syndrome. This finding is in keeping with the well recognized clinical association between inflammatory bowel disease and the seronegative spectrum of arthritic disease. However, in two other independent studies psoriasis has not been associated with *NOD2/CARD15.* It is possible that *CARD15* segregates with features of the arthropathic component of the PsA disease spectrum. It is of interest that Karason *et al.* (2003) report on unpublished data suggesting that chromosome 16 overlaps with a peak observed in families with osteoarthritis (OA). They postulate that some articular susceptibility locus may exist on this chromosome, although this remains to be proven. It is noteworthy also that only patients with psoriasis *a priori* were studied in the Icelandic cohort. Given the relatively unique nature of the populations studied, it will be important to confirm the association between *CARD15* and PsA in other independent clinical cohorts.

Novel treatments

A significant problem in providing evidence-based treatment for PsA patients is the lack of good quality placebo-controlled randomized trials to support the use of commonly employed DMARDs such as SASP, leflunomide and MTX. The level of evidence as of 2003 has been reviewed by Pipitone *et al.* [7]. The need for novel therapies also remains considerable. Two papers that provide potential alternative approaches to treatment are reviewed below.

Efficacy of infliximab in resistant psoriatic arthritis

Salvarani C, Cantini F, Olivieri I, *et al. Arthritis Rheum* 2003; **49**: 541–5

BACKGROUND. A recent feature of pathogenetic investigations in rheumatology has been rapid translation to clinical intervention. This is best exemplified in the use of TNF-α inhibiting agents in RA. Several groups have identified high levels of TNF-α expression in PsA synovial membrane. In a recent phase II study, etanercept has been shown to be effective in PsA patients and also showed efficacy in reducing skin disease activity (Psoriasis Area and Severity Index score, PASI) [1]. Until 2003, however, there was little published evidence for efficacy of infliximab, although there is no *a priori*

reason to believe that anything other than a class effect might be observed in PsA. This study is an open-label pilot study of 'add-on' design, in which infliximab was given to patients with active PsA despite MTX therapy.

Interpretation. Sixteen patients with PsA that exhibited ongoing disease activity (>5 swollen and tender joints, erythrocyte sedimentation rate >25 mm/h, visual analogue score >25 mm) despite at least 6 months' MTX therapy were given infliximab in a multicentre, open-label pilot study. Three patients also exhibited axial disease. Psoriasis was confirmed by a dermatology investigator. Infliximab was administered at 0, 2, 6, 14, 22 and 30 weeks in combination with MTX. At week 14 ACR20, ACR50 and ACR70 responses were observed in nine of 16, seven of 16 and seven of 16 patients respectively. By week 30 ACR20, ACR50 and ACR70 responses were observed in nine of 16, eight of 16 and eight of 16 patients, respectively. No withdrawals resulted from efficacy failure. Adverse events were observed in four of 16 patients. Severe infusion reactions led to withdrawal of two patients. No severe infections occurred.

Comment

Prior to this study, infliximab was studied in one small, open-label loading dose study in spondyloarthropathy |**8**| in which eight patients with PsA were included. Improvement in signs and symptoms of PsA were observed. A second placebo-controlled, double-blind study using infliximab in spondyloarthropathy also included 13 patients with PsA some of whom exhibited significant improvement. The present study provides preliminary evidence for efficacy in severe PsA selected on the basis of peripheral arthritis (mean joint counts at entry 10 TJC, 6.5 SJC) resistant to MTX. Many patients included had also failed other conventionally used drugs, including CyA, and SASP. Although informative, there are significant shortcomings in a study that is uncontrolled and in which numbers are small. However, a recent large randomized placebo-controlled study to define response rates to be expected in PsA to infliximab has been reported by Kavanaugh *et al.* |**9**| in abstract form. The Infliximab Multinational Psoriatic Arthritis Controlled Trial (IMPACT 2) enrolled 200 patients with active PsA and tested the activity of infliximab (5 mg/kg) versus placebo on a stable background of existing NSAID, methotrexate and corticosteroid therapy if taken. The primary outcome, namely ACR20, was achieved in proportions similar to those reported for etanercept. It is noteworthy that improvements in PASI were observed in all PsA TNF blockade studies performed thus far and it seems likely that cytokine inhibition will prove an efficient way of targeting both tissue compartments in the disease. However, PASI improvement representing skin disease activity reduction in IMPACT 2 was impressive: PASI 50 achieved in 100%, PASI 75 achieved in 68%. Interestingly, these response rates appear higher than those previously seen with etanercept for the skin component of the disease suggesting that there may be local mode of action differences that have clinical significance. Confirmation of this observation will require a directly comparative, appropriately controlled study. The earlier studies of Mease *et al.* using etanercept have provided proof of principle for the effect of TNF blockade in PsA and indeed psoriasis |**1**|. Several issues are now outstanding. It is unclear at what stage in the treatment algorithm for PsA biologics should be introduced or whether there is a preference for one agent over another beyond the obvious, namely currently available, peer reviewed, controlled data. A further issue concerns the longevity of the clinical response that requires to be confirmed in follow-up studies. In this respect, it is unclear what response criteria will be useful in clinical practice in determining which patients should receive ongoing therapy. Finally, decisions regarding therapy may be made on the basis of responses in peripheral arthritis, axial disease or skin disease or a combination of these. This provides a level of clinical decision making complexity not yet addressed in registry and guidelines emerging for the use of biologics in other inflammatory arthropathies.

Lymphocyte depletion with fludarabine in patients with psoriatic arthritis: clinical and immunological effects

Takada K, Danning CL, Kuroiwa T, *et al. Ann Rheum Dis* 2003; **62**: 1112–15

Background. Although cytokine targeting has received most attention recently, there remains a persuasive evidence base supporting the pathophysiological role of T cells in PsA. The present report utilized the halogenated adenosine analogue, fludarabine to deplete lymphocytes and thereby achieve long-lasting immunosuppression. Emphasis was given not only to clinical effects but also to alterations in host immune response parameters.

Interpretation. Fifteen patients with active PsA were admitted to a randomized placebo controlled (1 : 1) trial in which fludarabine or placebo was infused every 4 weeks for four cycles. ACR20 responses were observed in three of seven active and none of eight placebo-treated patients at 16 weeks. PsA response criteria (PsARC) were met in four of seven active and two of eight placebo-treated patients at 16 weeks. Three of seven active, but no placebo recipients, sustained a >20% improvement in PASI. These observed differences did not reach significance. Skin and joint responses were not concordant. No significant toxicities were observed. Peripheral lymphocyte depletion was observed in both naive and memory cell subsets with particular effects on the former. Examination of synovial biopsies obtained prior to and after treatment available on five patients revealed reduction but not ablation of synovial lymphocyte subsets. Most lymphocyte depletion was observed in tissues obtained from ACR20 responders. Significant effects on synovial E-selectin (an endothelial activation marker), but not P-selectin, expression were also noted.

Comment

T cells have been long associated with the pathogenesis of psoriasis and PsA. T cells are prominent in PsA synovial membrane where they exhibit an activated phenotype, T-cell targeting therapies such as CyA and mycophenolate have some efficacy at least in psoriasis and T-cell oligoclonality in PsA skin and synovial biopsies suggests that a local autoimmune response is ongoing. However, therapeutic effects of targeting T cells are most prominent in psoriasis and less marked in treating arthritis. For example, no controlled data support the efficacy of CyA in PsA. One open-label study has targeted T cells in PsA using OKT3 with marginal benefit only [10]. A further pilot study employed interleukin (IL)-10 to suppress, among other inflammatory pathways, T-cell activation but achieved immunological suppression without convincing clinical effects [11]. The present study exemplifies a depletion approach. This has proved unsuccessful in general in treating autoimmunity, but has rather more success in managing lymphoproliferative disorders. Although there is some trend to efficacy, it seems unlikely that the profound lymphodepletion will be desirable against the relatively safe profile currently emerging for the use of cytokine inhibitors in inflammatory arthritis. The present study does, however, provide pathogenetic information. Responses appeared to correlate with changes in synovial membrane, in particular, in lymphocyte counts. Altered E-selectin but not P-selectin (a lymphocyte adhesin) may account for the partial success in achieving responses. Similarly, macrophage function and numbers were not significantly altered and this may be important in ameliorating a disease process even if T cells have an upstream physiological role. Of interest, circulating CD3+, CD25+ subsets (putative regulatory T cells) were reduced, further emphasizing the need for very specific T-cell targeting regimens that account for functionally distinct T-cell subsets. This study therefore provides important pathological information but probably not a novel therapy for PsA.

The predominant advance in managing AS has been the emergence of biological agents that provide amelioration of not only peripheral joint but also axial disease. Critical studies in this area are reviewed below.

Six month results of a double-blind placebo-controlled trial of etanercept treatment in patients with active ankylosing spondylitis

Brandt J, Khariouzov A, Listing J, *et al. Arthritis Rheum* 2003; **48**: 1667–75

Background. TNF-α is implicated in the pathogenesis of AS. It is elevated in AS serum, expressed in inflamed synovium and sacroiliac joints and is implicated in models of spondyloarthropathy. Infliximab has been shown in a phase II placebo-controlled trial to be efficacious in AS. Although infliximab has been shown also to be effective in treating Crohn's disease, no effect of etanercept has been noted in that disease. Etanercept has been shown to be effective in suppressing clinical and MRI parameters of inflammation in a small open label study in AS. The present study sought placebo-controlled data to extend these observations.

Interpretation. Thirty-three patients with active AS (>85% HLA-B27+) of 49 screened were randomized to receive either etanercept or placebo for 6 weeks. Etanercept recipients received 12 weeks of therapy and were followed up for a further 12 weeks. After 6 weeks, placebo recipients entered an open-label phase in which they received 12 weeks etanercept and were then followed up for a further 12 weeks. Fourteen patients were evaluated at week 6 in the active versus 16 patients in the placebo group. Fifty-seven per cent of AS patients receiving etanercept exhibited at least 50% improvement in Bath AS Disease Activity Index (BASDAI) at week 6 compared with 6% in placebo-treated patients. After 12 weeks of etanercept, 71% of patients achieved BASDAI 50 improvement. Moreover, upon receipt of etanercept, 56% of initial placebo recipients exhibited clinical improvement. Only one patient achieved a BASDAI 70% improvement. ASAS Working Group criteria responses were noted at 20% improvement in 78% vs 25% of etanercept- and placebo-treated patients, respectively, and at 50% improvement in 43% vs 12% of patients, respectively. Pain, function, quality of life and mobility scores all improved in etanercept-treated patients. Mean C-reactive protein levels also significantly reduced. Non-steroidal anti-inflammatory drug (NSAID) use was reduced in etanercept recipients. Responses were sustained throughout 12 weeks of therapy and until 6 weeks post-cessation but waned thereafter. Relapse occurred a mean of 6.2 weeks after discontinuation of therapy. No serious adverse events were recorded in the trial.

Comment

This investigator driven study provides evidence for efficacy in AS for etanercept given subcutaneously 25 mg twice weekly. It is remarkable for the short placebo arm that nevertheless clearly allowed differentiation from active drug. The duration of placebo was selected initially on the basis of study medication shortage but compares favourably with the duration of previous flare design NSAID studies in AS. The data are of interest at several levels. Most importantly they provide further justification for the use of TNF inhibition in treating AS. The effects on axial disease are particularly striking given the paucity of benefit from other available treatments. The study extends the data from Gorman *et al.* in which early efficacy for etanercept in AS was provided but without the use of the validated endpoints reported here, e.g. BASDAI [**12**]. Patients were withdrawn from DMARD and corticosteroid treatment 4 weeks prior to screening and the possibility that further benefit can be achieved in combination treatment regimens remains open. This has been observed now in several RA studies using TNF inhibitors, in particular with MTX. The lack of effect reported for etanercept in bowel inflammation is intriguing. The present report argues against a role for bowel inflammation in the axial compartment in AS—the authors propose that these data separate the pathogenesis of bowel inflammation from axial pathology in AS. This remains to be formally explored in future studies. A further consideration arises in the health economic benefit in achieving true disease modulation and indeed remission induction in AS. AS contributes substantial direct and indirect health costs and as such the cost–benefit evaluation will be of considerable interest.

Recombinant human tumour necrosis factor receptor (etanercept) for treating ankylosing spondylitis

Davis JC Jr, Van Der Heijde D, Braun J, *et al.* *Arthritis Rheum* 2003; **48**: 3230–6

BACKGROUND. The justification for TNF inhibition in AS has been sustained in pre-clinical studies together with several open-label and placebo-controlled trials. The present study represents the largest study performed thus far to determine the effects and safety of etanercept in the treatment of moderate to severe AS.

Interpretation. Three hundred and thirty patients with moderate to severe AS were screened of which 277 were randomized to receive either etanercept (25 mg s.c. twice weekly; $n = 138$) or placebo ($n = 139$) for 24 weeks. Unlike the Brandt *et al.* study, patients remained on their existing DMARD but randomization was stratified to ensure balanced allocation of subjects. In all, 126 of 138 and 120 of 139 patients completed the study in active and placebo groups respectively. At 12 weeks, the ASAS20 was achieved in 59% of etanercept and 28% of placebo recipients. At 24 weeks the ASAS20 was achieved in 57% of etanercept and 22% of placebo recipients. ASAS50 and ASAS70 responses were also greater in actively treated patients. Partial remission was achieved in 17% of etanercept but only 4% of placebo-treated patients. Significant reduction in C-reactive protein and erythrocyte sedimentation rate was observed in etanercept-treated patients. Injection site reactions occurred more commonly in etanercept recipients as did accidental injuries.

Comment

This study provides a large, multicentre, controlled study upon which to base decision making in the treatment of AS. The study included contributions from the authors of the report highlighted above. The magnitude and proportion of responders is broadly similar to that observed in the previously reported Brandt *et al.* study and suggests consistency of response across different AS populations (Europe and USA). The issues of long-term safety and of true disease modification, particularly at the entheses and within the spine remain open and are being addressed in registries and sophisticated imaging studies at this time. Those studies addressing structural modification will be of particular import in considering the long-term prevention of spinal deformity and maintenance of functional performance.

It should be noted also that similar evidence for efficacy for infliximab in AS has been reported (Van der Heijde *et al.* |**13**|). The AS Study for the Evaluation of Recombinant Infliximab Therapy (ASSERT) enrolled 279 patients with AS and compared the effect of infliximab (5 mg/kg) or placebo in reducing disease activity. At 24 weeks, 61% of infliximab recipients were ASAS20 responders compared with 19% that received placebo. Moreover, 22% of actively treated patients met criteria for partial remission. Significant improvements in components of the ASAS response, and in measures of quality of life (Braun *et al.* |**14**|) were observed in response to infliximab. Taken together, therefore, it appears that TNF inhibition is effective in the treatment of the articular components of AS. By contrast, there appear to be discrete effects when TNF inhibitors are compared for efficacy in distinct tissue compartments, particularly the gastrointestinal tract (see below).

Efficacy of etanercept for treatment of Crohn's related spondyloarthritis but not colitis

Marzo-Ortega H, McGonagle D, O-Connor P, Emery P. *Ann Rheum Dis* 2003; **62**: 74–6

Background. There remains considerable uncertainty as to the primary mechanism of action of TNF blocking agents and indeed whether different agents employ similar

modes of action. Although superficially acting through a common target, namely membrane and soluble TNF-α, significant differences are emerging in the bioeffects of etanercept and infliximab. The former is a TNFR:Fc fusion protein that binds not only TNF-α but also lymphotoxin, the clinical significance of which is unclear. Infliximab is a chimeric antibody that retains many Fc-mediated accessory functions and importantly may induce apoptosis in cells upon which TNF-α is targeted as a membrane cytokine. The significance of this is most evident in Crohn's disease in which infliximab is effective but etanercept apparently is not. The authors provide an intriguing clinical vignette in which patients with Crohn's spondylitis were targeted with etanercept with distinct subsequent effects in different disease compartments.

INTERPRETATION. Previous studies and those reported above have clearly shown efficacy for etanercept in AS. Two patients with HLA B27, Crohn's spondylopathy are described. One male patient with a 10-year history of Crohn's followed by onset of inflammatory spondyloarthritis received etanercept 25 mg twice weekly. Ten weeks after commencing therapy, he exhibited rapid improvement in articular symptoms, but thereafter developed progressive onset of bowel disease (quiescent prior to this), accompanied by elevation of acute phase response. At 6 months, whereas musculoskeletal symptoms were settled, gastrointestinal symptomatology remained highly active. MRI scanning at outset and completion confirmed the remission of articular signs. A second male with juvenile onset AS developed iritis, psoriasis and, finally, Crohn's disease subsequent to articular disease onset. Commencement of etanercept induced prompt suppression of articular symptoms and signs with no effect noted on gastrointestinal disease up to 6 months.

Comment

This short report provides an intriguing insight to the distinct modes of action of etanercept and infliximab (and probably adalimumab, although data are as yet sparse for the latter). Infliximab is recognised to be effective in treating both bowel inflammation in Crohn's disease and inflammatory arthritis and spondyloarthritis. Whereas etanercept is clearly capable of relieving symptoms and signs associated with enthesitis in the above patients, there was no effect manifest in gastrointestinal inflammatory disease. These data clearly show that the mode of action of these TNF blocking agents is distinct—there is no apparent class effect in inflamed bowel. Whether they also suggest that the pathogenesis of tissue involvement in these patients is distinct between bowel and synovium/functional enthesis is less clear. The failure of etanercept despite effective TNF-α blockade in the periphery to alter outcome in the bowel suggests that features of TNF effector function in lamina propria or epithelium are most amenable to antibody mediated inhibition. Apoptosis induction in LP lymphocytes has been suggested as the most likely mode of action—such an effect has not yet been demonstrated in inflammatory synovium post-TNF-α blockade. A final implication from these observations is the fascinating possibility that tractable 'public' pathways exist across a range of tissues that are generally accessible, but in addition local features may exert profound 'private' (tissue-specific) influence upon either the pathways themselves or inhibitors employed for therapeutic effect. Identification of such pathways and their synergistic interactions will likely lead to further therapeutic opportunity.

Magnetic resonance imaging examinations of the spine in patients with ankylosing spondylitis before and after successful therapy with infliximab

Braun J, Baraliakos X, Golder W, *et al Arthritis Rheum* 2003; **48**: 1126–36

BACKGROUND. AS comprises inflammation leading to new bone formation and to ankylosis over time that is characteristic of the clinical presentation. Significant limitations arise in existing plain radiographic imaging measurements particularly with low sensitivity in detecting change. Infliximab has been shown to be effective in the treatment of signs and symptoms of AS. Infliximab is effective in reducing radiographic progression in RA, but this has not been addressed in AS. MRI is increasingly used to detect spinal lesions in AS both as a diagnostic tool and for assessment of activity over time in established disease. This study takes advantage of a cohort of patients included in a multicentre, placebo-controlled trial that attended one centre and had MRI performed at outset and after 3 months of treatment. The investigators address a novel scoring system for spinal manifestations of AS.

INTERPRETATION. Nine patients received infliximab and 11 patients received placebo. Three MRI sequences and two scoring systems were evaluated. Chronic lesions were measured by a T1 weighted turbo spin-echo (TSE) sequence and assigned a chronicity score. Activity of these lesions was determined by further TSE imaging after injection of gadolinium (Gd)-DTPA or by short tau inversion recovery (STIR) sequences. The 40 images were read twice by two readers blind to clinical details. Active lesions were detected in 15 of 20 patients included in the study. They were recorded using the ASspiMRI tool (for details see Braun and van der Heijde 2002 [**15**]). MRI changes corresponded to improvements in BASDAI indicating some correlation with clinical parameters. Measurement of spinal lesion activity using Gd-DTPA or STIR sequences were reliable and determined to have face validity. Both were sensitive to change over 3 months. The inter-rater variance and the intrarater variance for both Gd-DTPA and STIR were small compared with the variance between patients. Gd-DTPA scores improved by 40% in infliximab and by 6% in placebo recipients. STIR determined active lesion score improved by 60% in infliximab recipients and deteriorated by 21% in placebo-treated patients. The chronic score determined by T1 images was improved by 7% in infliximab and reduced by 35% in placebo-treated patients.

Comment

This paper is notable not only for providing data informing the use of MRI in measurement of chronicity and activity indices in AS, but also for providing evidence that infliximab might significantly modify such radiological indices and thereby structural damage. The authors point out that MRI performed better in measuring activity than chronicity measurements. This they attributed to lack of sensitivity of MRI in detecting chronic changes especially thin syndesmophytes, but also a discrepancy between rheumatology and radiology trained observers in assessing the presence of syndesmophytes. Several studies now demonstrate that TNF inhibition reduces features of inflammation on MRI, including bone marrow oedema and contrast enhancement. The present study suggests that STIR or contrast enhancement techniques may be employed to address this question in clinical practice. As yet no conclusion can be drawn as to the preference between Gd-DTPA and STIR as one apparently exhibits more specificity and sensitivity than the other, respectively. As the STIR technique is cheaper and shorter, the authors conclude that in clinical practice this should be the preferred technique. Further studies will be required to confirm this proposal. A further benefit in MRI imaging over conventional approaches is the opportunity to evaluate the thoracic skeleton in more detail than previously possible with existing scoring systems. Long-term studies are now required to compare and contrast the performance of MRI against conventional radiographic scoring systems. These will run in parallel to studies addressing the relationship of inflammatory activity and chronic bone and tissue damage.

Down regulation of the non-specific and antigen specific T cell cytokine response in ankylosing spondylitis during treatment with infliximab

Zou J, Rudwaleit M, Brandt J, *et al. Arthritis Rheum* 2003; **48**: 780–90

Background. Biological drugs that very specifically target mediators in the inflammatory cascade provide a unique opportunity to understand disease processes. The mode of action of TNF blocking agents is unknown but likely includes endothelial deactivation, modification of leucocyte trafficking into inflamed synovium and inhibition of cytokine networks within the inflammatory lesion. It should not be assumed, however, that the mode of action of different TNF inhibitors will be identical in similar or indeed discrepant disease processes. Mechanistic studies performed as an adjunct to clinical trials are therefore of considerable interest. Zou *et al.* provide an example of such a study in which mechanistic questions have been addressed in patients receiving either infliximab or placebo. They use a non-specific T-cell stimulus (phorbol myristate acetate/ionomycin) and also a specific putative autoantigen stimulus, namely an 18mer peptide derived from the G_1 domain of aggrecan to activate blood lymphocytes to test the capacity for immune activation during infliximab therapy. To test monocyte function during therapy, they used lipopolysaccharide (LPS) to stimulate monocytes *in vitro*.

Interpretation. Peripheral blood cells were derived from patients receiving either infliximab or placebo, before treatment and then 6 and 12 weeks after therapy. Cell subsets were identified using anti-CD4 and anti-CD8 antibodies and the capacity for these cells to upregulate cytokines (interferon [IFN]-γ, TNF-α, IL-4, IL-10) was measured within each cell using fluorescent activated cell scanning after stimulation with either phorbol myristate acetate/ionomycin or G_1-derived peptides. Cytokine release by monocytes following addition of LPS *in vitro* was measured by enzyme-linked immunosorbent assay. Infliximab treatment reduced the number of CD4+ and CD8+ cell subsets that expressed IFN-γ and TNF-α upon stimulation. No similar effect was noted with placebo. Moreover, when the autoantigen-specific response was measured, G_1-derived peptide stimulation of

IFN-γ and TNF-α in CD8+ T cells was reduced after infliximab treatment. Infliximab mediated no consistent effect on the expression of IL-4 or IL-10 in stimulated T cells, nor in the production of TNF-α or IL-10 by LPS-stimulated monocytes throughout treatment.

Comment

Elucidating the mode of action of TNF inhibitors in AS is paramount. A significant problem in this respect is the lack of well-validated parameters of immune function that can be tested throughout a clinical trial that will be consistent both within a given patient over time and in comparison between groups. The assays employed in this study have been evolved to address this issue, particularly in storing cells until simultaneous assay to reduce experimental error. The data appear to show a trend to reduced inducible T-cell cytokine expression mainly in T-helper (Th)1 cells, rather than enhanced Th2-cell cytokine expression (characterized by IL-4 or IL-10 expression). The data showing suppression of responses to G_1-derived peptides is of particular interest, although the suppression of mitogen responses suggests that the phenomenon observed is not specific. Moreover, others have suggested that infliximab may increase the number of circulating regulatory T cells in a non-antigen-specific manner—this was not addressed in the current study. The data are consistent with observations in biopsies from Crohn's patients following infliximab treatment [16] that reveal reduction in IFN-γ+ T cells. There is, however, a peculiar inconsistency with data from the same group that show increased numbers of IFN-γ+ T cells following administration of etanercept to AS patients. The explanation for this is currently unclear. A final footnote lies in the requirement for a strong Th1 response in combating tuberculosis. It is possible that the Th1 suppression by infliximab renders the host more susceptible to mycobacterial infection.

Elevated levels of synovial fluid antibodies reactive with the small proteoglycans biglycan and decorin in patients with rheumatoid arthritis and other joint diseases

Polgar A, Falus A, Koo E, *et al.* *Rheumatology* 2003; **42**: 522–7

BACKGROUND. An elusive search in rheumatology remains that for the autoantigens that are crucial to initiation or perpetuation of synovial disease. These may not be synonymous. Evidence has been presented previously for autoantibody responses in inflammatory arthropathies against type II collagen, aggrecan, fibronectin, citrinullated cyclic peptides, HCgp39 and heat shock proteins. The present study sought evidence for immune reactivity in serum or synovial fluid against small proteoglycans of cartilage matrix. These represent a small component of mass but are present in equivalent molar amount to large proteoglyans in cartilage and contain leucine-rich sequences in their homologous core proteins. Their capacity to promote autoreactivity has not previously been explored.

Interpretation. Sera and synovial fluid samples were obtained from 60 patients in a prospective study (28 RA, 10 PsA, 10 seronegative spondyloarthritis, 12 OA). Enzyme-linked immunosorbent assay methodology was employed to detect immune reactivity to bovine type II collagen, biglycan, decorin, aggrecan and fibronectin. Prevalence of reactivity was defined as those above the mean + 2SD value of OA samples. Patients with RA displayed novel reactivity (IgM) against biglycan. In contrast, patients with seronegative arthropathies exhibited elevated titres of IgG antibodies recognizing decorin. Anti-type II collagen antibodies were elevated in RA, seronegative and PsA patients. Overall the prevalence of autoantibodies recognizing cartilage components was lower than for RA or seronegative spondyloarthropathy patients.

Comment

This paper does not provide (and does not claim to provide) definitive evidence for a pathogenetic role for cartilage autoantibodies in pathogenesis of synovitis. The nature of the study design cannot distinguish between primary and secondary antibody generation. The presentation of neoepitopes and of previously privileged antigens is postulated as one means whereby autoimmunity can contribute to the inflammatory milieu in inflammatory arthritis. Seronegative disease seems no exception and indeed the propensity for cartilage immune reactivity seems most correlated with articular destruction in the context of inflammation rather than a specific diagnostic clinical group. An important caveat to this study also is the lack of normal controls but rather presentation of data as a relative expression with OA tissues that themselves may exhibit some inflammation and cartilage damage. Nevertheless the data provide interesting insights to mechanisms of perpetuation of tissue damage and perhaps to factors that can promote the switch to chronicity. Moreover, if remission is to be maintained in such patients it is likely that some kind of tolerizing regimen will be required to prevent recurrence of disease promoted by this secondary reactivity. It is in such a role that co-stimulator therapeutics, e.g. CTLA4 immunoglobulin, may find utility in due course. A final comment lies in the activities of decorin itself. Although contained in immune complexes it seems likely that it can contribute to local immune modulation through binding C1q, inhibiting the C1 complex and perhaps inhibiting the effects of local cytokines, e.g. transforming growth factor-β.

Expression of the pro-inflammatory protein S100A12 (EN-RAGE) in rheumatoid and psoriatic arthritis

Foell D, Kane D, Bresnihan B, *et al. Rheumatology* 2003; **42**: 1383–9

Background. Neutrophil, macrophage and lymphocytic infiltration are characteristic of the inflamed synovium in psoriatic and seronegative disease. Factors that regulate this inflammatory response have been much more poorly characterized than in RA. S100A12 (calgranulin C; or EN-RAGE), a member of a family of proteins that share EF hand domains, is produced predominantly by granulocytes and once secreted acts as a

chemotactic factor. Via binding to its reciprocal receptor, RAGE, it leads in turn to activation of several signalling cascades associated with inflammatory synovitis, particularly NF-κB. Prior studies have not identified S100A12 in human tissues, most work having been performed in rodent models.

Interpretation. Forty-two patients contributed a variety of serum and synovial tissue and fluid biopsies with a range of diseases including RA, PsA and seronegative arthritis. In four patients synovial biopsies were performed before and after commencement of MTX therapy. S100A12 levels were highest in synovial fluid compared with serum. SA levels were higher than either RA or PsA levels. Of interest, S100A12 levels correlated with erythrocyte sedimentation rate and Ritchie index. Levels in synovial fluid did not correlate with neutrophil counts locally. S100A12 was localized histologically to diffuse distribution throughout infiltrates, representing degranulation of neutrophils. Distinct perivascular staining was noted as was staining within neutrophils. Finally, S100A12 levels were observed to reduce significantly in serum from 14 patients and in four synovial biopsies obtained after commencement of MTX therapy.

Comment

These are the first data to identify this family of proteins within inflamed synovial membrane. The association with erythrocyte sedimentation rate in serum and the prompt resolution of expression in tissues following successful MTX administration point to a close correlation with disease activity. NF-κB modulation in rodent models of arthritis and in human synovial cultures using small molecule inhibitors and adenoviral dominant negative mutants of the NF-κB signalling components, clearly link the RAGE effector pathway to perpetuation of inflammation and to tissue destruction. The capacity of S100A12 to promote this pathway therefore immediately assigns it a pro-inflammatory effector function. Moreover, polymorphisms in the RAGE gene have been associated with predisposition to arthritis |**17**|. An intriguing feature of this study is the distinct distribution of S100A12 in PsA versus RA and seronegative synovia particularly surrounding small blood vessels. S10012A may represent a novel mode of endothelial cell activation in PsA that in turn is characteristic of the inflamed psoriatic synovium in excess of that noted in other inflammatory disease states. This seems more plausible than an effect manifest only via neutrophil effector function. In murine studies RAGE or S10012A inhibition leads to anti-inflammatory effects. Such inhibition studies are now awaited in models of arthritis and in *ex vivo* human synovial culture systems to provide proof of concept for this potential novel therapeutic target.

Identification of Naf1/ABIN-1 among TNFα induced expressed genes in human synoviocytes using oligonucleotide microarrays

Gallagher J, Howlin J, McCarthy C, *et al. FEBS Lett* 2003; **551**: 8–12

Background. The utility of gene array technology has only recently been introduced to understand synovitis. This study is an example of the application of microarray

technology capable of identifying thousands of genes upregulated within a single cell lineage under specific *in vitro* conditions. This technique allows confirmation of candidate but also identification of novel moieties that may be associated with inflammation.

Interpretation. Fibroblast-like synoviocytes from inflammatory arthritis patients were examined for gene expression following exposure to TNF-α *in vitro*. The transcriptosome was probed using oligonucleotide microarray analysis. Differential expression at different time-points after TNF-α exposure was measured to identify genes that were altered in expression by TNF-α. Two hundred and thirty-one genes were induced at 4 and 24 h, whereas 148 and 184 genes were induced at 4 or 24 h respectively. Families of genes emerged of potential interest, including cytokine subsets (IL-8, IL-6, RANTES, MCP-1), matrix metalloproteinases and interferon γ responsive genes. Specific validation was performed using the *Naf1* gene, that codes for Naf1, a human homologue for the murine A20 NF-κB inhibitor ANIN-1. Confirmatory studies using Northern blot and Taqman polymerase chain reaction analysis validated the differential expression arising from the gene array analysis. Moreover, increased expression of Naf1 was measured in biopsies from seronegative and RA synovial tissues.

Comment

These studies provide initial proof of concept that novel gene expression in synovial tissue can be identified using the strategy of microarray analysis and follow-up in synovial biopsy material. The studies provide little pathogenetic information but rather serve to 'discover' moieties in context of synovitis that may not otherwise be recognized to have a role. Subsequent functional analyses are clearly essential as part of any such investigational design. Whether Naf1 truly represents an endogenous attempt in the synovium to regulate NF-κB will now require functional evaluation in separate studies. Nevertheless, the report provides insight as to the potential for discovery for microarray technology.

Conclusion

The foregoing represents a selection of clinically based papers of interest in the seronegative field in 2003. New data continue to highlight the progressive nature of seronegative disease, with associated functional decline and increasing disability. This highlights the requirement for more effective therapies. A short selection of basic papers relevant to seronegative disease is also highlighted to illustrate directions from which such novel therapies might arise. The clinical studies selected provide novel therapies and insights to their mode of action that in turn provoke further insight to underlying pathogenesis of disease. Moreover, they challenge the current treatment paradigms and raise expectations for physician and patient alike in the management of these chronic inflammatory disorders.

References

1. Mease PJ, Goffe BS, Metz J, VanderStoep A, Finck B, Burge DJ. Etanercept in the treatment of psoriatic arthritis and psoriasis: a randomised trial. *Lancet* 2000; **356**: 385–90.
2. Moll JM, Wright V. Psoriatic arthritis. *Semin Arthritis Rheum* 1973; **3**: 55–78.
3. Helliwell PS, Hetthen J, Sokoll K, Green M, Marchesoni A, Lubrano E, Veale D, Emery P. Joint symmetry in early and late rheumatoid and psoriatic arthritis: comparison with a mathematical model. *Arthritis Rheum* 2000; **43**: 865–71.
4. Marsal S, Armadans-Gil L, Martinez M, Gallardo D, Ribera A, Lience E. Clinical, radiographic and HLA associations as markers for different patterns of psoriatic arthritis. *Rheumatology* 1999; **38**: 332–7.
5. Gladman DD, Stafford-Brady F, Chang CH, Lewandowski K, Russell ML. Longitudinal study of clinical and radiological progression in psoriatic arthritis. *J Rheumatol* 1990; **17**: 809–12.
6. Stafford L, Kane D, Murphy E, Duffy T, Lassere M, Youssef PP, Bresnihan B, Fitzgerald O. Psoriasis predicts a poor short-term outcome in patients with spondylarthropathy. *Arthritis Rheum* 2001; **45**: 485–93.
7. Pipitone N, Kingsley GH, Manzo A, Scott DL, Pitzalis C. Current concepts and new developments in the treatment of psoriatic arthritis. *Rheumatology* 2003; **42**: 1138–48.
8. Van den Bosch F, Kruithof E, Baeten D, De Keyser F, Mielants H, Veys EM. Effects of a loading dose regimen of three infusions of chimeric monoclonal antibody to tumour necrosis factor alpha (infliximab) in spondyloarthropathy: an open pilot study. *Ann Rheum Dis* 2000; **59**: 428–33.
9. Kavanaugh A, Krueger G, De Vlam K, Birbara C, Beutler A, Guzzo C, Zhou B, DeWoody K, Antoni C. Infliximab improves arthritis and psoriasis in patients with active polyarticular psoriatic arthritis: results of the IMPACT 2 trial. *Ann Rheum Dis* 2004; **63** (Suppl 1): Abstr. No. SAT0050.
10. Utset TO, Auger JA, Peace D, Zivin RA, Xu D, Jolliffe L, Alegre ML, Bluestone JA, Clark MR. Modified anti-CD3 therapy in psoriatic arthritis: a phase I/II clinical trial. *Arthritis Rheum* 2001; **44**(9S): S92.
11. McInnes IB, Illei GG, Danning CL, Yarboro CH, Crane M, Kuroiwa T, Schlimgen R, Lee E, Foster B, Flemming D, Prussin C, Fleisher TA, Boumpas DT. IL-10 improves skin disease and modulates endothelial activation and leukocyte effector function in patients with psoriatic arthritis. *J Immunol* 2001; **167**: 4075–82.
12. Gorman JD, Sack KE, Davis JC Jr. Treatment of ankylosing spondylitis by inhibition of tumor necrosis factor alpha. *N Engl J Med* 2002; **346**: 1349–56.
13. Van der Heijde D, Dijkmans B, Geusens P, Sieper J, DeWoody K, Williamson P, Braun J. Efficacy and safety of infliximab in patients with ankylosing spondylitis: results of a 24-week randomized, placebo-controlled trial (ASSERT). *Ann Rheum Dis* 2004; **63** (Suppl 1): Abstr. No. SAT0053.

14. Braun J, Kellner H, Deodhar A, Inman R, Han CL, DeWoody K, Williamson P, Bala M, van der Heijde D. Infliximab improves quality of life in patients with ankylosing spondylitis: results of a randomized, placebo-controlled trial (ASSERT). *Ann Rheum Dis* 2004; **63** (Suppl 1): Abstr. No. SAT0049.

15. Braun J, van der Heijde D. Imaging in ankylosing spondylitis. *Best Pract Res Clin Rheumatol* 2002; **16**: 573–604.

16. Plevy SE, Landers CJ, Prehn J, Carramanzana NM, Deem RL, Shealy D, Targan SR. A role for TNF-alpha and mucosal T helper-1 cytokines in the pathogenesis of Crohn's disease. *J Immunol* 1997; **159**: 6276–82.

17. Hoffman MA, Drury S, Hudson BI, Gleason MR, Qu W, Lu Y, Lalla E, Chitnis S, Monteiro J, Stickland MH, Bucciarelli LG, Moser B, Moxley G, Itescu S, Grant PJ, Gregersen PK, Stern DM, Schmidt AM. RAGE and arthritis: the G82S polymorphism amplifies the inflammatory response. *Genes Immunity* 2002; **3**: 123–35.

Part III

Connective tissue disorders

Connective tissue disorders

RAJAN MADHOK

Introduction

In advising contributors to this section we were restrictive, but restrictive only in the sense that the papers chosen had to be patient centred; we asked that the information should be useful to the practising clinician. However, as Uribe, Toloza and Alarcón point out, it is only by obtaining a better understanding of the molecular and cellular basis that new therapies will emerge. Hence, in the subsections on systemic lupus erythematosus (SLE), scleroderma, myositis and vasculitis, the contributors have selected papers that will help clinicians add to their fundamental knowledge in order to understand the role of emerging therapies and the consensus that is arising in the management of these conditions.

When it comes to rheumatologists with an interest in managing the connective tissue diseases, there are the 'lumpers' and the 'splitters'. The splitters clearly seem to be having the day. In all three disorders, a better understanding and hence better treatment approaches have evolved by looking at the subcategories of disease. In SLE, the utility of modifying the diagnostic criteria is discussed and, although this had little impact, the reviewers highlight the importance of recording the number of American College of Rheumatology criteria at enrolment and those achieved. Herrick highlights the importance of recognizing the difference between limited and diffuse systemic sclerosis, a distinction of particular importance as management of isolated pulmonary hypertension becomes more amenable, and therefore of identifying those at risk early. Miller records that a retrospective review of muscle biopsies showed the importance of major histocompatibility complex class I staining in recognizing inflammatory myopathies.

Herrick also notes in her introduction that these are exciting times for rheumatologists and that this excitement is not only confined to the management of rheumatoid arthritis (RA). In the connective tissue diseases as well as the vasculitides, methods for meaningful clinical trials are evolving, thus further developing the evidence base for the management of these complex disorders. This is particularly important as most evidence to date has been based on trials only a few of which meet the rigorous criteria required to remove uncertainty from our decision making. As new therapies emerge, clinical trials rather than empirical theory must remain the strategy of choice. In this regard, in all four sections the contributors highlight the importance of the tools developed in order to undertake meaningful studies.

Finally, as in RA, it is accepted that premature cardiovascular disease is a frequent contributor to late mortality in SLE. Like RA, SLE appears to be an independent risk factor in addition to the effects of traditional cardiovascular risk factors. As in RA, the results of treatments that modify traditional cardiac risk factors are awaited.

As this collection of patient-centred contributions highlights, rheumatologists now have a better chance of making a significant difference in improving patient outcome. These are indeed exciting times in rheumatology.

7

Systemic lupus erythematosus

AMÉRICA URIBE, SERGIO TOLOZA, GRACIELA ALARCÓN

Introduction

In selecting the papers that will have the greatest lasting impact in systemic lupus erythematosus (SLE), we have used a patient-centred approach; that is, we have primarily chosen those papers that may, directly or indirectly, translate into better patient outcomes.

There is significant heterogeneity in the prevalence and incidence of SLE and on its clinical expression among different world populations: non-Caucasians experience the disease more frequently and have less favourable outcomes. These differences have been regarded as genetically and/or socio-economically determined. The possible role of African ancestry as a risk factor for the occurrence of SLE has been examined by studying admixture proportions in a mixed (European and African) population in the Caribbean island of Trinidad (Molokhia *et al.*). The role of specific gene polymorphisms in predisposing to the occurrence of SLE or to some of its manifestations continues to be the focus of intense investigation; the meta-analysis by Karassa *et al.* of the role of low-binding alleles of Fc gamma IIIA receptor (R) gene polymorphisms in predisposing to lupus nephritis (LN) has been chosen as the prototype within a vast group of such papers, given that it systematically summarizes pertinent world literature (Karassa *et al.*). Only by understanding the scientific basis of SLE can better treatments be devised and implemented.

In diseases of unknown aetiology, such as SLE, we must rely on defined criteria to identify patients suffering from it; any modification of established criteria will therefore affect patient recruitment in longitudinal observational studies and randomized controlled trials (RCTs). Thus, the effect of the modification of the 1982 American College of Rheumatology (ACR) criteria for the classification of patients with SLE is discussed (Feletar *et al.*). The next four papers reviewed address either poorly understood disease manifestations (fatigue) (Tench *et al.*), or manifestations that occur as a consequence of the disease or its treatments (damage); one such paper (Ravelli *et al.*) addresses the use in children of the instrument developed to measure damage in adult SLE patients |**1**|, whereas the other two papers describe specific 'damage' items, such as the identification of risk factors for accelerated atherosclerosis (Al-Herz *et al.*) and the proper follow-up of patients receiving hydroxychloroquine (Mavrikakis *et al.*).

The last group of papers deals primarily with the design and quality of available lupus RCTs (Karassa *et al.*), with treatment outcomes (LN and renal transplantation) (Deegens *et al.*; Fiehn *et al.*) and with newer treatment options for the lupus patient (an anti-DNA non-immunogenic immunomodulatory tolerogenic agent [LJP 394] and haematopoietic stem-cell transplantation [HSCT]) (Traynor *et al.* and [**2**]). The last two papers are not definitive; however, both are quite meritorious. The first points out that selection of patients based on specific laboratory parameters may be needed if biological treatments are going to be effective, and the second provides the largest and longest follow-up data on HSCT in lupus.

We hope the reader finds this selection of papers as interesting and informative as we have found it.

Relation of risk of systemic lupus erythematosus to West African admixture in Caribbean populations

Molokhia M, Hoggart C, Patrick AL, *et al. Hum Genet* 2003; **112**: 1–9

BACKGROUND. The phenotypic expression of SLE is quite variable among human populations: non-Caucasians around the world exhibit more serious disease manifestations and poorer outcomes than Caucasians. The extent to which these differences are genetically or socio-economically/demographically based remains a matter of intense investigation and controversy. The rarity of SLE among Africans contrasts with its increased frequency (and severity) among individuals of African ancestry residing in the Caribbean islands or in the Americas. A possible approach to deconfounding the effects of ethnicity and socio-economic/demographic factors is to examine admixture proportions among ethnically diverse populations.

INTERPRETATION. One hundred and twenty-four SLE patients and 219 matched controls from the Caribbean island of Trinidad were studied; the analyses were, however, restricted to patients without an Indian (from the Indian subcontinent) or Chinese genetic background as the frequencies of ancestry-informative markers (AIMs) in the corresponding founding populations were not available. Patients and controls were typed for AIMs (markers showing large allelic differences between European and West African populations). African admixture was found to be greater (0.81) in cases than in controls (0.74) and the difference between these two rates was significant ($P = 0.01$) (Fig. 7.1). The estimated risk of the development of SLE for each unit of admixture was 32.5. Adjustments for measures of socio-economic status did not significantly alter this risk.

Comment

The study by Molokhia *et al.* is the first in which admixture proportions are used to estimate the risk of developing SLE (admixture has been used in other diseases). Admixture and two measures of socio-economic status were included to determine their independent contributions to the risk of SLE. In fact, the risk ratio of SLE due to African admixture was found to be 32.5 by univariable analyses but was reduced only to 28.4 in multivariable analyses in which socio-economic measures were included, very strongly suggesting that their contribution to the risk of SLE was not as important as the genetic component. Admixture can also be used to pursue genetic mapping and to determine the precise gene(s) that explain the large difference in the risk of SLE between Caucasians and populations of African ancestry. Numerous candidate genes (HLA, complement, MBL, GST, ACE, *Fc gamma R* polymorphisms) have been examined in SLE, but they do not by themselves explain this different risk. It is important to know that the use of admixture in populations from founding populations that are poorly defined genetically, in which the frequency of AIMs is unknown, is not possible. When more than two founding populations are present, it may not be as straightforward to study their admixture estimates as when only two are present. The time seems right to study admixture proportions as means of exerting genetic control in heterogeneous populations. This may prove useful in the USA, where admixture between Caucasians (European), Amerindians (native to the American continent) and Africans has occurred. The parcelling of patients and controls into

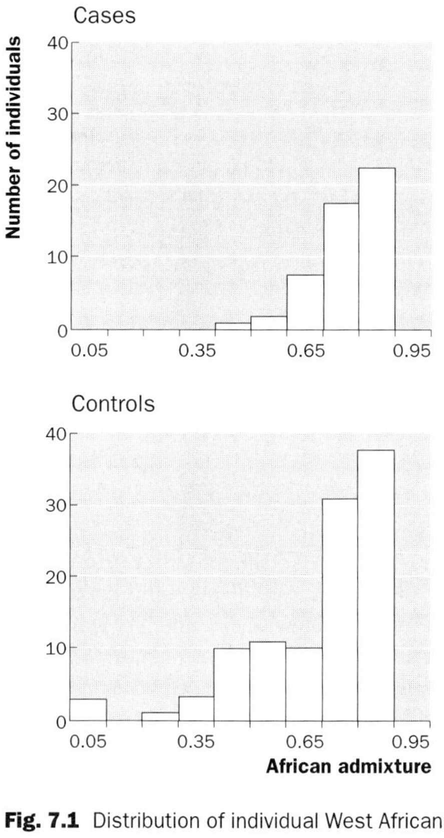

Fig. 7.1 Distribution of individual West African admixture estimates in cases (*top*) and controls (*bottom*). Source: Molokhia *et al.* (2003).

arbitrarily or self-defined ethnic groups may no longer be acceptable in studying the genetics of SLE (and other disorders) [**3,4**].

The Fc gamma RIIIA-F158 allele is a risk factor for the development of lupus nephritis: a meta-analysis

Karassa FB, Trikalinos TA, Ioannidis JP; Fc gamma RIIIA-SLE meta-analysis investigators. *Kidney Int* 2003; **63**: 1475–82

BACKGROUND. The role of genetic factors in the occurrence of SLE and its clinical expression (phenotype) is now considered to be essential. The Fcγ R gene polymorphisms have been considered important for both disease susceptibility and severity. The data published so far regarding Fcγ RIIIA emanate from relatively small studies; not surprisingly, the results have not been uniform regarding the role of 158 V/F polymorphism in susceptibility to LN. An international meta-analysis was conducted to rigorously quantify the existing evidence.

INTERPRETATION. After reviewing the published literature (to August 2002) and data presented at pertinent meetings (or obtained from the authors), a total of 16 comparisons from eleven studies in which *V/F158* genotyping had been performed were included; these studies included 154 patients with LN, 1261 with SLE and 1455 healthy controls. There was no significant heterogeneity between studies when examining the LN data. Low-binding alleles of *F158* were over-represented among LN patients, with an odds ratio (OR) of 1.20 (95% confidence interval [CI] 1.06–1.36, $P = 0.003$). *FF* homozygotes had a greater risk than *VV* homozygotes (OR 1.47, 95% CI 1.11–1.93, $P = 0.006$) (Fig. 7.2a). However, susceptibility to SLE in patients with the low-binding alleles of *F158* was uncertain given that the CI included 1, even though the OR was 1.19. In contrast with the LN studies, there was significant heterogeneity between SLE susceptibility studies (Fig. 7.2b). The authors conclude that the Fcγ *RIIIA-V/F158* polymorphism has a significant effect on the development of LN but not of SLE.

Comment

This international meta-analysis supports the role of homozygosity for the low-binding alleles of *Fc gamma RIIIA* in predisposing to LN. This was true regardless of the population in which this association was examined. These findings contrast with data generated from a meta-analysis examining the role of low-binding alleles of *Fc gamma RIIA*, in which no association between these alleles and LN was found. This discrepancy probably relates to the IgG subclass of pathogenic autoantibodies in LN; anti-double-stranded (ds) DNA and anti-nucleosome antibodies, the auto-antibodies most commonly associated with LN, are of the IgG1 and IgG3 subclasses, which bind to *Fc gamma RIIIA*; individuals with the low-binding alleles of *Fc gamma RIIIA-F158* are therefore expected to clear immune complexes containing such pathogenic antibodies with difficulty, leading to their deposition in the glomerular basement membrane and subsequent tissue injury. In contrast, those of IgG2 sub-class are cleared by *Fc gamma RIIA* and are not associated with LN; thus, low-binding

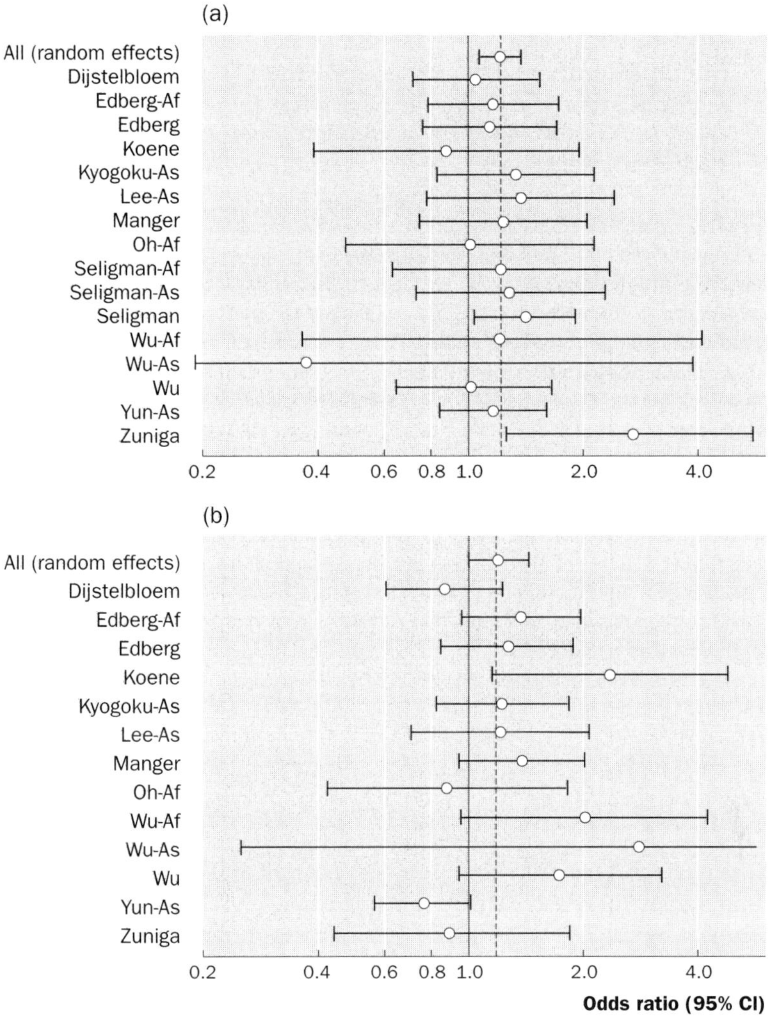

Fig. 7.2 Meta-analysis of the effects of the *FcγRIIIA-V/F158* polymorphism on the risk of (a) lupus nephritis and (b) systemic lupus erythematosus (SLE). Source: Karassa *et al.* (2003).

alleles of *Fc gamma RIIA* do not influence the occurrence of LN, although they are enriched in patients with SLE in general |**5**|. Haplotypes of *Fc gamma RIIA* and *Fc gamma RIIIA* have been found to be associated with SLE, but the data are not consistent across all studies and a meta-analysis regarding this association is not possible (there are relatively few studies and patients). Other polymorphisms of *Fc gamma RIIA* and *Fc gamma RIIIA* may also be important, but these data are just emerging.

The impact of the 1997 update of the American College of Rheumatology revised criteria for the classification of systemic lupus erythematosus: what has been changed?

Feletar M, Ibanez D, Urowitz MB, Gladman DD. *Arthritis Rheum* 2003; **48**: 2067–9

BACKGROUND. The 1982 ACR revised criteria for SLE were updated in 1997 (removing the lupus erythematosus [LE] cell test from the immunological criterion and including instead a test for antiphospholipid [aPL] antibodies; the serological false-positive test for syphilis remained). Recently, Feletar *et al.* examined the performance of the ACR revised criteria and its effect in lupus studies. They examined an inception cohort (1992–2002) of SLE patients ($n = 154$) including only patients fulfilling four 1982 ACR criteria (immunological criterion being one of them). Thirty-six patients were identified. All patients had been tested for LE cells and aPL antibodies (IgG and/or IgM anticardiolipin antibodies and/or lupus anticoagulant). They examined the effect on patient classification of removing the LE cell test and adding the test for aPL antibodies.

INTERPRETATION. By removing the LE cell test, two patients could no longer be classified as having SLE (they did not exhibit aPL antibodies); thus, they did not regain their SLE classification status. One patient with a negative LE cell test but who was positive for aPL antibodies was found (but this patient already met the immunological criterion of positivity for anti-dsDNA).

Comment

Feletar *et al.* have addressed a timely and important issue by examining the performance of the recent changes made by the ACR to the 1982 criteria. Neither the addition nor the removal of one immunological feature from the immunological criterion seem to affect the identification of patients with SLE significantly; this has obvious implications for research studies, but not so much for clinical care. Although a small number of patients were studied, the removal of the LE cell test altered the classification status only in two patients (1.3%), whereas the inclusion of aPL antibodies had no effect.

Extrapolating these findings to more contemporary lupus cohorts will be difficult because the LE cell test is rarely done nowadays, having been replaced by testing for antinuclear antibodies, a more sensitive and simple alternative. Any modification to the ACR classification criteria needs to be tested using appropriate controls (patients with other connective tissue disorders, for example). Only after determining that a given modification improves the criteria's performance, could the revised criteria be adopted.

To allow meaningful interpretation of SLE studies, researchers should provide not only the number of criteria met at enrolment but also the number of criteria ever met. Another consideration is the time it takes to accrue four ACR criteria [6]; Hispanics (of Mexican ancestry) may accrue ACR criteria more rapidly than patients from other ethnic groups. This information may help clinicians to follow these patients closely in order to identify the disease during its initial stages and to introduce therapeutic interventions early.

Fatigue in systemic lupus erythematosus: a randomized controlled trial of exercise

Tench CM, McCarthy J, McCurdie I, White PD, D'Cruz DP. *Rheumatology* 2003; **42**: 1050–4

BACKGROUND. Fatigue is a poorly understood and relatively common complaint of patients with SLE and one for which no successful therapeutic interventions currently exist. Thus, any manoeuvre that proves to be beneficial for such patients should be viewed very favourably. Tench *et al.* performed an RCT with promising results.

INTERPRETATION. Ninety-three patients with SLE according to the ACR classification criteria, without active disease in a major organ system (Systemic Lupus Activity Measure scores between 3 and 8) and on stable therapy, were randomized to exercise, relaxation or a minimal intervention (control). The protocol lasted 12 weeks. Patients in the exercise group were asked to exercise at home at least three times a week, for 30–50 min on each occasion, to a heart rate of 60% of their peak oxygen consumption; patients in the relaxation group listened to an audiotape three times a week, 30 min each time, and patients in the control group were asked to continue their normal daily life activities, avoiding extraneous physical exercise. By intention-to-treat analysis, a higher proportion of patients in the exercise group (16/33, 49%) improved compared with the relaxation group (8/29, 28%) and the control group (5/32, 16%) ($\chi^2 = 8.3$, df = 2, $P = 0.02$).

Comment

The authors powered the study on the basis of their experience with fibromyalgia; nevertheless, the study is relatively small. Before it can be concluded that this exercise technique will work in all lupus patients, a large and more diverse patient population needs to be studied and patients need to be followed up longer to be sure that the intervention has lasting effects. Furthermore, patients certainly need to continue to exercise to maintain the benefits attained; this requirement in itself may necessitate drastic changes in the patient's lifestyle, which are not always easy to accomplish. Fatigue in lupus is one of a series of poorly understood clinical manifestations for which we have no successful treatment, as it occurs in patients who otherwise appear not to have evidence of active disease and/or of organ system involvement. A recent small study suggests that patients with SLE have evidence of aerobic insufficiency, which in turn is associated with fatigue |**7**|. Whether aerobic insufficiency could be modified by the graded exercise programme described by Tench *et al.* can only be surmised, since it was not ascertained in their patients. Another relatively common and baffling manifestation present in lupus patients is that of cognitive impairment; if properly ascertained, cognitive impairment is found in a large proportion of SLE patients. Although some patients may have overt neurocognitive impairment, others may have only very mild impairment (impairment that is only apparent to them). Like fatigue, the underlying pathological correlate of neurocognitive impairment is unclear at the moment; recently, however, it has been shown that global brain damage (ascertained by magnetization transfer imaging), but not disease duration, is highly correlated with neurocognitive impairment [8]. It is certain that, with increasing understanding of why these poorly defined symptoms occur so frequently in lupus patients, our treatment approaches will become more scientifically based and probably more successful. For the time being, however, graded exercise therapy may be all we have to offer to manage these patients' fatigue (but not their impaired cognition).

Assessment of damage in juvenile-onset systemic lupus erythematosus: a multicenter cohort study

Ravelli A, Duarte-Salazar C, Buratti S, *et al. Arthritis Rheum (Arthritis Care Res)* 2003; **49**: 501–7

BACKGROUND. This international multicentre study investigated the prevalence and associated factors (demographic, clinical and quality of life) of cumulative organ damage, as measured by the Systemic Lupus International Collaborating Clinics (SLICC) Damage Index (SDI), in patients with juvenile-onset SLE. Damage in lupus has a tremendous impact in all patients, but perhaps a greater effect in the very young. Three hundred and eighty-seven patients with juvenile-onset (before 18 years of age) SLE, from eight institutions or national study groups from Europe, the USA, Mexico and Japan, with disease duration of at least 12 months were enrolled between January and October 1999.

INTERPRETATION. In this study half the patients had accrued some damage; 5.7 years from disease onset the mean SDI score was 1.1. In decreasing order of frequency, damage occurred in the renal (22%), neuropsychiatric (16%), musculoskeletal (12%), ocular (11%) and cutaneous (10%) systems (Table 7.1). Damage was associated with the presence of neuropsychiatric involvement (by ACR criteria) at diagnosis, longer disease duration and a greater number of cyclophosphamide pulses received; gender and ethnicity were not predictive of damage. School work performance decreased in patients who had accrued any damage; this was related to physical rather than to emotional or behavioural problems.

Comment

Over the last two decades, the life expectancy of patients with juvenile-onset SLE has improved notably; consequently, these young people face considerable damage accrual that is secondary to disease activity and the medications used. The appropriateness of the SDI for the assessment of damage in children and adolescents with SLE has been discussed in the literature. Most researchers acknowledge the fact that some modifications are needed; for example, proteinuria should be referred to body

Table 7.1 Frequency of damage in the twelve organ systems/domains of the SDI

System/domain	No. (%)
Renal	21.8
Musculoskeletal	11.7
Ocular	10.9
Skin	9.6
Pulmonary hypertension	2.3
Cardiovascular	3.1
Peripheral vascular	6.2
Gastrointestinal	3.9
Premature gonadal failure	3.9
Diabetes	0.5
Malignancy	0

Source: Ravelli *et al.* (2003).

surface area, gonadal failure should be based on hormonal studies, and growth abnormalities should be considered. Work along these lines is in progress [**9**].

Previously identified risk factors for damage accrual among these patients are younger age at diagnosis, male gender, non-Caucasian ethnicity, greater disease activity, the presence of antiphospholipid antibodies, acute thrombocytopenia or diffuse proliferative glomerulonephritis, and the cumulative dose and length of use of corticosteroids. Most frequently affected are the renal, musculoskeletal, neuropsychiatric, ocular, skin and gastrointestinal organ systems; however, these data come primarily from small studies (i.e. studies that include relatively few patients). The article reviewed includes a large number of patients from different countries, continents and ethnicities; even though the analyses were limited to one time-point, the data carry more weight. It is important to note that disease duration, neuropsychiatric involvement and cyclophosphamide pulse therapy, but not ethnicity, age or gender, were identified as predictors of damage. Cyclophosphamide pulses and the presence of neuropsychiatric involvement at diagnosis are likely proxies of disease activity. It is of interest that, although cyclophosphamide therapy predicted overall damage, premature gonadal failure was uncommon in this study (3.9%); this probably reflects the age of these patients as well as their limited time of follow-up. Work is in progress towards preserving ovarian function in these young women [**10**].

Cardiovascular risk factor screening in systemic lupus erythematosus

Al-Herz A, Ensworth S, Shojania K, Esdaile JM. *J Rheumatol* 2003; **30**: 493–6

Background. Cardiovascular (CV) disease is the leading cause of late mortality in SLE. Traditional and non-traditional cardiovascular risk factors contribute to CV events

in SLE. Al-Herz *et al.* studied the extent to which CV risk factor screening is performed by university and community-based rheumatology practices. Medical records of SLE patients were reviewed to determine whether screening for traditional and disease lupus-related risk factors for CV disease had been performed. Screening was considered appropriate if a family history of CV disease, smoking and menstrual histories were obtained, body habitus or weight and blood pressure measured, and lipid profile, blood glucose, serum homocysteine, urinalysis, anticardiolipin antibody and/or partial thromboplastin time documented at the initial visit.

Interpretation. One hundred and eighty-three SLE patients were studied (about one-third were from a university-based practice and two-thirds from community-based practices). Thirty-one per cent (56/183) of these patients had at least a screening for hyperlipidaemia. This was more commonly performed by the university-based practice than by the community-based practices (62 versus 15%; $P<0.001$) (Fig. 7.3a). Twenty-six of the 56 screened patients had an increase in serum cholesterol; five additional patients had instead abnormal results for high-density lipoprotein (HDL), triglycerides and/or very low-density lipoprotein (VLDL) (total abnormal results, 31/56 or 55%). However, only one-third of the patients (mostly from the university-based practice) with an abnormal test received appropriate therapy (diet, antihyperlipidaemic therapy and/or hydroxychloroquine initiation) (Fig. 7.3b). Screening for hyperlipidaemia in SLE patients was performed infrequently, regardless of the clinic setting, and was not followed by an adequate treatment plan. Nine non-lipid CV risk factors were also documented infrequently (a median of eight were assessed in the university-based practice versus three in the community-based practices ($P = 0.31$); those more commonly assessed were nephrotic syndrome, hypertension and smoking.

Comment

The increased frequency of CV events in SLE has become evident in the last few years |**11**| and the predisposing risk factors have been identified |**12**|. Who is responsible for screening for these factors and implementing therapies? An answer is not readily available. This study from Al-Herz *et al.* shows that screening for CV risk factors in SLE is done infrequently; moreover, it is not always followed by therapy. It is likely that the data from this study are not unique but rather are representative of practices worldwide. What are the underlying factors that explain these findings? Several distinct possibilities are likely to intertwine. First, lupus patients may present other pressing problems in any given clinic visit; secondly, limited clinic visit time may preclude caring time for preventive practices; and thirdly, rheumatologists may feel that preventive practices are the realm of general practitioners, who may feel they are the realm of rheumatologists.

Given the relationship between SLE and CV disease, we believe it is the responsibility of the rheumatologist to ascertain the presence of CV risk factors and to implement decisive interventions to modify those factors that are amenable to treatment. In the long run such a practice may be as beneficial as treating a disease flare.

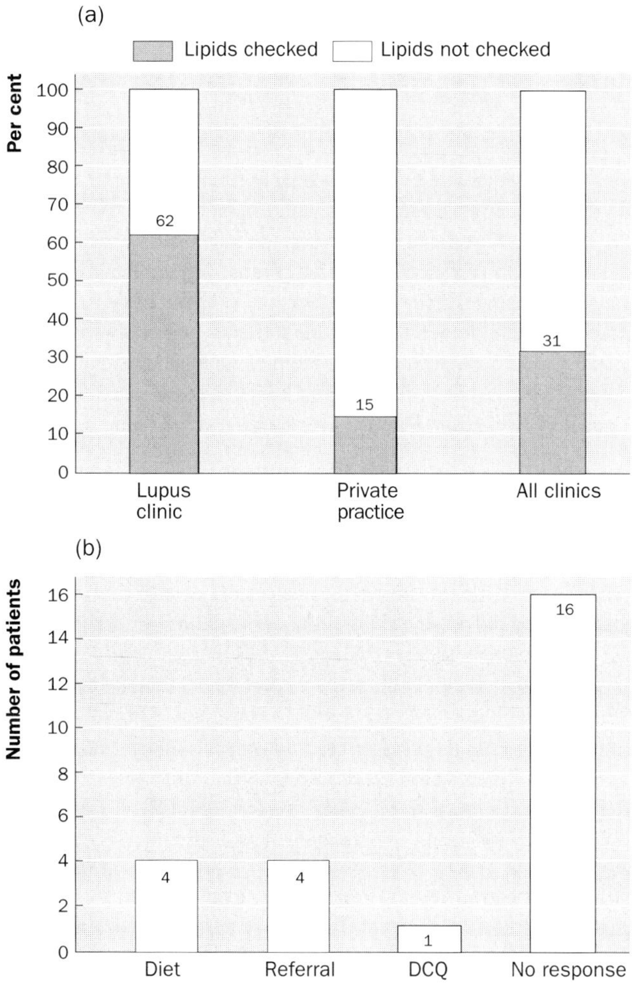

Fig. 7.3 (a) Percentage of SLE patients screened for hyperlipidaemia in the lupus clinic and in private practices (P <0.001). (b) Charted responses of rheumatologists to elevated lipid test results. Source: Al-Herz *et al.* (2003).

The incidence of irreversible retinal toxicity in patients treated with hydroxychloroquine: a reappraisal

Mavrikakis I, Sfikakis PP, Mavrikakis E, *et al. Ophthalmology* 2003; **110**: 1321–6

BACKGROUND. Antimalarials have proved to be beneficial in the treatment of different rheumatological and skin disorders but are associated with retinal toxicity. The authors describe a 15-year (1985–2000) cohort study to ascertain the risk of retinopathy in 526 patients (rheumatoid arthritis, $n = 335$; SLE, $n = 191$) receiving the recommended doses of hydroxychloroquine ($\leq$6.5 mg/kg/day). Four hundred of these patients had received long-term treatment, ranging from 6 to 16 years. Patients were followed up at 6-month intervals from 1985 to 1995, then yearly. Ophthalmological assessment included the following: funduscopy, visual acuity (Snellen best-corrected), colour vision (Farnsworth D-15 panel test), central visual field (Rodenstock), and full-field electroretinography.

INTERPRETATION. Retinal toxicity appears to be exceedingly rare in patients receiving the recommended doses of hydroxychloroquine (adjusted to their ideal body weight) during the first years of treatment. A baseline ophthalmological examination to exclude pre-existing retinal pathologies and to identify known risk factors of possible retinal toxicity (older age, previous exposure to antimalarials, liver or renal dysfunction) is indicated. Retinal toxicity occurred only in two patients after 6.5 and 8 years of treatment. Although the lesions were irreversible, vision stabilized. The authors recommend that yearly ophthalmological monitoring should not commence sooner than 6 years after initiation of the drug.

Comment

In its 1996 guidelines, the ACR recommends a baseline eye examination for patients older than 40 years who have a personal or family history of eye disease and who are to start antimalarial therapy; subsequent monitoring is recommended every 6–12 months or more frequently if liver or renal dysfunctions are present or after 10 years of use. In 2002, the American Academy of Ophthalmology (AAO) updated their recommendations on screening for chloroquine and hydroxychloroquine retinopathy [**13**]. According to their recommendations, all patients starting antimalarials should have a baseline ophthalmological evaluation (funduscopy and central visual fields at the least). For low-risk patients, eye evaluations should be scheduled as follows: at least once during treatment for patients aged 20–29 years, at least twice for patients aged 30–39, every 2–4 years for patients aged 40–64, and yearly for patients 65 and older. For high-risk patients, yearly screening is recommended. Although these guidelines are probably correct for most patients, they may fail patients who, despite not having any of the known risk factors, develop retinal toxicity relatively soon after therapy initiation [**14**]. It is conceivable that these patients have a genetic predisposition to the development of retinopathy (mutation of the photoreceptor-specific ATP-binding cassette transporter gene [*ABCR* or *ABCA4*] [15]), but this has not been determined to date.

In this publication, Mavrikakis and collaborators report data on the largest cohort of hydroxychloroquine-treated patients followed regularly for the presence of retinal toxicity. Given the very low incidence of retinal toxicity (0.5%), they suggest that ophthalmological monitoring should not be done as frequently as recommended by the ACR (i.e. that monitoring should be more in line with the AAO's recommendations). Rheumatologists should exercise their judgement in the follow-up of antimalarial-treated patients.

Design, quality and bias in randomized controlled trials of systemic lupus erythematosus

Karassa FB, Tatsioni A, Ioannidis JPA. *J Rheumatol* 2003; **30**: 979–84

BACKGROUND. Rheumatologists base SLE treatment decisions on clinically accepted therapeutic interventions as well as on the results of RCTs. There are, for the most part, substantial differences between RCT patients and those from ordinary clinical practice. Therefore, when applying the results of RCTs to a particular clinical situation, possible deficiencies in their development and conduct need to be considered.

INTERPRETATION. The authors searched, retrieved and reviewed medical literature (between 1966 and April 2002) in four languages (English, French, German and Italian) from three major databases (MEDLINE, EMBASE and the Cochrane Library Controlled Trials Register). Publications reporting studies with at least five SLE patients (regardless of the inclusion of patients with other rheumatic diseases) were included. Pseudorandomized and substudies were excluded. For duplicate reports, only that with the longest follow-up and/or additional arms was retained. Structured data extraction was performed and the following were assessed: (1) study design; (2) quality of data; and (3) trial results (LN and other SLE manifestations). Of the 174 studies reviewed, 94 were selected for analysis; all but two were in English. Thirty-seven were of LN. The RCTs included 2257 SLE patients (795 from LN trials). Half were double-blind; only one-third described the randomization scheme used. Interestingly, only 20% (19 trials) of all trials described allocation concealment and only 7.5% of them (seven trials) had adequate power. In general, two-thirds of the RCTs described adequately the reasons for withdrawals; those with the highest quality standards were those with a large sample. Other indicators of high-quality publications were complete reporting of withdrawals along with adequate descriptions of outcomes and intention-to-treat analyses. RCTs showing efficacy or a trend to efficacy were those published recently. In contrast, none of the LN trials were adequately powered; they were more likely to have a longer follow-up and to include younger patients with short disease duration compared with the other trials. LN trials were also less likely to be double-blinded, to have a comparison group (either placebo or no treatment) and to describe patient withdrawal adequately. These data are shown in Table 7.2.

Table 7.2 Quality and results of randomized controlled trials

Characteristics	All trials (n = 94)	Nephritis trials (n = 37)	Other trials (n = 57)
Quality			
Sample size per arm specified, n (%)	78 (83)	30 (81.1)	48 (84.2)
Randomization mode specified, n (%)	31 (33)	11 (29.7)	20 (35.1)
Allocation concealment specified, n (%)	19 (20.2)	7 (18.9)	12 (21.1)
Withdrawals described, n (%)	76 (80.9)	25 (67.6)*	51 (89.5)*
Withdrawals described per arm, n (%)	63 (67)	19 (51.4)*	44 (77.2)*
Power calculations mentioned, (%)	22 (23.4)	8 (21.6)	14 (24.6)
Power 80% at a = 0.05, n (%)	7 (7.5)	0 (0)**	7 (12.3)**
Outcomes well specified, n (%)	55 (58.5)	20 (54.1)	35 (61.4)
Intention-to-treat analyses used, n (%)	50 (53.2)	23 (62.2)	27 (47.4)
Results of the experimental intervention			
Significant efficacy, n (%)	50 (53.2)	17 (45.9)	33 (57.9)
Trend for efficacy, n (%)	22 (23.4)	12 (32.4)	10 (17.5)
No effect, n (%)	20 (21.3)	8 (21.6)	12 (21.1)
Trend of harm, n (%)	1 (1.1)	0	1 (1.8)
Significant harm, n (%)	1 (1.1)	0	1 (1.8)

*P <0.01 for nephritis trials vs other trials; **P <0.05 for nephritis trials vs other trials.
Source: Karassa *et al.* (2003).

Comment

Current SLE RCTs are methodologically flawed. Limitations have occurred at several steps during their development or execution |**16**|. Most commonly, RCTs are not adequately powered and the follow-up is not long enough; in addition, there may be bias in reporting their results |**17**|. More importantly, RCTs may lack generalizability if they do not include patients from a diverse socio-economic and ethnic background. The recent introduction of standardized outcome measures has made a great contribution to SLE RCTs, improving their likelihood of being of high quality. Karassa's findings should be kept in mind when RCTs are in the early planning stages. Similar considerations apply to longitudinal observational studies.

Improved clinical outcome of lupus nephritis during the past decade: importance of an early diagnosis and treatment

Fiehn C, Hajjar Y, Mueller K, Waldherr R, Ho AD, Andrassi K. *Ann Rheum Dis* 2003; **62**: 435–9

Background. Approximately half of the patients with SLE will experience signs of renal involvement at any time during their disease course; renal failure, when it occurs,

usually develops during the first decade after renal involvement is detected. This work aimed to ascertain the differences in outcome in patients with biopsy-proven LN diagnosed between 1980 and 1989 (Group I) and between 1990 and 2000 (Group II) being treated and followed up at a single German referral centre. Patients' characteristics at diagnosis, treatment regimens and renal outcome were obtained by reviewing all available medical records. End-stage renal disease (ESRD) or death was considered the end-point in all analyses.

INTERPRETATION. LN was demonstrated in 15 patients in Group I and 41 patients in Group II; most were classified as having WHO class IV LN. Group I patients had a longer time from the first detection of proteinuria until a kidney biopsy was performed, a higher frequency of nephrotic-range proteinuria, renal failure (high serum creatinine concentration), arterial hypertension, and high chronicity indices on their kidney biopsies compared with Group II patients, who in turn, showed higher activity indices on their biopsies. Treatment schemes were not significantly different between the two groups. No Group II patients developed ESRD (median observation time of 24 months), whereas six of 15 (40%) of patients from Group I did so (median observation time of 94 months) (Fig. 7.4). One patient in each group succumbed to an infection.

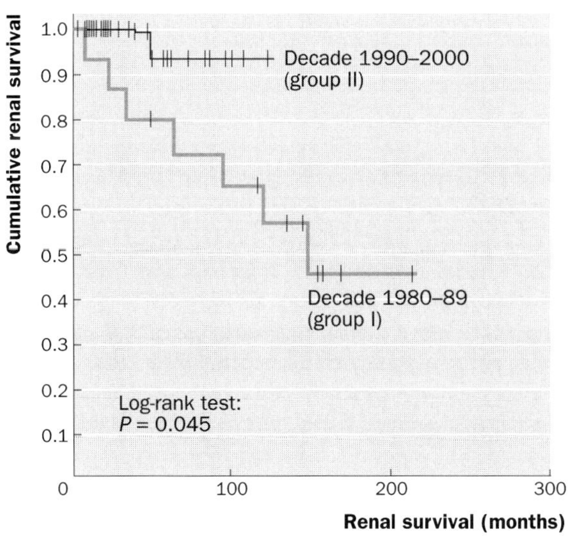

Fig. 7.4 Renal survival curve of patients with lupus nephritis diagnosed in the decade 1990–2000 (Group II, $n = 41$) in comparison with those diagnosed during the decade 1980–1989 (Group I, $n = 15$). Whereas six patients of the earlier decade had terminal renal failure in the follow-up, no patients of the later decade had the same event, which is a significant difference ($P = 0.045$). In both groups one patient died from infection. Source: Fiehn *et al.* (2003).

Comment

The prognosis of LN has gradually improved over the last few years, as clearly noted in this German paper. Prompt recognition of the presence of LN is crucial if long-term renal survival is to be accomplished; features suggestive of advanced renal involvement (high chronicity index, arterial hypertension and high serum creatinine were the strongest predictors of ESRD). Of interest, although the median follow-up time in Group I patients was substantially longer than in Group II patients, Kaplan–Meier survival curves still showed a significantly better outcome in Group II patients. Although the therapeutic approach was similar in the two groups, Group II patients may not have been treated as early as Group II patients as there was a delay in performing kidney biopsies in these patients.

These data contrast with data involving non-Caucasian populations, in whom progression to renal failure may occur despite the institution of aggressive treatment regimens. Dooley *et al.* have suggested that conventional treatment (pulse intravenous cyclophosphamide plus corticosteroids) is probably less effective in African-Americans [**18**]. A recent study from Jamaica extends the observations of Dooley *et al.* to Afro-Caribbean patients [**19**]. Whether this differential response is related to socio-economic-demographic, cultural and behavioural characteristics or is genetically based (angiotensin-converting enzyme [**2**], *Fc gamma R* polymorphisms [**20**], other genes) remains to be determined. Clinicians need to be aware of these differences and to be more vigilant when treating patients with LN who are at high risk of ESRD.

Outcome of renal transplantation in patients with systemic lupus erythematosus

Deegens JK, Artz MA, Hoitsma AJ, Wetzels JFM. *Transplantation Int* 2003; **16**: 411–18

BACKGROUND. LN is one of the most serious clinical manifestations of SLE; currently accepted therapeutic strategies do not always prevent the occurrence of ESRD in these patients. In the past, LN patients were not offered a renal transplant in the belief that the transplanted kidney will also develop LN. More recent data cast some doubt on this assertion.

INTERPRETATION. The outcome of renal transplantation in patients with LN was studied at a single centre in The Netherlands between 1968 and 2001. Patients less than 15 years of age were excluded. Post-transplant immunosuppressive therapy consisted of prednisone and azathioprine before 1983, cyclosporin or azathioprine in 1983 and 1985, and cyclosporin thereafter. Graft survival and patient survival were compared with those of a matched control group. Of 23 patients who were identified with LN (21 women, two men) only one patient developed post-transplant renal failure in the context of extra-renal lupus activity; two additional patients exhibited some evidence of extra-renal lupus activity but had no decrement in their renal function. Patient and graft survival at 5 years were 86 and 68%, respectively, which were not different from the survival figures for the control group

(95 and 78%, respectively) (Fig. 7.5). The authors conclude that transplantation is adequate renal replacement therapy for LN.

Comment

The data from this single Netherlands centre are quite encouraging. However, they contrast with data from other centres suggesting that renal flares are common in lupus patients undergoing renal transplantation. These were also the conclusions of Goral *et al.* after examining data at a single US centre [**21**]. In contrast to the work from The Netherlands, the US authors suggest that unless renal biopsies in the

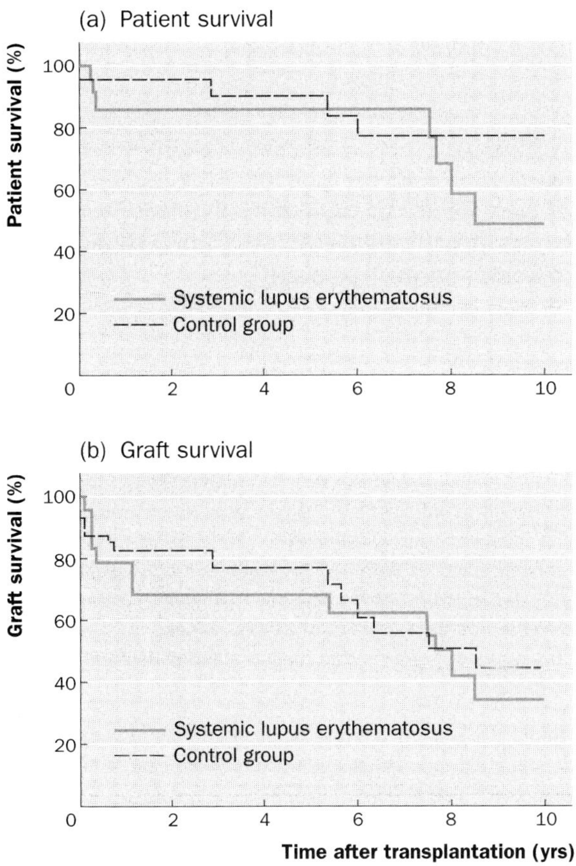

Fig. 7.5 Patient (a) and graft (b) survival rates after renal transplantation in patients with systemic lupus erythematosus (solid line) and in the control group (dashed line). Source: Deegens *et al.* (2003).

transplanted kidney are done systematically and are examined by immunofluorescence and electron microscopy, recurrent LN (RLN) is missed. In their series, RLN was detected in 52% of patients in whom renal biopsy was performed and in 30% overall (50 patients were studied, 29 underwent renal biopsies, 15 developed RLN). Patient survival was 82% at 5 years and graft survival was 60%; however, there was no difference in graft survival between those patients who developed RLN and those who did not. No predictive features of RLN were identified among these 50 patients. RLN was not necessarily serious, accompanied by extra-renal lupus manifestations or treated differently. Whether the rate of RLN will be the same with current immunosuppressive therapy is unknown. The data from these two papers, taken together, suggest that renal transplantation is a definitive option for LN ESRD; although flares may occur, they do not appear to affect graft or patient survival. A larger number of African-American patients and others at high risk of developing ESRD may be needed before these data can be generalized.

LJP 394 for the prevention of renal flare in patients with systemic lupus erythematosus. Results from a randomized, double blind, placebo-controlled study

Alarcón-Segovia D, Tumlin JA, Furie RA, *et al. Arthritis Rheum* 2003; **48**: 442–54

Background. LJP 394 is a synthetic molecule consisting of four double-stranded oligodeoxyribonucleotides conjugated to a pharmacologically inert, non-immunogenic polyethylene glycol that selectively reduces anti-dsDNA antibodies and their parent B cells by forming antigen–antibody complexes and the development of B-cell tolerance. This study was aimed at determining the effect of LJP 394 on renal flares among patients with SLE and kidney involvement. During 76 weeks, 230 patients (114 receiving LJP 394 and 116 receiving placebo) with SLE (at least four ACR criteria) were randomized to receive 16 weekly doses of LJP 394 or placebo, followed by alternating 8-week drug-free periods and twelve weekly doses of LJP 394 or placebo for the remaining 60 weeks. Affinity assays were performed to measure anti-dsDNA antibody levels.

Interpretation. Overall, time to renal flare and number of renal flares were comparable between the two treatment groups; however, patients receiving LJP 394 had a longer time to establishment of high-dose corticosteroids and/or cyclophosphamide (HDCC), required lower doses of corticosteroids and presented a significant reduction of anti-dsDNA antibody levels. Patients with high-affinity anti-dsDNA treated with LJP 394 experienced fewer renal flares, a longer time to flare, a longer time to institution of HDCC and less frequent use of these treatments compared with patients receiving placebo (Fig. 7.6). In contrast, these parameters were comparable among patients with low-affinity anti-dsDNA.

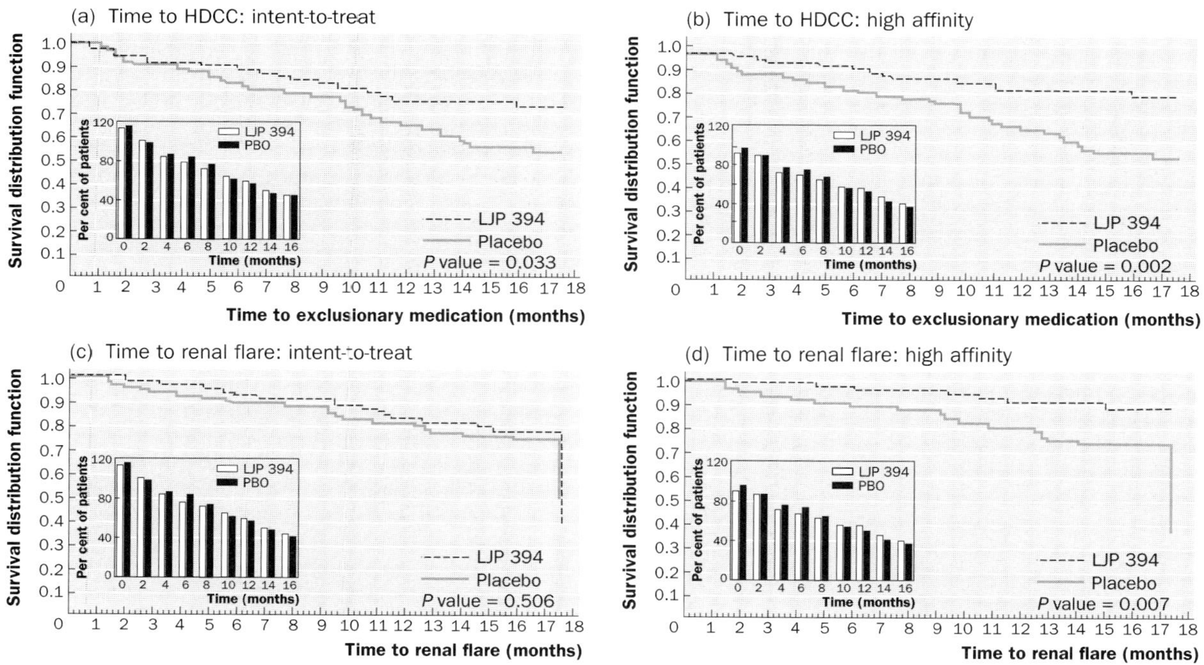

Fig. 7.6 Analysis of time to first administration of high-dose corticosteroids and/or cyclophosphamide (HDCC) in the LJP 394-treated and the placebo-treated groups in the (a) intention-to-treat population and (b) high-affinity population. Analysis of time to first renal flare in the LJP 394-treated and the placebo-treated groups of (c) the intention-to-treat population and (d) the high-affinity population. The terminal decrease in the proportion of patients who did not experience a renal flare was a result of the premature termination of the trial. **Insets** show the number of patients in each group at 2-month intervals over the course of the 18-month trial. PBO = placebo. Source: Alarcón-Segovia *et al.* (2003).

Comment

Aggressive immunosuppressants are indicated for severe SLE manifestations; however, the usefulness of this approach is frequently limited by the toxicity associated with these compounds. During the last few years there has been increased interest in novel targeted molecules designed to modify the immune response. These new agents ideally have minimal adverse effects with maximum clinical efficacy. Examples of the use of these agents include the modulation of co-stimulatory molecules on immune cells (anti-CD40L), the manipulation of cytokines (anti-interleukin-10), the induction of tolerance (LJP 394), the use of anti-idiotype antibodies (intravenous immunoglobulins) and the depletion of specific cellular populations (anti-BLyS or anti-CD20 monoclonal antibodies). Most of these molecules are still in Phase I–II trials; some have already been noted to produce moderate or severe adverse effects [22], and others have produced negative results [23]. Nevertheless, the future treatment of lupus will probably include one or more biological compounds.

The authors present the results of a multicentre RCT. This RCT was terminated after an interim analysis had suggested that the trial was unlikely to reach statistical significance for differences in time to renal flare between treatment groups in the intention-to-treat population. With almost 60% of patients completing 12 months of treatment, the study showed that LJP 394 significantly reduced the time and number of renal flares and the use of HDCC, primarily in patients with high affinity anti-dsDNA. The number and severity of adverse effects were comparable in the two treatment groups, although there was a slightly higher frequency of thromboembolic events in the LJP 394 arm. A multinational RCT to assess time to renal flare in patients with high baseline affinity antibodies is ongoing.

Hematopoietic stem cell transplantation for severe and refractory lupus: analysis after five years and fifteen patients

Traynor AE, Barr WG, Rosa RM, *et al. Arthritis Rheum* 2002; **46**: 2917–23

BACKGROUND. SLE is a chronic disease that can severely affect vital organ systems such as the kidneys and the central nervous system; the survival of these patients has improved dramatically over recent decades. There are, however, some SLE patients who exhibit severe and sometimes life-threatening disease manifestations despite appropriate therapy. The study of Traynor *et al.* examines the safety and long-term outcome of HSCT, which is currently considered the last treatment resort for patients with refractory SLE.

INTERPRETATION. The safety and long-term efficacy of HSCT was assessed in an open-label study that included 15 SLE patients (ACR criteria) from a single US centre. Patients had at least one of five refractory manifestations (to cyclophosphamide) attributable to SLE: (1) Class III/IV LN; (2) heart or lung involvement (biopsy-proven vasculitis); (3) cerebritis or transverse myelitis; (4) refractory autoimmune cytopenias; or

(5) catastrophic antiphospholipid syndrome. LN treatment failure required 6 months of cyclophosphamide therapy; for other organs 3 months was required. The transplantation protocol consisted of stem-cell mobilization (cyclophosphamide at 2000 mg/m^2 and granulocyte colony-stimulating factor), depletion of lymphocytes from the graft (selecting $CD34^+$ cells) and the conditioning regimen (cyclophosphamide 200 mg/kg, antithymocyte globulin 90 mg/kg and methylprednisolone 3 mg/kg). SLE status was assessed (at 2 and 6 months) after HSCT with the SLE disease activity index (SLEDAI), serum complement, immunological tests, function of affected organs and immunosuppressive requirements. Fifteen patients (seven critically ill) underwent HSCT (median follow-up, 36 months [range 12–66]); all of them had a gradual but marked and sustained improvement in the SLEDAI, which reached less than 5 points in twelve of the 15 patients. Immunological tests, serum complement and organ involvement surrogates improved significantly in all patients. Ten of twelve patients who were followed up for at least 1 year discontinued all immunosuppressants; of those who had been followed up for more than 18 months, only two continued taking prednisone. Two patients experienced clinical recurrences, which were controlled with both intermittent cyclophosphamide and prednisone; one of these patients was previously refractory to these therapies but responded adequately after HSCT. The most common complication was neutropenic fever (80%, $n = 12$). Other complications were uncommon, self-limited and non-fatal.

Comments

Innovative strategies for the treatment of severe SLE manifestations are desperately needed. Few therapeutic options are available for patients with such manifestations, and they are based on immunosuppressive therapy that includes primarily intravenous cyclophosphamide. HSCT is the currently available therapy for refractory SLE |**24**|. The data provided by Traynor *et al.* bring new hope to these patients; the findings are quite relevant since remission was achieved in all patients with a reasonable safety profile. Of major importance, prednisone and immunosuppressive medications were discontinued in almost all patients. Additionally, significant improvement of relevant clinical and laboratory features occurred. However, because this trial was relatively small in size its results may not be generalizable.

Conclusion

It is impossible to summarize the entire pertinent lupus literature for the year in these few pages. We wanted to give the reader an idea of the breadth and depth of the most relevant clinical publications. Progress made in the laboratory, coupled with better trial design and outcome assessment, should translate into better treatment modalities and ultimately into better patient outcomes. There is significant interest by the pharmaceutical industry, advocacy (and funding) private groups, funding and regulatory governing agencies and researchers that should move this field forward. Exciting data that may significantly change the manner in which we view and treat SLE are forthcoming.

References

1. Gladman DD, Urowitz MB, Goldsmith CH, Fortin P, Ginzler E, Gordon C, Hanly JG, Isenberg DA, Kalunian K, Nived O, Petri M, Sanchez-Guerrero J, Snaith M, Sturfelt G. The reliability of the Systemic Lupus International Collaborating Clinics/American College of Rheumatology Damage Index in patients with systemic lupus erythematosus. *Arthritis Rheum* 1997; **40**: 809–13.
2. Parsa A, Peden E, Lum RF, Seligman VA, Olson JL, Li H, Seldin MF, Criswell LA. Association of angiotensin-converting enzyme polymorphisms with systemic lupus erythematosus and nephritis: analysis of 644 SLE families. *Genes Immun* 2002; **3**(Suppl 1): S42–6.
3. Parra EJ, Marcini A, Akey J, Martinson J, Batzer MA, Cooper R, Forrester T, Allison DB, Deka R, Ferrell RE, Shriver MD. Estimating African American admixture proportions by use of population specific alleles. *Am J Hum Genet* 1998; **63**: 1839–51.
4. Shriver MD, Parra EJ, Dios S, Bonilla C, Norton H, Jovel C, Pfaff C, Jones C, Massac A, Cameron N, Baron A, Jackson T, Argyropoulos G, Jin L, Hoggart CJ, McKeigue PM, Kittles RA. Skin pigmentation, biogeographical ancestry and admixture mapping. *Hum Genet* 2003; **112**: 387–99.
5. Karassa FB, Trikalinos TA, Ioannidis JPA. Role of the Fcγ receptor IIa polymorphism in susceptibility to systemic lupus erythematosus and lupus nephritis. *Arthritis Rheum* 2002; **46**: 1563–71.
6. Fessler BJ, McGwin G Jr, Roseman JM, Bastian HM, Friedman AW, Lisse JR, Alarcón GS, Reveille JD. Characteristics of ACR criteria accrual for systemic lupus erythematosus in 3 ethnic groups for the LUMINA Study Group. *Arthritis Rheum* 2000; **43**: S525.
7. Keyser RE, Rus V, Cade WT, Kalappa N, Flores RH, Handwerger BS. Evidence for aerobic insufficiency in women with systemic lupus erythematosus. *Arthritis Rheum* 2003; **49**: 16–22.
8. Bosma GP, Middlekoop HA, Rood MJ, Bollen EL, Huizinga TW, van Buchem MA. Association of global brain damage and clinical functioning in neuropsychiatric systemic lupus erythematosus. *Arthritis Rheum* 2002; **46**: 2665–72.
9. Ruperto N, Ravelli A, Murray KJ, Lovell DJ, Andersson-Gare B, Feldman BM, Garay S, Kuis W, Machado C, Pachman L, Prieur AM, Rider LG, Silverman E, Tsitsami E, Woo P, Giannini EH, Martini A, for the Paediatric Rheumatology International Trials Organisation (PRINTO), The Pediatric Rheumatology Collaborative Study Group (PRCSG). Preliminary core sets of measures for disease activity and damage assessment in juvenile systemic lupus erythematosus and juvenile dermatomyositis. *Rheumatology* 2003; **42**: 1–8.
10. Blumenfeld Z, Shapiro D, Shteinberg M, Avivi I, Nahir M. Preservation of fertility and ovarian function and minimizing gonadotoxicity in young women with systemic lupus erythematosus treated by chemotherapy. *Lupus* 2000; **9**: 401–5.
11. Manzi S, Meilahn EN, Rairie JE, Conte CG, Medsger TA Jr, Jansen-McWilliams L, D'Agostino RB, Kuller LH. Age-specific incidence rates of myocardial infarction and angina in women with systemic lupus erythematosus: comparison with the Framingham study. *Am J Epidemiol* 1997; **145**: 408–15.

12. Esdaile JM, Abrahamowicz M, Grodzicky T, Li Y, Panaritis C, Du Berger R, Cote R, Grover SA, Fortin PR, Clarke AE, Senecal JL. Traditional Framingham risk factors fail to fully account for accelerated atherosclerosis in systemic lupus erythematosus. *Arthritis Rheum* 2001; **44**: 2331–7.
13. Marmor MF, Carr RE, Easterbrook M, Farjo AA, Mieler WF, for the American Academy of Ophthalmology. Recommendations on screening for chloroquine and hydroxychloroquine retinopathy: a report by the American Academy of Ophthalmology. *Ophthalmology* 2002; **109**: 1377–82.
14. Alarcón GS. How frequently and how soon should we screen our patients for the presence of antimalarial retinopathy? *Arthritis Rheum* 2002; **46**: 561.
15. Shroyer NF, Lewis RA, Lupski JR. Analysis of the ABCR (ABCA4) gene in 4-aminoquinoline retinopathy: is retinal toxicity by chloroquine and hydroxychloroquine related to Stargardt disease? *Am J Ophthalmol* 2001; **131**: 761–6.
16. Hill CL, LaValley MP, Felson DT. Secular changes in the quality of published randomized clinical trials in rheumatology. *Arthritis Rheum* 2002; **46**: 779–84.
17. Begg C, Cho M, Eastwood S, Horton R, Moher D, Olkin I, Pitkin R, Rennie D, Schulz KF, Simel D, Stroup DF. Improving the quality of reporting of randomized controlled trials; the CONSORT statement. *JAMA* 1996; **276**: 637–9.
18. Dooley MA, Hogan S, Jennette C, Falk R. Cyclophosphamide therapy for lupus nephritis: poor renal survival in black Americans. Glomerular Disease Collaborative Network. *Kidney Int* 1997; **51**: 1188–95.
19. Williams W, Bhagwandass A, Sargeant LA, Shah D. Severity of systemic lupus erythematosus with diffuse proliferative glomerulonephritis and the ineffectiveness of standard pulse intravenous cyclophosphamide therapy in Jamaican patients. *Lupus* 2003; **12**: 640–5.
20. Zuñiga R, Ng S, Peterson MG, Reveille JD, Baethge BA, Alarcón GS, Salmon JE. Low-binding alleles of Fcγ receptor types IIA and IIIA are inherited independently and are associated with systemic lupus erythematosus in Hispanic patients. *Arthritis Rheum* 2001; **44**: 361–7.
21. Goral S, Ynares C, Shappell SB, Snyder S, Feurer ID, Kazancioglu R, Fogo AB, Helderman JH. Recurrent lupus nephritis in renal transplant recipients revisited: it is not rare. *Transplantation* 2003; **75**: 651–6.
22. Boumpas DT, Furie R, Manzi S, Illei GG, Wallace DJ, Balow JE, Vaishnaw A; BG9588 Lupus Nephritis Trial Group. A short course of BG9588 (anti-DC40 ligand antibody) improves serologic activity and decreases hematuria in patients with proliferative lupus glomerulonephritis. *Arthritis Rheum* 2003; **48**: 719–27.
23. Kalunian KC, Davis JC, Merrill JT, Totoritis MC, Wofsy D; IDEC-131 Lupus Study Group. Treatment of systemic lupus erythematosus by inhibition of T cell costimulation with anti-CD154; a randomized, double-blind, placebo-controlled trial. *Arthritis Rheum* 2002; **46**: 3251–8.
24. Burt RK, Traynor AE. Hematopoietic stem cell transplantation for systemic lupus erythematosus. *Arthritis Res Ther* 2003; **5**: 207–9.

8

Systemic sclerosis

ARIANE HERRICK

Introduction

A large number of systemic sclerosis (SSc)-related publications of interest to the clinician has been published in the last year. This is an exciting time for rheumatologists caring for patients with SSc: although there is still no treatment known to modify the underlying disease process, several drugs are in development or in clinical trial, and there are effective therapies for several of the organ-based manifestations of the disease.

These new approaches to therapy are being driven by advances in our understanding of the molecular and cellular biology of the underlying disease process. The pathogenesis of SSc includes excessive fibrosis, vascular dysfunction and immune aberration, but how these interact remains unclear. Thus, therapies are being developed which are antifibrotic and/or induce vasodilation/vascular remodelling |**1**| and/or suppress immune activation. Many papers have been published on basic disease mechanisms, many of which have implications for new approaches to therapy, for example those elucidating the roles of transforming growth factor β (TGF-β), endothelin-1 and nitric oxide.

A major advance in the study of SSc has been the recognition that the two major subtypes of disease—limited cutaneous and diffuse cutaneous SSc—have different natural histories, different autoantibody associations and different prognoses |**2**|. The ability to classify and subtype disease has provided an infrastructure for studies examining risk factors for particular manifestations, for example pulmonary arterial hypertension and renal crisis, as discussed below. Better understanding of these predictors allows us to identify and treat problems at an early stage. Advances have also been made in the measurement of the disease process—a key issue, especially now that several new therapies are entering clinical trial.

This chapter will consider some of the recent literature of interest to clinicians under four headings: (1) Pathogenesis; (2) Disease progression and risk factors; (3) Outcome measures; and (4) Treatment.

Pathogenesis

Much of the SSc literature published in the past year relates to basic disease mechanisms. Three papers have been selected for comment, to illustrate the enormous advances which have been made in our understanding of the molecular and cellular biology of SSc. Many others could have been chosen, for example studies examining subjects as diverse as the role of T cells [3], the regulation of collagen gene expression [4] and of TGF-β receptor expression [5], the effects of TGF-β on fibrillin-1 matrix formation [6], and the role of monocyte chemoattractant protein 3 [7]. Our increased understanding of the SSc disease process is now being translated into new therapeutic options, as seen with endothelin-1 receptor antagonists, now licensed for use in pulmonary arterial hypertension and being investigated in SSc-related digital vascular disease.

Genome-wide association study for regions of systemic sclerosis susceptibility in a Choctaw Indian population with high disease prevalence

Zhou X, Tan FK, Wang N, *et al. Arthritis Rheum* 2003; **48**: 2585–92

BACKGROUND. Genetic contributions to SSc are now well recognized, but these are complex and it is likely that multiple genetic loci are involved in disease susceptibility and expression. Studying the genetics of SSc is complicated by the rarity and heterogeneity of the disease and by the lack of knowledge of candidate loci. In this study, a case–control approach was applied in the unique population of Oklahoma Choctaw Indians, who have a high prevalence and relatively homogeneous clinical expression of SSc (most affected patients have diffuse cutaneous disease with pulmonary fibrosis and autoantibodies to topoisomerase 1). The authors conducted a genome-wide screen using 400 microsatellite markers, followed up by higher-density scanning in regions in which associations with SSc were suggested. Twenty Choctaw patients and 76 ethnically matched controls were studied.

INTERPRETATION. The genome-wide screen identified 12 markers that were highly significantly associated with SSc ($P < 0.01$) and five that were significantly associated ($0.01 < P < 0.05$). These markers included loci near the genes for secreted protein, acidic and rich in cysteine (SPARC) or osteonectin, fibrillin-1, the major histocompatibility complex and topoisomerase 1 (confirming the results of previous studies), and loci previously reported to show linkage to systemic lupus erythematosus and other autoimmune diseases. Fourteen potential haplotypes were identified with significant frequency differences between cases and controls. The authors suggested that, in the Choctaw population, SSc may share some common genetic loci with other autoimmune diseases.

Comment

The authors are careful to point out that their results, obtained from a relatively small number of Choctaw Indians, may not be applicable to SSc in more outbred populations and that the results should be considered preliminary. Therefore, this study needs to be followed up by linkage and association studies in outbred populations. Nonetheless, a number of biologically relevant susceptibility markers have been identified, suggesting that multiple genetic factors are involved and that these overlap with other autoimmune diseases. Identification of key candidate loci is likely to be a crucial step in furthering our understanding of the disease's pathogenesis.

Expression and regulation of intracellular SMAD signaling in scleroderma skin fibroblasts

Mori Y, Chen S-J, Varga J. *Arthritis Rheum* 2003; **48**: 1964–78

BACKGROUND. TGF-β has become strongly implicated in the pathogenesis of SSc—its expression is increased in SSc fibroblasts, as are levels of its type I and type II receptors (TGF-βRI and TGF-βRII). There has been considerable recent interest in the intracellular signalling mechanisms which mediate its profibrotic effects and it is now recognized that, after receptor binding, the effects of TGF-β are propagated downstream via SMADs, recently characterized intracellular effectors. Nuclear import is necessary for SMAD-dependent transcriptional responses but the mechanisms relating to SMAD nuclear–cytoplasmic shuttling are unclear. The authors of this paper used a variety of methods to further examine the expression and function of SMADs. Dermal fibroblasts from 14 patients with SSc and four healthy controls were studied.

INTERPRETATION. Protein and messenger RNA (mRNA) levels of SMAD3 (a substrate for activated TGF-βRI) were increased in most scleroderma fibroblasts, but not those of SMAD4 (the common signalling partner for SMAD2 and SMAD3) or of SMAD7 (which is inhibitory). When intracellular expression of SMAD proteins was examined in the presence and absence of TGF-β, TGF-β repressed expression of SMAD3 mRNA in both control and SSc fibroblasts, suggesting that the elevated steady-state levels of SMAD3 seen in some SSc fibroblasts cannot be attributed to failure of a SMAD3-related negative feedback mechanism. In the absence of exogenous TGF-β, SMAD3 and 4 had a predominantly cytoplasmic localization in control fibroblasts, whereas they showed elevated nuclear localization in SSc fibroblasts. Also, the levels and nuclear localization of phosphorylated SMAD2/3 were increased in SSc fibroblasts (in the absence of TGF-β), suggesting activation of the SMAD pathway. TGF-β blockade failed to correct the subcellular localization of SMAD in SSc fibroblasts. This suggests that the increased nuclear localization of SMADs is due to alterations downstream of the TGF-β receptors and is therefore ligand-independent. Thus, abnormalities in SMAD signalling may contribute to the abnormal SSc fibroblast phenotype and therefore to fibrosis.

Comment

This paper provides further information on the complexities of the TGF-β/SMAD signalling pathway in SSc fibroblasts. The studies described provide evidence for constitutive SMAD activation in SSc fibroblasts which is likely to be independent of autocrine signalling by endogenous TGF-β. Through a series of experiments, the authors demonstrate how it is possible to delineate the different roles of the different effectors/receptors involved in TGF-β signalling. The paper is relevant to clinicians because the more precise we can be in localizing the site of fault(s) in the TGF-β/SMAD signalling pathway in SSc, the nearer we come to developing targeted therapies.

Elevated levels of leukotriene B_4 and leukotriene E_4 in bronchoalveolar lavage fluid from patients with scleroderma lung disease

Kowal-Bielecka O, Distler O, Kowal K, *et al.* *Arthritis Rheum* 2003; **48**: 1639–46

BACKGROUND. Leukotrienes, a family of lipid mediators derived from arachidonic acid via the action of 5-lipoxygenase, have both proinflammatory and profibrotic effects. Leukotrienes have been little studied in SSc, and the aim of this study was to analyse the roles of leukotriene B_4 (LTB_4) and LTE_4 in scleroderma lung disease. Levels of LTB_4 and LTE_4 were assayed in bronchoalveolar lavage (BAL) fluid from 30 patients with SSc (19 with and eleven without scleroderma lung disease) and ten healthy control subjects. In a subset of six patients with scleroderma lung disease, LTB_4 and LTE_4 were measured before and after 6 months of treatment with cyclophosphamide.

INTERPRETATION. Levels of LTB_4 and LTE_4 were significantly increased in the 19 patients with scleroderma lung disease (251 ± 170 and 479 ± 301 pg/ml respectively) compared with the eleven patients without lung disease (114 ± 86 and 159 ± 149 pg/ml) and the ten healthy controls (86 ± 49 and 110 ± 67 pg/ml) (Fig. 8.1). In the patients with SSc, these levels of LTB_4 and LTE_4 correlated positively with the total number of cells on BAL and negatively with the forced vital capacity. Levels of LTB_4, but not of LTE_4, fell significantly after treatment with cyclophosphamide. These findings were interpreted as suggesting that leukotrienes are implicated in the pathogenesis of scleroderma lung disease and could therefore be a therapeutic target.

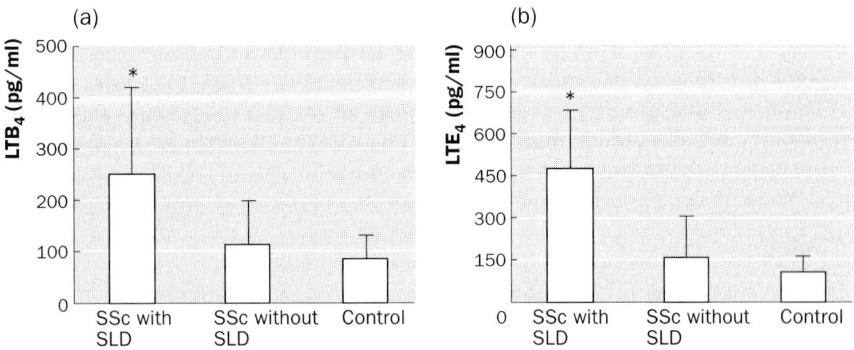

Fig. 8.1 Levels of (a) leukotriene B_4 (LTB_4) and (b) LTE_4 in bronchoalveolar lavage (BAL) fluid from patients with systemic sclerosis (SSc) with and without scleroderma lung disease (SLD) and from healthy control subjects. *$P < 0.05$ versus SSc patients without SLD and versus controls. Source: Kowal-Bielecka *et al.* (2003).

Comment

It is perhaps surprising that leukotrienes have not attracted more interest in SSc, as there is good theoretical evidence supporting a role for leukotrienes in fibrosis. In their discussion the authors cite studies of the bleomycin mouse model, in which fibrosis was attenuated in mutant mice lacking the gene encoding cytosolic phospholipase A_2 but enhanced in mice deficient in cyclooxygenase 2. These findings in the mouse model suggest that specific inhibition of the leukotriene pathway might be beneficial, but that inhibition of the upstream phospholipase A_2 might be less effective, or even detrimental, as this would also block the cyclooxygenase pathway.

In the small subgroup of patients who were studied both before and after cyclophosphamide treatment, LTB_4 levels fell in parallel with the cell count. While cyclophosphamide is fairly widely used in the treatment of scleroderma lung disease, its benefit has yet to be confirmed in controlled clinical trials and it has the potential for severe toxicity. Thus the prospect of being able to suppress inflammation and fibrosis with inhibitors of leukotriene synthesis and/or leukotriene receptor antagonists is extremely attractive, and this is an area meriting further investigation.

Disease progression and risk factors

With improvements in our ability to detect internal organ involvement early (for example, the detection of early interstitial lung disease by high-resolution computed tomography) we need to broaden our understanding of the natural history of the disease so as to better inform treatment decisions. Also, clinicians need to be aware of which patients are at increased risk of particular manifestations of disease, so that they can be appropriately monitored with a view to preventative and/or early treatment.

Much of the impetus for the early identification and treatment of patients with SSc-related pulmonary arterial hypertension comes from studies of patients with primary pulmonary hypertension, and it is therefore important to know whether the natural histories of these differ. This is the subject of the first paper selected. The second paper in this section also relates to SSc-related pulmonary hypertension, this time to the identification of predictors: early identification of at-risk patients is especially important now that prostanoids and endothelin-1 receptor antagonists are of proven benefit. Two further papers discuss predictors/risk factors for renal crisis and digital ischaemia.

Hemodynamics and survival in patients with pulmonary arterial hypertension related to systemic sclerosis

Kawut SM, Taichman DB, Archer-Chicko CL, Palevsky HI, Kimmel SE.
Chest 2003; **123**: 344–50

BACKGROUND. The aim of this retrospective cohort study was to determine whether patients with SSc-related pulmonary arterial hypertension (SScPH) have a higher

mortality than those with pulmonary hypertension that is sporadic, familial or related to anorexigen use (primary pulmonary hypertension [PPH]). The cohort comprised 33 patients with PPH and 22 patients with SScPH who underwent pulmonary artery catheterization and vasodilator studies over a 4.5-year period (January 1997 to June 2001) at the University of Pennsylvania.

INTERPRETATION. The two groups of patients had similar haemodynamics and received similar treatments during the study periods. Percentages of predicted total lung capacity (80 vs 92%; $P = 0.06$) and of diffusion capacity for carbon monoxide (42 vs 68%; $P = 0.0002$) were lower in the SScPH group. The risk of death during the study period was significantly higher in the SScPH group than in the PPH group (unadjusted hazard ratio 2.9, 95% confidence interval [CI] 1.1–7.8; $P = 0.03$), and this increased risk persisted after adjustment for age, haemodynamic and treatment variables (although it fell below statistical significance after adjustment for right atrial pressure, digoxin and epoprostenol treatment).

Comment

The study has the limitations of a retrospective cohort, and the authors discuss these. Also, the relatively small sample size, leading to wide confidence intervals, limits the precision of the hazard ratios. Nonetheless, the study does strongly point to increased mortality in patients with pulmonary arterial hypertension when this is associated with SSc (Fig. 8.2). The reasons for this cannot be determined from this study. A key point is that, although patients with significant restrictive lung disease were excluded, forced vital capacity, total lung capacity and diffusion were reduced in the SSc cohort, reflecting multisystem fibrotic/vascular disease. Since the recruitment of the cohort of patients described in this study, there has been enormous interest in the treatment of pulmonary arterial hypertension, driven by the new therapeutic approaches

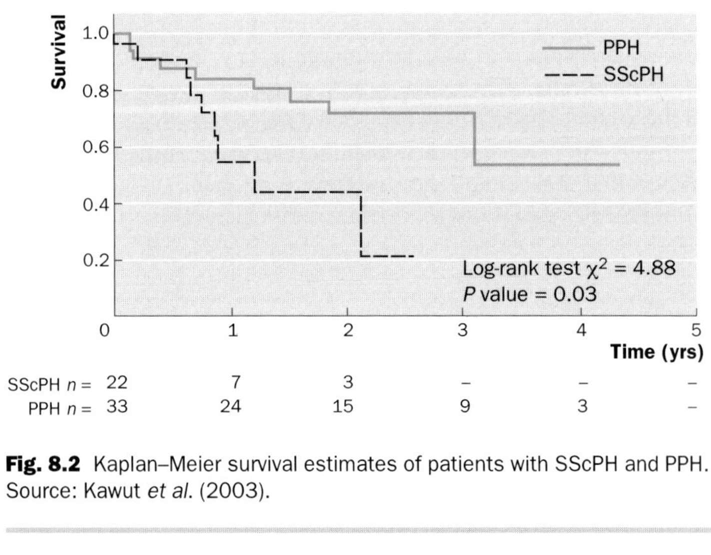

Fig. 8.2 Kaplan–Meier survival estimates of patients with SScPH and PPH. Source: Kawut *et al.* (2003).

becoming available, including endothelin-1 receptor antagonists. This study emphasizes the importance of subgrouping patients with pulmonary arterial hypertension according to the underlying disease process in studies of pathophysiology and treatment |**8**|.

Predictors of isolated pulmonary hypertension in patients with systemic sclerosis and limited cutaneous involvement

Steen V, Medsger TA. *Arthritis Rheum* 2003; **48**: 516–22

BACKGROUND. The aim of this study was to determine whether there are factors which are predictive of the development of pulmonary hypertension in patients with SSc. One hundred and six patients from the Pittsburgh Scleroderma Databank in whom a diagnosis of isolated pulmonary hypertension was made after January 1982 were compared with 106 matched controls from the same database ('isolated' refers to pulmonary hypertension not associated with pulmonary fibrosis, renal crisis or cardiomyopathy). All 106 cases had an estimated pulmonary artery systolic pressure of >30 mmHg on echocardiogram, mild to moderate exertional dyspnoea, and at least one additional objective finding of pulmonary hypertension. Asymptomatic patients were not included.

INTERPRETATION. Diffusing capacity for carbon monoxide (DL_{CO}), measured on average 4.5 years before the diagnosis of pulmonary hypertension, was significantly lower in the 62 cases in whom data were available than DL_{CO} measured on average 6.0 years before the time of matching in the 47 controls in whom data were available (52 vs 81% predicted, $P < 0.0001$). In the 40 cases in whom estimated pulmonary artery pressure (PAP) measurements on echocardiogram were available a mean of 3.9 years before diagnosis, mean systolic PAP was only slightly higher (34 mmHg) than in 27 controls studied a mean of 3.5 years before matching time (29 mmHg). In 19 patients in whom serial DL_{CO} measurements were available before diagnosis, there was a linear fall in DL_{CO} (Fig. 8.3). Patients with pulmonary hypertension had more severe Raynaud's phenomenon and more severe digital tip ulcers (as assessed on a patient-generated visual analogue scale [VAS]) and used calcium channel blockers less frequently (37% of cases used calcium channel blockers vs 61% of controls, $P < 0.001$). Pulmonary hypertension was not associated with anticentromere antibodies but there was an association with the presence of antinucleolar antibodies (anti-U3 RNP) and the absence of anti-Scl-70 antibodies. The authors interpreted their findings as showing that a falling DL_{CO} is a good predictor of isolated pulmonary hypertension and that calcium channel blockers may be protective.

Comment

This was a retrospective cohort study, the cohort being drawn from a large database of patients who, after initial evaluation, were followed up at different centres. This means that the investigative follow-up was not fully standardized, as reflected by the differing proportions of patients in whom lung function and echocardiographic data were available before diagnosis or matching time. The criteria for referral for investigation

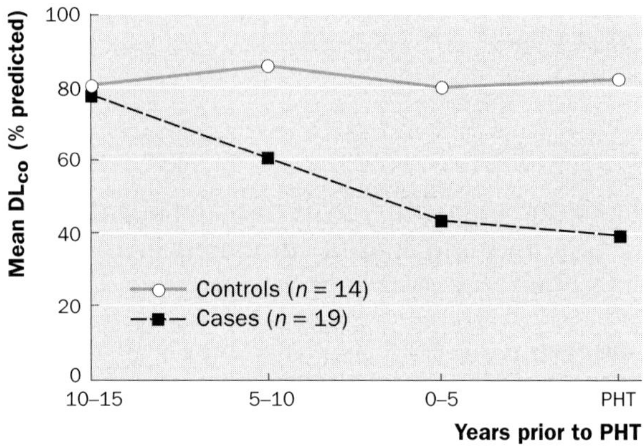

Fig. 8.3 Distribution of the mean diffusing capacity for carbon monoxide (DL_{CO}; in % of predicted [% Pred.]) among patients with limited scleroderma with (cases) or without (controls) a subsequent diagnosis of pulmonary hypertension (PHT) who underwent at least one pulmonary function test in each of the four time periods over 15 years prior to the diagnosis of PHT (or matching time in controls). Source: Steen *et al.* (2003).

of suspected pulmonary hypertension are not clear. However, these limitations of the study are balanced by the advantages of a very large database which allowed a sizeable cohort of patients with clinically significant pulmonary hypertension to be included. The key finding of the study—that a falling DL_{CO} predicts pulmonary hypertension—is well demonstrated in Fig. 8.3, and is of major practical relevance to the clinician. Thus, pulmonary hypertension should be suspected if the transfer factor falls.

The other findings of the study, while of interest, are of less clinical importance. The calcium channel blocker data should be interpreted with some caution, given that it is unlikely that patients were treated according to specific protocols.

Finally, the association between a falling transfer factor and pulmonary hypertension raises interesting pathophysiological questions.

Predictors and outcomes of scleroderma renal crisis: the high-dose versus low-dose D-penicillamine in early diffuse systemic sclerosis trial

DeMarco PJ, Weisman MH, Seilbold JR, *et al. Arthritis Rheum* 2002; **46**: 2983–9

Background. Although the incidence of scleroderma renal crisis has fallen, this remains a significant cause of morbidity and mortality in SSc. This paper examines prognostic factors for and the outcome of scleroderma renal crisis in the 134 patients

(from 17 centres) with diffuse cutaneous SSc recruited into the high-dose versus low-dose penicillamine study |9|. All patients had a disease duration of less than 18 months at the time of recruitment into the study. Because there was no difference in outcome between the two groups, for the purpose of this retrospective analysis data from both treatment groups were pooled.

Interpretation. The mean duration of follow-up was 4.0 years (SD 1.1 years). Eighteen patients developed scleroderma renal crisis (at a mean of 11 months after study entry), of whom nine died. Univariate logistic regression and life-table methods suggested four baseline predictors for scleroderma renal crisis: modified Rodnan skin score ≥20 ($P < 0.01$), enlarged heart on radiograph ($P = 0.04$), large joint contractures ($P = 0.008$) and prednisone use at entry ($P = 0.001$). Ten (56%) of the 18 patients who developed renal crisis were taking prednisone at study entry compared with 30 (26%) of the 115 without renal crisis. In the 40 patients taking prednisone, the mean daily dose at study entry was 7.4 mg; it was 9.7 ± 10.8 mg in the ten patients developing renal crisis and 6.0 ± 5.4 mg in the 30 patients without renal crisis. The authors found that low-dose prednisone alone was not associated with the onset of scleroderma renal crisis, but that prednisone increased the risk of renal crisis in patients with both a high skin score and contractures (from 21 to 43%).

Comment

The penicillamine study afforded a unique opportunity to examine predictors and outcome of scleroderma renal crisis; here was a large cohort of patients with early diffuse disease that was well documented and carefully followed prospectively over a 4-year period. The fact that as many as 13% of patients developed renal crisis reflects the early, aggressive disease of the cohort studied and highlights to the clinician that renal crisis remains a common clinical problem, and one with a high mortality rate despite the use of angiotensin-converting enzyme (ACE) inhibitors (17 of the 18 renal crisis patients received ACE inhibitors). A key message for clinicians is that even low dosages of prednisone (7–8 mg daily) should only be used with extreme caution in patients with high skin scores and joint contractures. An editorial accompanying this paper provides further comment for the interested reader |**10**|.

Cigarette smoking as a significant risk factor for digital vascular disease in patients with systemic sclerosis

Harrison BJ, Silman AJ, Hider SL, Herrick AL. *Arthritis Rheum* 2002; **46**: 3312–16

Background. In patients with SSc, Raynaud's phenomenon can progress to irreversible tissue ischaemia and some patients come to amputation. Cigarette smoking is a risk factor for vascular disease. The aim of this study was to investigate whether cigarette smoking was associated with the severity of digital vascular disease in a cohort of 101 patients with SSc. Digital ischaemic events were classified as digital debridements, requirement for intravenous vasodilators, and digital amputation.

Interpretation. Twenty-one of the 101 patients were current smokers, 37 were ex-smokers and 43 had never smoked. Results were adjusted for age, sex and disease duration. Current smokers were significantly more likely than never-smokers to have had digital debridement (odds ratio [OR] 4.5, 95% CI 1.1–18.3) or admission for intravenous vasodilators (OR 3.8, 95% CI 1.1–12.9). The data for amputations showed a similar trend (OR 3.4, 95% CI 0.8–15.1). In ex-smokers compared with never-smokers, there were increased risks of debridement (OR 1.5, 95% CI 0.4–6.1) and amputation (OR 2.0, 95% CI 0.5–7.9), but these differences were not statistically significant. Patients who smoked at a higher intensity (23–51 pack-years) were more likely to require admission for intravenous vasodilators.

Comment

While it might seem intuitive that a double vascular insult (smoking and SSc) will be associated with a high risk of digital vascular disease, this association has not been reported previously. It has obvious practical implications: smoking should be strongly discouraged in patients with SSc and resources should be directed to the support of smoking cessation. The study also prompts speculation about the pathophysiology of vascular injury in SSc and in smokers.

Outcome measures

Measurement of the SSc disease process presents major challenges. The lack of reliable outcome measures which are sensitive to change has presented difficulties in clinical trials in the past. The identification of robust outcome measures of organ-specific involvement and of disease activity/severity is the subject of much ongoing research. Interested readers are referred to the report from the OMERACT 6 Workshop on Systemic Sclerosis |**11**| and the proceedings of an international symposium held in Portonovo, Italy in February 2002, entitled 'The assessment of the patient with systemic sclerosis' |**12**|. The report from the OMERACT 6 Workshop (which focused on early diffuse disease) describes the current status of assessment tools for skin, lung and heart involvement, and for digital ischaemia, renal disease, gastrointestinal involvement, musculoskeletal disease, function and health-related quality of life |**11**|. The proceedings from the Portonovo symposium outline the findings of nine subcommittees, each of which had one particular brief. These briefs were the assessment of skin and musculoskeletal disease, peripheral vascular disease, digestive tract, lung, heart, kidney, non-organ based laboratory markers, activity, and severity/prognosis |**12**|. As a result of the symposium, a core set of variables for assessment was proposed (Table 8.1); bear in mind that this list does not include certain useful investigations, such as high-resolution computed tomography, because these are not routine in all centres |**12**|.

In recent years, there has been increasing focus in SSc (as in other rheumatic diseases) on measuring the impact of disease on functional capacity and on lifestyle. Two studies are discussed.

Table 8.1 Core set variables to be assessed to define each organ system involvement

Skin	Modified Rodnan skin score
Vessels	Raynaud; digital ulcers (active/healed)
Joints	FTP (finger tip distance) measurement
	DAS28 when synovitis occurs
Tendons	Number of tendon friction rubs at hands, wrists, elbows, knees, ankles
Muscles	Proximal weakness; serum CPK
GI tract	Dysphagia, heartburn, early satiety, bloating, vomiting, diarrhoea, constipation, malabsorption, intestinal distension, barium oesophageal and intestinal X-ray
Lung	Dyspnoea, lung fibrosis (chest X-ray), restrictive defect (by FVC, DL_{CO}), pulmonary hypertension (by Echocolour Doppler, DL_{CO})
Heart	Dyspnoea, palpitatons, chest pain
	Dizziness/pre-syncope/syncope
	Heart rate, conduction defects, arrhythmias
	Oedema/venous congestion
	Pericardial effusion
	Ejection fraction; E/A ratio
Kidney	Arterial pressure, serum creatinine, urinalysis

Source: Valentini *et al.* (2003) [12].

A cross-sectional comparison of three self-reported functional indices in scleroderma

Smythe AE, MacGregor AJ, Mukerjee D, Brough GM, Black CM, Denton CP.
Rheumatology 2003; **42**: 732–8

BACKGROUND. The Disability Index of the Health Assessment Questionnaire (HAQ-DI) measures physical disability, predicts survival [13], and has the potential of being sufficiently sensitive to change to be used in the clinical trial setting. In this study, HAQ-DI was compared with two recently developed scleroderma-specific indices: the scleroderma VAS and the UK scleroderma Functional Score (UKFS) [14]. These three functional indices are all self-administered. The scleroderma VAS has five scales: pain, vascular symptoms (Raynaud's and digital ulcers), gastrointestinal symptoms, shortness of breath and overall disease severity. Nine of the eleven questions on the UKFS relate to upper limb function and two to muscle strength and lower limb function. Predictors of disease severity were also studied. The study population comprised 115 consecutive patients with SSc (40 diffuse cutaneous, 75 limited cutaneous).

INTERPRETATION. The mean HAQ-DI and mean UKFS were higher in patients with diffuse cutaneous disease than in those with limited cutaneous disease (1.23 vs 0.79, $P = 0.005$ and 14.7 vs 10.6, $P = 0.02$ respectively). There was good correlation between the HAQ-DI and the UKFS ($r = 0.9$, $P < 0.001$), and also between both these scores and (1) the pain VAS ($r = 0.66$ for each) and (2) the overall severity VAS ($r = 0.68$ for HAQ-DI and $r = 0.72$ for UKFS). Multivariate regression analysis showed that fist closure and elevation of C-reactive protein (CRP) were independent predictors for higher HAQ-DI, and fist closure, elevated CRP and impaired hand spread were predictors for higher UKFS scores. Higher HAQ-DI and UKFS scores were found in patients with more severe disease, as judged by a variety of clinical and laboratory parameters. For example, both scores were higher in patients with modified Rodnan skin scores of ≥15. The authors concluded that these simple, easily administered tools correlate well, reflect disease severity, and assess both organ-specific and more general symptoms.

Comment

This paper describes the background to three different functional assessments (HAQ-DI, the UKFS and the scleroderma VAS) and, by applying them in a large cohort of well-described patients with SSc, gives the reader an understanding of how these three outcome measures perform, at least in cross-sectional studies. The HAQ-DI has the advantage that most rheumatologists are familiar with this from its application in patients with rheumatoid arthritis; it gives a global assessment of physical disability. The fact that the UKFS, specially designed for patients with SSc and with an emphasis on hand function, correlates well with the HAQ-DI probably reflects, as suggested by the authors, that six of the HAQ categories are influenced by hand function (albeit also by other factors). An advantage of the UKFS is that it is extremely easy to complete and to score; it is an eleven-item questionnaire, each item being scored from 0 (able to perform in a normal manner) to 3 (impossible to achieve).

Measurement of function should now be considered part of the routine assessment of patients with SSc. Because the three indices discussed are complementary, patients should ideally complete all three. However, if this is not feasible in a busy clinic setting, one of them can be chosen because they all correlate.

Measuring disease activity and functional status in patients with scleroderma and Raynaud's phenomenon

Merkel PA, Herlyn K, Martin RW, *et al.* *Arthritis Rheum* 2002; **46**: 2410–20

BACKGROUND. The aim of this study was to document disease activity and functional status in patients with SSc-related Raynaud's phenomenon, and to examine a set of outcome measures with respect to sensitivity to change, reliability, ease of use, and validity. Two hundred and eighty-one patients (48% limited cutaneous, 52% diffuse cutaneous disease) were studied. All were participating in a multicentre, randomized, placebo-controlled trial of oral iloprost [15] and underwent assessments at baseline, 6 weeks (after 6 weeks of treatment) and 12 weeks (6 weeks after stopping treatment). Twenty-one per cent had digital ulcers. The following were measured/documented for each patient at each visit (18 outcome measures in total): number and duration of Raynaud's attacks over the preceding 2 weeks, a Raynaud's Condition Score (ordinal scale, 0–10), digital tip ulcers/infarcts, a Health Assessment Questionnaire (HAQ), the scleroderma VAS (already referred to above), physician's and patient's global and

symptom-specific (for Raynaud's and digital ulcers) assessments of disease activity, and the Arthritis Impact Measurement Scales 2 (AIMS2) for mood and tension.

Interpretation. In this group of patients, selected on the basis that all were experiencing problems with Raynaud's, fairly high levels of depressed mood and tension were identified and HAQ scores showed significant disability at baseline, especially in those subscales relating to hand function. Patients with digital ulcers scored higher on a number of parameters, including the Raynaud's Condition Score. Patients' VAS scores for digital ulcers were not consistent with physicians' scores. When examining effect sizes, results from both study arms (active and placebo) were considered together as similar improvements were found in both treatment groups. Effect sizes and standardized response means (measuring relative sensitivity to change) were highest for the Raynaud's-related variables (Raynaud's Condition Score, frequency and duration of attacks, scleroderma VAS, and physician's and patient's assessment). There were clear differences in consistency (reliability) between the 18 study measures, as assessed during the post-trial period (examining results from the baseline and 12-week visits). The most reliable measures were Raynaud's Condition Score and the frequency and duration of attacks. The VAS measures were the least reliable. The AIMS2 scales and the disability score of the HAQ had intermediate values. From these results the authors proposed a core set of measures for use in clinical trials in patients with Raynaud's phenomenon (Table 8.2).

Comment

Clinical trials in patients with Raynaud's phenomenon have tended in the past to rely upon the frequency and duration of Raynaud's attacks as end-points. However, Raynaud's phenomenon, especially when severe, as in many patients with SSc, is functionally disabling and affects quality of life. This study is probably the first to

Table 8.2 Proposed core set of outcome measures for studying RP in scleroderma*

Core area	Specific measure
Primary outcome measures	
Patient's assessment of RP activity	Raynaud's Condition Score
Physician's assessment of RP activity	Physician's assessment of RP activity (by VAS)
Patient's assessment of digital ulcer activity	SHAQ Digital ulcer VAS†
Pain	HAQ pain VAS†
Disability	HAQ disability VAS†
Psychological measures	AIMS2 mood and tension scales
Supplementary outcome measures	
RP attack frequency	Inherent in Raynaud's Condition Score
RP attack duration	Inherent in Raynaud's Condition Score
Overall scleroderma disease assessment	SHAQ Scleroderma disease VAS†

*RP, Raynaud's phenomenon; VAS, visual analogue scale; HAQ, Health Assessment Questionnaire; AIMS2, Arthritis Impact Measurement Scales 2.
†Part of the Scleroderma HAQ (SHAQ) developed by Steen and Medsger |**13**|.
Source: Merkel *et al.* (2002).

examine the feasibility of developing a core/global set of outcome measures for Raynaud's phenomenon which could be used in clinical trials. A large patient cohort was examined and a large amount of data was collected prospectively. The study confirms the impression of many clinicians that Raynaud's phenomenon in the patient with SSc has effects on function and on mood, evidenced by the HAQ and AIMS2 scores. As the authors state, outcome measures should therefore cover several domains and the core set of outcome measures proposed includes the HAQ pain and disability scales and the AIMS2 mood and tension scales (Table 8.2).

A key feature of the study is that it addresses the issue of the reliability of 18 different measures. Interestingly, the three which performed best included the frequency and duration of Raynaud's attacks, which supports the continued use of the time-honoured diary card. In this study, the authors suggest that the small size and portability of the diary contributed to its high acceptance and completion rate. Also, patients filled this in over periods of not more than 2 weeks at a time, in other words not over the full 12-week period. These practical points should be taken into account when designing clinical trials.

Finally, as the authors point out, the study indicates the need for the development of more robust outcome measures for digital ulceration, evidenced by the lack of consistency between patient's and physician's assessments of ulcer symptoms. Digital ulcers, as shown in this study, in themselves cause pain and disability. The definition and measurement of digital ulcers is a major challenge to clinicians and an area in need of further research.

Treatment

It is disappointing that more papers on treatment have not been published in the last year. However, this is counterbalanced by the fact that trials are ongoing. Only one paper is discussed here.

Sacral nerve stimulation for faecal incontinence due to systemic sclerosis

Kenefick NJ, Vaizey CJ, Nicholls RJ, Cohen R, Kamm MA. *Gut* 2002; **51**: 881–3

BACKGROUND. Faecal incontinence is a common symptom in SSc, occurring in approximately one-third of patients. Several factors may contribute, including diarrhoea (for example, relating to malabsorption), decreased rectal capacity and compliance, and faecal leakage through a weak internal anal sphincter. Faecal incontinence is difficult to treat. The aim of this study was to evaluate sacral nerve stimulation in SSc-related faecal incontinence. Five female patients were studied. All had severe incontinence that had not responded to other measures, including antidiarrhoeal agents and biofeedback. A 3-week bowel diary, quality of life assessment (SF-36) and anorectal physiology were completed at baseline and after temporary and permanent sacral nerve stimulation.

INTERPRETATION. Four patients benefited from temporary stimulation. The fifth patient experienced premature lead dislodgement after 24 h and was not permanently implanted. Permanent implantation was performed 1 month after temporary stimulation in the other four patients. The follow-up period ranged from 6 to 60 months (60, 36, 24 and 6 months). Weekly incontinent episodes fell from 15, 11, 23 and 7 episodes per week to none. Urgency resolved. Responses in quality of life assessments were reported as showing 'variable' improvement, with the most consistent improvements in physical and social function. There were also benefits in terms of anorectal physiology. For example, maximal anal resting pressure rose from a median of 37 cm H_2O (range 16–39) to 65 cm H_2O (range 47–85). There were no major complications.

Comment

Recent years have brought increasing recognition that anorectal dysfunction, leading to faecal incontinence, is a common and distressing feature of the SSc disease process. This was a small study in a selected group of patients (all patients had an atrophic anal sphincter and none had evidence of malabsorption, megacolon or secondary pseudo-obstruction). The results therefore need to be reproduced in a larger number of patients. Nonetheless, the results in the four implanted patients are impressive. The authors report that both temporary and permanent stimulator implantation are relatively minor procedures, which therefore warrant further evaluation in patients with SSc.

Conclusion

The ten papers summarized and discussed above were chosen primarily to update clinicians on clinical research which is influencing current practice, but also to give an insight into the scope of ongoing basic science research. For example, the studies by Mori *et al.* suggest that further elucidation of the TGF-β/SMAD signalling pathway may inform and refine treatment strategies aimed at blocking the effects of TGF-β.

The papers discussed by Kawut *et al.* and DeMarco *et al.* provide further insight into survival in patients with pulmonary hypertension and renal crisis respectively (the latter also discussing predictors) and serve to remind us of the significant mortality of SSc. From the papers by Steen and Medsger, De Marco *et al.* and Harrison *et al.*, a number of points emerge which are directly relevant to clinical practice:

1. if the DL_{CO} falls, consider a diagnosis of pulmonary arterial hypertension;
2. be very cautions about using even low-dose steroids in patients with diffuse cutaneous disease who have a high skin score and contractures;
3. emphasize the importance of stopping smoking.

Regarding outcome assessment, one of our aims should be to include at least one index of function in the routine clinical assessment of patients with SSc, in the same way as the HAQ is used in rheumatoid arthritis. The paper by Smythe *et al.* is therefore relevant to all clinicians with an interest in SSc. This and the paper by Merkel *et al.* will guide those of us involved in clinical trial work in our choice of outcome measures.

The paper by Kenefick *et al.* on sacral nerve stimulation described only a very small number of patients and a technique which will be restricted to specialist centres, but it demonstrates that we must continue to research new treatment approaches for the different organ-based manifestations of disease, as well as potential disease-modifying therapies.

A key point from the papers discussed is that two of them (those by DeMarco *et al.* and Merkel *et al.*) are based upon analysis of outcome measures collected during large multicentre double-blind studies, demonstrating how large-scale studies, in which data are carefully collected prospectively, generate important data on predictors and outcome.

In conclusion, publications from the last year demonstrate the broad spectrum of clinical and laboratory-based research and how research opportunities are being maximized.

References

1. Maddison PJ. Prevention of vascular damage in scleroderma with angiotensin-converting enzyme (ACE) inhibition. *Rheumatology* 2002; **41**: 965–71.
2. LeRoy EC, Black C, Fleischmajer R, Jablonska S, Kreig T, Medsger TA, Rowell N, Wollheim F. Scleroderma (systemic sclerosis): classification, subsets and pathogenesis. *J Rheumatol* 1988; **15**: 202–5.
3. Sakkas LI, Xu B, Artlett CM, Lu S, Jininez SA, Platsoucas CD. Oligoclonal T cell expansion in the skin of patients with systemic sclerosis. *J Immunol* 2002; **168**: 3649–59.
4. Kubo M, Czuwara-Ladykowska J, Moussa O, Markiewicz M, Smith E, Silver RM, Jablonska S, Blaszczyk M, Watson DK, Trojanowska M. Persistent down-regulation of Fli1, a suppressor of collagen transcription, in fibrotic scleroderma skin. *Am J Pathol* 2003; **163**: 571–81.
5. Yamane K, Ihn H, Kubo M, Tamaki K. Increased transcriptional activities of transforming growth factor beta receptors in scleroderma fibroblasts. *Arthritis Rheum* 2002; **46**: 2421–8.
6. Kissen EY, Lemaire R, Korn JH, Lafyatis R. Transforming growth factor beta induces fibroblast fibrillin-1 matrix formation. *Arthritis Rheum* 2002; **46**: 3000–9.
7. Ong VH, Evans LA, Shiwen X, Fisher IB, Rajkumar V, Abraham DJ, Black CM, Denton CP. Monocyte chemoattractant protein 3 as a mediator of fibrosis: overexpression in systemic sclerosis and the type 1 tight-skin mouse. *Arthritis Rheum* 2003; **48**: 1979–91.
8. Badesch DB, Tapson VF, McGoon MD, Brundage BH, Rubin LJ, Wigley FM, Rich S, Barst RJ, Barrett PS, Kral KM, Jobsis MM, Loyd JE, Murali S, Frost A, Girgis R, Bourge RC,

Ralph DD, Elliott CG, Hill NS, Langleben D, Schilz RJ, McLaughlin VV, Robbins IM, Groves BM, Shapiro S, Medsger TA Jr. Continuous intravenous epoprostenol for pulmonary hypertension due to the scleroderma spectrum of disease. A randomized, controlled trial. *Ann Intern Med* 2000; **132**: 425–34.

9. Clements PJ, Furst DE, Wong WK, Mayes M, White B, Wigley F, Weisman MH, Barr W, Moreland LW, Medsger TA Jr, Steen V, Martin RW, Collier D, Weinstein A, Lally E, Varga J, Weiner S, Andrews B, Abeles M, Seibold JR. High-dose versus low-dose D-penicillamine in early diffuse systemic sclerosis: analysis of a two-year, double-blind, randomized, controlled clinical trial. *Arthritis Rheum* 1999; **42**: 1194–203.
10. Strand V. Predictors and outcome of scleroderma renal crisis: data from the high-dose versus low-dose penicillamine in early diffuse systemic sclerosis trial [editorial]. *Arthritis Rheum* 2002; **46**: 2836–37.
11. Merkel PA, Clements PJ, Reveille JD, Suarez-Almazor ME, Valentini G, Furst DE. Current status of outcome measure development for clinical trials in systemic sclerosis. Report from OMERACT 6. *J Rheumatol* 2003; **30**: 1630–47.
12. Valentini G, Medsger TA, Silman AJ, Bombardieri S (eds). The assessment of the patient with systemic sclerosis [proceedings of a symposium]. *Clin Exp Rheumatol* 2003; **21**(Suppl 29).
13. Steen VD, Medsger TA. The value of the Health Assessment Questionnaire and special patient-generated scales to demonstrate change in systemic sclerosis patients over time. *Arthritis Rheum* 1997; **40**: 1984–91.
14. Silman A, Akesson A, Newman J, Henriksson H, Sandquist G, Nihill M, Palfrey S, Lomas R, Wollheim F, Black C. Assessment of functional ability in patients with scleroderma: a proposed new disability assessment instrument. *J Rheumatol* 1998; **25**: 79–83.
15. Wigley FM, Korn JH, Csuka ME, Medsger TA Jr, Rothfield NF, Ellman M, Martin R, Collier DH, Weinstein A, Furst DE, Jimenez SA, Mayes MD, Merkel PA, Gruber B, Kaufman L, Varga J, Bell P, Kern J, Marrott P, White B, Simms RW, Phillips AC, Seibold JR. Oral iloprost treatment in patients with Raynaud's phenomenon secondary to systemic sclerosis: a multi-center, placebo-controlled, double-blind study. *Arthritis Rheum* 1998; **41**: 670–7.

9

Vasculitis

RAASHID LUQMANI

Introduction

Vasculitis remains a diagnostic and therapeutic challenge in the 21st century and it is essential to continue the task of understanding the pathophysiology and possibly the genetic or environmental basis for this set of unusual but potentially life-threatening conditions in order to make significant advances in managing and, hopefully, curing the vasculitis. Until then, however, we continue to refine the available therapeutic measurements and develop existing or newer agents to suppress the major manifestations of these diseases. In the absence of a simple reproducible biological marker of disease activity, it has been important to develop robust clinical tools to evaluate disease activity and disease damage, which in turn has allowed us to test new and existing therapeutic agents. This is because the current therapeutic strategies have resulted in over 80% survival in vasculitis |**1–3**| compared with over 80% mortality without them |**4**|. However, the search for the least toxic and most effective agent has to be guided by measurement of the efficacy of these regimens, and this is best achieved using developed tools such as the Birmingham Vasculitis Activity Score (BVAS) |**5**| and the Vasculitis Damage Index (VDI) |**6**|. The role of antineutrophil cytoplasmic antibody (ANCA) |**7**| in the pathophysiology of the vasculitides has remained controversial despite many publications on the subject. A clearer picture of the specific subtypes of ANCA is emerging which should lead to greater understanding of vasculitis. Not all vasculitides are associated with ANCA but the ANCA-associated vasculitides do represent an important subset with greater predisposition to serious organ involvement, such as significant kidney disease. Other pathophysiological mechanisms in vasculitis include viruses, drugs and other antibodies (including failure of immune complex clearance, complement consumption and direct antibody attack).

Epidemiology and aetiology of vasculitis

The controversial role of the leukotriene receptor antagonists in Churg-Strauss syndrome may help to increase our understanding of the relationship between asthma and vasculitis and may also suggest a novel pathogenetic mechanism for the

Table 9.1 Disease manifestations for Churg-Strauss syndrome in patients in the present series and other large series

	Present series 1990–2000 (*n* = 91)	**Chumbley 1950–1974 (*n* = 30)**	**Lanham 1976–1982 (*n* = 138)**	**Reid 1982–1995 (*n* = 23)**	**Guillevin 1963–1995 (*n* = 96)**	**Solans 1977–1999 (*n* = 32)**
	Mean ± 6 SD, number (%), or range					
Characteristic						
Age at diagnosis (years)	49 ±16	47	38	57	48 ± 14	43
Male sex	51 (56)	21 (70)	76 (55)	15 (65)	44 (46)	9 (28)
Asthma	90 (99)	30 (100)	138 (100)	22 (96)	96 (100)	32 (100)
Peripheral eosinophilia						
>10%*	88 (97)	30 (100)	NA	21 (91)	87 (91)	32 (100)
>1.5 × 10^9/l†	81 (89)	NA	138 (100)	21 (91)	80 (83)	32 (100)
Organ involvement						
Paranasal sinus	67 (74)	NA	97 (70)	12 (52)	59 (61)	NA
Peripheral nerve	69 (76)	NA	91 (66)	16 (70)	75 (78)	23 (72)
Skin	52 (57)	20 (67)	97 (70)	14 (61)	49 (51)	26 (81)
Lung	53 (58)	8 (27)	99 (72)	11 (48)	36 (38)	20 (63)
Joint	27 (30)	6 (20)	70 (51)	13 (57)	40 (42)	6 (19)
Kidney	23 (25)	6–9 (20–30)	80 (58)	13 (57)	25 (26)	NA
Gastrointestinal	28 (31)	10 (33)	81 (59)	10 (43)	32 (33)	4 (13)
Endomyocardial	12 (13)	NA	65 (47)	4 (17)	14 (14)	14 (44)
Pericardial	7 (8)	NA	44 (32)	6 (26)	22 (23)	9 (28)
Central nerve	10 (11)	NA	37 (27)	9 (39)	8 (8)	2 (6)

* Used in American College of Rheumatology criteria.
† Used in Lanham criteria.
NA, not available.
Source: Keogh and Specks (2003).

induction of disease. Epidemiological data have illustrated differences between the incidence of systemic vasculitis in different parts of the world (Wegener's granulomatosis showing a predilection for northern European countries compared with southern European countries) and a possible link between Churg-Strauss syndrome and farming |**8**|. Viruses such as hepatitis C and hepatitis B are closely associated with certain types of vasculitis (mixed essential cryoglobulinaemic vasculitis and hepatitis B-related polyarteritis nodosa). In fact the incidence of hepatitis B is falling, as a result of which hepatitis B-related polyarteritis nodosa (PAN) has become a rare disease |**9**|.

Churg-Strauss syndrome: clinical presentation, antineutrophil cytoplasmic antibodies, and leukotriene receptor antagonists

Keogh KA, Specks U. *Am J Med* 2003; **115**: 284–90

Background. In this observational study of patients with Churg-Strauss syndrome, the role of ANCA and the use of leukotriene receptor antagonists were recorded.

Interpretation. Of the 98 patients identified at the Mayo Clinic between 1990 and 2000, 70–75% had ANCA before treatment compared with only 16% of patients at times of disease inactivity. The use of leukotriene receptor antagonists was recorded in 23 patients, and in 16 cases it was started before the diagnosis of Churg-Strauss syndrome was made. However, in trying to establish a link between the introduction of a leukotriene antagonist and the appearance of vasculitis, there is no clear pattern to suggest that the leukotriene antagonist was the cause of the vasculitis. Therefore, the conclusion from this study is that there is still a significant amount of uncertainty about whether leukotriene antagonists do indeed induce Churg-Strauss syndrome or whether or not they are responsible for exacerbation of an underlying Churg-Strauss syndrome.

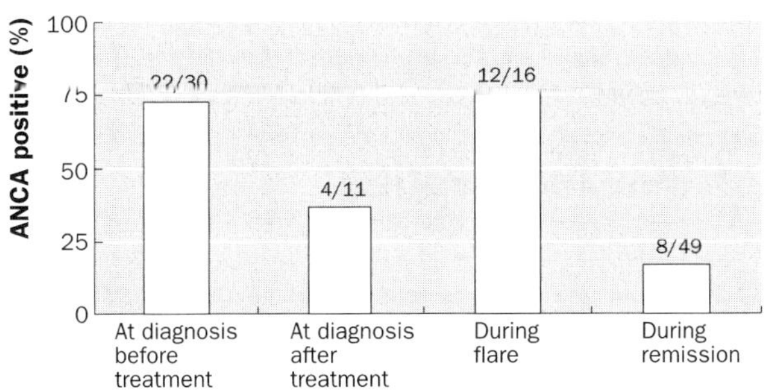

Fig. 9.1 Association of antineutrophil cytoplasmic antibodies (ANCA) with Churg-Strauss syndrome disease activity. Source: Keogh and Specks (2003).

Comment

The role of leukotriene receptor antagonists in inducing Churg-Strauss syndrome remains controversial. One suggestion is that the drug simply unmasks underlying Churg-Strauss syndrome by allowing patients to reduce or stop their corticosteroids for asthma, these corticosteroids having been used previously to treat their low-grade vasculitis symptoms. However, there may still be a pathogenic role for drugs in the development of Churg-Strauss syndrome and other forms of vasculitis.

Kawasaki syndrome hospitalizations and associated costs in the United States

Belay ED, Holman RC, Maddox RA, Foster DA, Schonberger LB. *Public Health Reports* 2003; **118**: 464–9

BACKGROUND. The childhood vasculitic syndrome Kawasaki disease is a significant clinical problem in young children. A comparison between the cost of hospitalization for Kawasaki syndrome and that for other acute diseases in childhood was the subject of this study.

INTERPRETATION. By reviewing all records in a proportion of children's units throughout the USA during the period from 1997 to 1999, the authors identified over 7000 hospital discharges related to Kawasaki syndrome (approximately 2500 per annum). Most of the children were male (60%) and over 75% were under the age of 5. The extrapolated hospitalization rate for children with Kawasaki disease varied from 8.3 per 100 000 per annum for girls to 12 per 100 000 per annum for boys. The median cost per stay for children under the age of 5 years with Kawasaki syndrome was greater than that for children with respiratory syncytial virus-associated bronchiolitis or acute diarrhoeal illness.

Comment

Kawasaki syndrome remains a significant cause of morbidity and, in some cases, mortality in undiagnosed children, particularly under the age of 5 years.

Prognosis and outcome in vasculitis

Traditionally, we have regarded Henoch–Schönlein purpura (HSP) as a less aggressive form of vasculitis than other small vessel vasculitides, such as Wegener's granulomatosis, microscopic polyangiitis and Churg–Strauss syndrome. However, long-term studies suggest that all is not well for adults and sometimes children who suffer from HSP.

Henoch–Schonlein purpura in children and adults: clinical differences in a defined population

Garcia-Porrua C, Valvino MC, Llorca J, Couselo JM, Gonzalez-Gay MA.
Semin Arthritis Rheum 2002; **32**: 149–56

BACKGROUND. This study reviewed the clinical and epidemiological differences between adult- and childhood-onset HSP in northern Spain. The aim was to describe the long-term features of HSP in both adults and children.

INTERPRETATION. By separately following patients who had developed HSP under the age of 14 years and those who developed it over the age of 20, 73 children and 31 adults were included in the study. More males suffered from HSP in adult-onset disease compared with childhood-onset disease and there was a seasonal difference in incidence, children being more commonly affected in autumn and winter and adults in summer and winter. Gastrointestinal manifestations were similar in the two groups but 19% of the adults had severe renal manifestations and a further 13% developed renal impairment. By 5–6 years of follow-up, most children had made a complete recovery but up to 40% of the adults had persistent haematuria and in 10% significant renal impairment was sustained.

The adult kidney 24 years after childhood Henoch–Schonlein purpura: a retrospective cohort study

Ronkainen J, Nuutinen M, Koskimies O. *Lancet* 2002; **360**: 666–70

BACKGROUND. This paper looked at a long-term observational cohort of children who had suffered from HSP for up to 24 years to observe the long-term outcome and natural history of this disease.

INTERPRETATION. Children were followed for between 16 and 36 years; 90% were reviewed by a clinician at the time of observation. Of children who had severe HSP with glomerulonephritis at onset, 35% went on to develop severe renal impairment compared with 7% of those who had mild or no renal symptoms at onset, giving a relative risk of poor outcome of 4.7 (95% confidence interval [CI] 1.3–18.7). This risk appeared to be higher in women (5.0, CI 1.1–32.5) than in men (2.0, CI 0.2–17.5). In women who achieved pregnancy 70% had hypertension or proteinuria, and in five out of nine women who had complicated pregnancies a poor renal outcome was the result. This suggests that, in childhood-onset HSP, renal disease develops in a significant proportion of patients.

Comment

These two studies demonstrate that HSP should be regarded as a serious and significant cause of renal disease in children who have severe-onset disease and, more particularly, in adults who have any evidence of renal impairment. Long-term

Table 9.2 Numbers of patients with poor outcome, by severity of renal symptoms at onset of Henoch-Schönlein purpura

	Number of patients reported	Follow-up (years)	Renal symptoms at onset		
			No symptoms	Mild symptoms	Severe symptoms
Series					
Our series	47	24.1 (mean)	0/9	2/18 (11%)	7/20 (35%)
Stewart and colleagues*	55	8.3 (mean)		0/37	3/18 (17%)
Goldstein and colleagues*	78	23.4 (mean)		5/39 (13%)	17/39 (44%)
Niaudet and colleagues*	151	>1		3/18 (17%)	50/133 (38%)
Schärer and colleagues*	63*	6.1 (mean)		2/25 (8%)	18/38 (47%)
Total	394		0/9	12/137 (9%)	95/248 (38%)

Mild symptoms = haematuria, proteinuria (<1 g/day), or both. Severe symptoms = nephritic syndrome, nephrotic syndrome, or both, proteinuria (>1 g/day), biopsy specimen grade III or more.
*One patient who died of an extra-renal cause is not included in this table.
Source: Ronkainen *et al.* (2002).

follow-up should be the norm for such patients in order to monitor renal function and manage the long-term effects of this disease.

Long-term follow-up studies are allowing us to understand the natural history of treated vasculitis and may provide clues to understanding the prognosis and the risk factors for poor outcome.

The long-term mortality and morbidity of Behcet syndrome: a 2-decade outcome survey of 387 patients followed at a dedicated centre

Kural-Seyahi E, Fresko I, Seyahi N, *et al. Medicine (Baltimore)* 2003; **82**: 60–76

Background. This is a 20-year observational study of patients with Behçet's syndrome attending a specialist outpatient clinic for this disease. The aim was to describe the natural history of Behçet's syndrome in this large cohort. The cohort contains over 387 patients and information is available on over 90% of them.

Interpretation. The mortality was approximately 10% (predominantly males; 39 male and three female deaths) as a result of neurological involvement or major vessel involvement. In young males there was an increase in standardized mortality ratio compared with healthy controls, but the difference became less significant in older patients. Morbidity was highest during the early course of the disease (especially eye involvement). Although most clinical problems became less apparent over time, the exceptions were central nervous system involvement and major vessel disease, which occurred after 5–10 years of disease. Late onset of eye involvement implied a better visual prognosis compared with early involvement of the eyes.

Determinants of outcome in ANCA-associated glomerulonephritis: a prospective histopathological analysis of 96 patients

Hauer HA, Bajema IM, Van Houwelingen HC, *et al.*, European Vasculitis Study Group (EUVAS). *Kidney Int* 2002; **62**: 1732–42

BACKGROUND. The renal histology in 96 patients with ANCA-associated glomerulonephritis was reviewed and compared with the clinical outcome in these patients, who formed part of the European Vasculitis Study Group trials of therapy in systemic vasculitis. The aim was to determine whether any specific histological features had predictive value in clinical outcome.

INTERPRETATION. Using 39 histological features obtained from 96 biopsies, hard clinical outcomes, such as renal function 18 months after the start of therapy, relapse or death, were compared with the histological abnormalities. There was a strong association between renal function at 18 months, measured in terms of glomerular filtration rate, compared with the initial renal function at diagnosis ($r = 0.67$). This would be expected. However, there were also correlations between 18-month glomerular filtration rate and interstitial fibrosis ($r = -0.45$), glomerulosclerosis ($r = -0.37$) and tubular atrophy ($r = -0.36$). Correlations with corrected glomerular filtration rate at 18 months were strong for segmental crescents ($r = 0.45$), cellular crescents ($r = 0.30$) and fibrinoid necrosis ($r = 0.46$). However, relapse or death could not be predicted using histological parameters. It is suggested that initial renal function and changes in chronic renal lesions were useful predictors of future renal function in systemic vasculitis, whereas active lesions were more likely to be associated with recovery of renal function, and therefore represent reversible disease activity.

Baseline features and initial treatment as predictors of remission and relapse in Wegener's granulomatosis

Koldingsnes W, Nosent JC. *J Rheumatol* 2003; **30**: 80–8

BACKGROUND. The use of disease activity and disease damage assessments in predicting remission and relapse in patients with Wegener's granulomatosis was the subject of this paper, which reports a retrospective analysis of 56 patients followed over a course of over 40 months. Patients were assessed using the BVAS and damage was measured with the VDI. The analysis of this study included an assessment of the cumulative amounts of therapy and a description of which initial therapies were used with particular regard to the use of cyclophosphamide and corticosteroid.

Interpretation. Evaluation of patients who had survived longer than 1 month showed that 85% achieved complete remission and 15% partial remission. At onset, a high BVAS increased the likelihood of achieving remission, so that a BVAS score of 23 out of 63 had a relative hazard ratio of 2.94 (CI 1.48–5.85) while achieving remission, compared with a level of BVAS below this figure. Sixty per cent of patients suffered a relapse at a median follow-up of around 18 months. The risk of relapse was predicted by lower doses of cyclophosphamide (less than 10 g) given during the first 6 months (relative hazard ratio 2.83, CI 1.33–6.02). Patients treated with higher doses of prednisolone (>20 mg/day for <2.75 months) had a higher likelihood of relapse (relative hazard ratio 2.41, CI 1.12–5.21). Presentation with cardiac involvement was also predictive of future relapse (relative hazard ratio 2.87, CI 1.09–7.58). The presence of a higher damage score at baseline (VDI >1) was associated with a higher likelihood of failure to achieve complete remission (odds ratio 1.53, CI 1.03–2.27). The conclusions were that, overall, in Wegener's granulomatosis, acute disease activity as measured by BVAS increased the likelihood of complete remission, whereas the presence of baseline organ damage had a significant negative effect on achieving remission. There was a relationship between less intensive initial treatment and a higher likelihood of relapse, as measured by lower amounts of cyclophosphamide and a shorter time on high-dose steroid.

Comment

These three studies looked at the clinical and histological features of vasculitis over a long period of time. In the study of Koldingsnes and Nosent the clinical behaviour of patients with Wegener's granulomatosis and their response to therapy was evaluated. The findings with regard to the use of cyclophosphamide and steroid are likely to have mirrored the need to adjust therapy according to disease severity since this was not in the context of a clinical trial. However, the authors report that, contrary to previous data, baseline disease activity as measured by BVAS did not predict mortality [**5,10**]. Renal histological findings of active vasculitis such as crescentic nephritis and fibrinoid necrosis have been previously shown to predict poor renal outcome. However, the novel findings in the paper by Hauer *et al.* suggest that fibrosis, scarring and tubular atrophy are important histological predictors of poor renal outcome. As the authors point out though, it is important to also include baseline clinical features in evaluating future disease activity. The large study by Kural-Seyahi and colleagues provides evidence of longevity, and therefore clinicity, in patients with Behçet's syndrome who continue to suffer problems in later life, particularly from the central nervous system lesions and major vessel disease which can occur in well-established disease. Prediction of future outcome in systemic vasculitis is a goal worthy of pursuit. If there are factors at onset that can be used to determine future outcome, this could help in fashioning appropriate therapies.

Renal transplantation in vasculitis

In patients who have end-stage renal disease due to vasculitis, renal replacement therapy is a significant benefit. However, there has always been a concern that this might be complicated by recurrence of the original disease.

Outcome of renal transplantation in patients with pauci-immune small vessel vasculitis or anti-GBM disease

Deegens JK, Artz MA, Hoitsma AJ, Wetzels JF. *Clin Nephrol* 2003; **59**: 1–9

BACKGROUND. There has always been concern that the use of renal transplantation in patients with small vessel vasculitis or anti-glomerular basement membrane (GBM) antibody disease might be complicated by a recurrence of the original disease or complications as a result of previous immunosuppression. The authors reviewed the outcome of renal transplantation for these conditions over a 32-year period in order to determine what the long-term outcome was for these patients.

INTERPRETATION. Forty-three patients were followed for up to 5 years from transplantation. Patients had a mixture of Wegener's granulomatosis (eight patients), microscopic polyangiitis (seven), renal limited vasculitis (18) and anti-GBM disease (ten). During the follow-up period only one patient had a relapse of Wegener's granulomatosis, which occurred 5 months after transplantation. The 5-year patient and graft survival rates were 77 and 60%, respectively (similar to figures from a matched control group of non-vasculitic patients, in which there was 79% patient survival and 56% graft survival). However, there was a clear increase in incidence of malignancies in patients with primary systemic vasculitis or anti-GBM disease as the cause of their renal failure compared with the control group ($P = 0.02$).

Relapse rate and outcome of ANCA-associated small vessel vasculitis after transplantation

Elmedhem A, Adu D, Savage CO. *Nephrol Dial Transplant* 2003; **18**: 1001–4

BACKGROUND. There is a concern that the development of end-stage renal failure in patients with ANCA-associated systemic vasculitis (five with Wegener's granulomatosis and four with microscopic polyangiitis [MPA]) may be complicated if patients receive a transplant by the recurrence of potentially fatal activity of the primary disease. The renal survival of nine patients with ANCA-associated systemic vasculitis was compared with that of a control group given renal transplantation for other causes (excluding diabetes).

INTERPRETATION. Two of the Wegener's granulomatosis patients suffered a relapse of their vasculitis affecting the upper respiratory tract between 40 and 50 months after transplantation. Comparison of the renal function of the transplant in vasculitis patients with that in 18 non-diabetic controls suggested that function was better in the vasculitis patients.

Comment

From these data we conclude that renal transplantation is safe and effective in patients with vasculitis compared with other patient groups. However, the increased risk of malignancy should be carefully observed; it may relate to prior use of immunosuppression to manage the primary disease. In terms of relapse, the evidence suggests that only a minority of patients will suffer recurrence of their original disease once they have reached end-stage renal failure.

Therapeutic trials of existing strategies

In terms of therapeutic advances, new agents are being trialled currently, but in the last 12 months the best evidence for therapies has emerged from measurements of the benefit of existing agents tested in controlled trials using standardized outcome measures.

A randomized trial of maintenance therapy for vasculitis associated with antineutrophil cytoplasmic autoantibodies

Jayne D, Rasmussen N, Andrassy K, *et al.* *N Engl J Med* 2003; **349**: 36–44

BACKGROUND. The induction of remission of systemic vasculitis with cyclophosphamide is well established but the longer-term use of cyclophosphamide as a maintenance agent remains controversial. It is common practice in a number of centres to switch from cyclophosphamide to an alternative, less toxic maintenance regimen, but this has not been the subject of a controlled trial until now. The European Vasculitis Study Group (EUVAS) group have undertaken a significant controlled trial involving 155 patients with systemic vasculitis who are new presentations with generalized disease and significant but not severe renal involvement. All patients were given a standardized regimen of oral cyclophosphamide for the first 3–6 months to induce remission and were then randomized to either continue receiving cyclophosphamide, but at a lower dose, or to switch to azathioprine for the subsequent 12–15 months.

INTERPRETATION. The results of this trial show that there was very little difference between the outcomes in the cyclophosphamide and azathioprine limbs. Overall, the remission rate was 93% during the induction regimen and mortality was 5%, particularly early in the course of the disease, as might be expected. The relapse rate was not significantly different between the azathioprine and cyclophosphamide groups (13.7 and 15.5%, respectively). Adverse events occurred equally in both groups; 10% of all patients experienced severe adverse events in the induction phase and a further 11% experienced them in the azathioprine group during the remission phase compared with 10% in the cyclophosphamide group. There did appear to be some difference between relapse rates in Wegener's granulomatosis and MPA, Wegener's granulomatosis patients having a higher relapse rate in their series; this is mirrored in other studies.

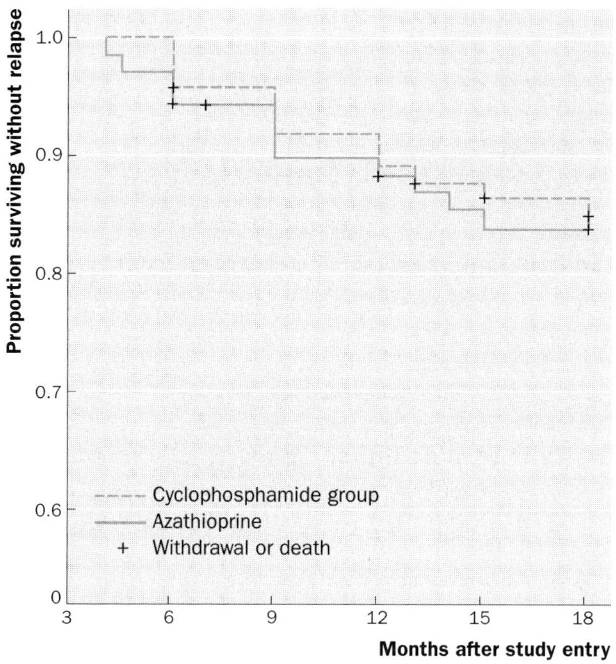

Fig. 9.2 Kaplan-Meier analysis of the time to first relapse in the azathioprine and cyclophosphamide groups. Plus signs represent withdrawals or deaths.
Source: Jayne *et al.* (2003).

Treatment of polyarteritis nodosa and microscopic polyangiitis with poor prognosis factors: a prospective trial comparing glucocorticoids and six or twelve cyclophosphamide pulses in sixty-five patients

Guillevin L, Cohen P, Mahr A, *et al. Arthritis Rheum* 2003; **49**: 93–100

Background. In this study of patients who had vasculitis with poor prognosis (PAN or MPA), a comparison was made between prolonged high-dose pulse therapy of twelve cycles of cyclophosphamide and steroid and a short high-dose therapy of six cycles.

Interpretation. Sixty-five new patients (18 with PAN and 47 with MPA) were randomized to either twelve or six pulses. All patients had at least one of the five factors indicating poor prognosis (proteinuria, impaired renal function, abdominal involvement,

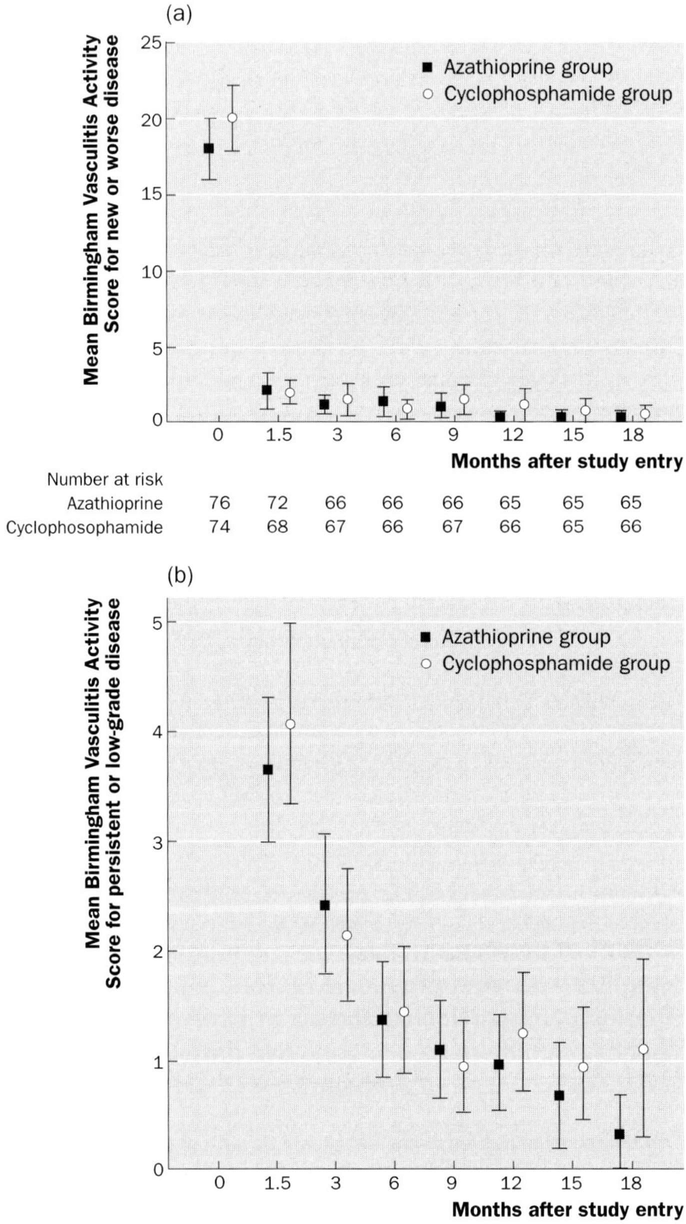

Fig. 9.3 Sequential Birmingham Vascular Activity Score for new or worse disease (a) and for persistent disease (b). Source: Jayne *et al.* (2003).

CNS involvement or cardiac involvement). The trial included fortnightly pulses for the first 2–3 weeks and thereafter every 4 weeks, and the end-point was relapse or death. The results showed that there was a significant difference of = 0.02 of event-free survival in the patients given more prolonged therapy with twelve cycles (hazard ratio 0.44), but there was no difference in mortality overall. This suggests that the quality of survival was enhanced by using twelve cycles of pulse therapy compared with six in this 1-year trial.

Comment

The paper by Jayne *et al.* supports the concept that it is safe to administer a short course of low-dose continuous oral cyclophosphamide and then substitute azathioprine without loss of efficacy in terms of disease control. Clearly it is possible that, in the long term, patients who are managed with azathioprine may have a higher rate of subsequent relapse and require further prolonged courses of cyclophosphamide. This may eliminate any benefit from azathioprine treatment, but this is probably the first study that has conclusively supported the use of a less aggressive treatment regimen in managing generalized systemic vasculitis. The protocols produced in the study are very suitable for the majority of patients presenting with systemic vasculitis, and this is an extremely important paper for rheumatologists and physicians caring for these patients. The French group compared the effectiveness of short courses of pulse therapy with intravenous cyclophosphamide with that of more prolonged courses, and have demonstrated the significant risk of undertreatment when only six pulses are used compared with twelve. However, long-term studies are required in this cohort because one group is being given twice the dose of cyclophosphamide, and this may have an effect in terms of long-term toxicity. The other important factor to bear in mind in this study is that no maintenance therapy was given after the end of the course of cyclophosphamide, and the study by Jayne *et al.* strongly supports the use of maintenance therapy, such as low-dose azathioprine, after induction of remission has been achieved. Nevertheless, it would be interesting to note whether the difference in relapse rates will be sustained between the two groups over a longer period of time, as previous studies have suggested that relapse tends to occur at a median of 3–4 years after the onset of disease |**2**|.

Anticytokine therapy in systemic vasculitis

The role of new agents in the management of vasculitis is being explored. The antitumour necrosis factor (TNF) therapies have a clear rationale in their application to vasculitic diseases, especially those with granulomatous involvement.

Effectiveness of TNF-alpha blockade with infliximab in refractory Wegener's granulomatosis

Lamprecht P, Voswinkel J, Lilienthal T, *et al. Rheumatology* 2002; **41**: 1303–7

BACKGROUND. Anti-TNF therapy has been tried in resistant Wegener's granulomatosis where all other remedies with conventional therapies, such as cyclophosphamide and steroid and additional intravenous gammaglobulin, have failed.

INTERPRETATION. Six patients were recruited to the study and were treated with between 3 and 5 mg/kg of infliximab per infusion every 2 weeks for the first two doses and then every 4 weeks until remission was obtained (using the BVAS as a measure of remission). Success was achieved in five out of the six cases. The higher dose of infliximab was more effective than the lower dose. Remission was maintained for up to 24 months in these patients.

Efficacy of the anti-TNF-alpha antibody infliximab against refractory systemic vasculitides: an open pilot study on 10 patients

Bartolucci P, Ramanoelina J, Cohen P, *et al. Rheumatology* 2002; **41**: 1126–32

BACKGROUND. Resistant systemic vasculitis patients were treated with anti-TNF therapy on the basis that TNF is a major agent in the pathogenesis of vasculitis.

INTERPRETATION. Out of ten patients with resistant disease, seven had Wegener's granulomatosis, two had rheumatoid-associated vasculitis and one had cryoglobulinaemia, with disease duration between 9 and 17 years prior to treatment. Patients were given 5 mg/kg infliximab at intervals of 8 weeks after the induction period and the treatment response was measured using the BVAS. There was complete or partial remission in all patients, with a reduction in mean BVAS from 9.1 at entry to 1.9 by day 42 and 1.3 by 6 months, which is a significant fall in disease activity. BVAS levels of zero were recorded in four patients, suggesting that complete remission had been achieved. Although the follow-up is short, the results are impressive.

Limited versus severe Wegener's granulomatosis: baseline data on patients in the Wegener's granulomatosis etanercept trial

Stone JH, Wegener's granulomatosis etanercept trial research group. *Arthritis Rheum* 2003; **48**: 2299–309

BACKGROUND. Etanercept as additional therapy for treatment of Wegener's granulomatosis was trialled in a randomized double-blind placebo-controlled trial of the

usual therapy for Wegener's with additional etanercept versus placebo. The full trial evaluation is ongoing; this paper presents the descriptive demographic pattern of these patients.

Interpretation. The 180 patients recruited into the trial were stratified according to whether they had severe disease (these patients tend to be younger at onset of disease compared with patients with severe disease) or limited disease. In patients with severe disease the majority were men (67%), whereas most of those with limited disease were women (58%). Patients with limited disease tended to have longer disease duration (as has been shown previously in other studies) and a higher risk of relapse following remission. There was also a tendency for more chronic grumbling, destructive upper respiratory lesions in patients with limited disease than in those with severe disease. The prevalence of ANCA related to proteinase-3 or myeloperoxidase was lower in patients with limited disease compared with those with severe disease. All of these findings suggest

Table 9.3 Baseline disease characteristics by disease severity*

Characteristic	**Limited (*n* = 52)**	**Severe (*n* = 128)**	**All paitnets (*n* = 180)**	***P*†**
Age at symptom onset, mean ± SD years	41 ± 16	50 ± 16	47 ± 16	0.005
Sex				0.002
Male, %	42.3	67.2	60.0	
Female, %	57.7	32.8	40.0	
Ethnicity				0.251
White, non-Hispanic, %	88.4	93.7	92.2	
African-American, non-Hispanic, %	1.9	1.6	1.7	
Hispanic, %	3.9	3.9	3.9	
Other, %	5.8	0.8	2.2	
Newly diagnosed at enrollment, %	32.7	49.2	44.4	0.043
Time since onset of symptoms, median (IQR) months	25.0 (7.7, 63.9)	14.2 (3.9, 46.7)	16.7 (5.0, 50.4)	0.057
Total patient-years, no.	199.1	368.4	567.5	
Time since diagnosis, median (IQR) months	13.3 (1.1, 44.0)	2.7 (0.7, 32.1)	4.7 (0.8, 35.8)	0.097
Total patient-years, no.	151.0	230.3	381.3	
BVAS/WG, mean ± SD	4.5 ± 2.1	7.9 ± 3.4	6.9 ± 3.4	<0.001
Physician's global assessment score, mean ± SD	4.2 ± 2.0	6.2 ± 2.2	5.6 ± 2.3	<0.001
Patient's global assessment score, mean ± SD	5.7 ± 2.7	6.7 ± 2.7	6.4 ± 2.7	0.011
VDI score, medan ± SD	1.5 ± 1.7	1.3 ± 1.7	1.3 ± 1.7	0.214

* IQR, interquartile range; BVAS/WG, Birmingham Vasculitis Activity Score for Wegener's granulomatosis; VDI, Vasculitis Damage Index.
† Determined by the chi-square test or Fisher's exact test for categorical data and Wilcoxon's rank sum test for continuous data.
Source: Stone, WGET Research Group (2003).

Table 9.4 Organ involvement at enrolment, as recorded on the BVAS/WG form, by disease severity*

	Limited (*n* = 52)	Severe (*n* = 128)	All patients (*n* = 180)	*P*†
General	76.9	70.3	72.2	0.370
Arthralgia/arthritis	69.2	64.8	66.1	
Fever	7.7	21.1	17.2	
Cutaneous	15.4	21.9	20.0	0.324
Purpura	13.5	18.8	17.2	
Ulcers	3.9	3.1	3.3	
Gangrene	0.0	0.8	0.6	
Mucous membranes/eyes	25.0	27.3	26.7	0.747
Mouth ulcers	7.7	11.7	10.6	
Conjunctivitis/episcleritis	13.5	14.8	14.4	
Retroorbital mass/proptosis	1.9	4.7	3.9	
Uveitis	0.0	0.0	0.0	
Scleritis	1.9	2.3	2.2	
Ear/nose/throat	88.5	71.9	76.7	0.017
Bloody nasal dischage/ nasal crusting/ulcer	67.3	56.3	59.4	
Sinus involvement	59.6	41.4	46.7	
Swollen salivary gland	1.9	3.1	2.8	
Subglottic inflammation	11.5	7.0	8.3	
Conductive deafness	25.0	22.7	23.3	
Sensorinoural deafness	1.9	3.1	2.8	
Cardiovascular	1.9	1.6	1.7	0.864
Pericarditis	0.0	0.8	0.6	
Gastrointestinal	1.9	2.3	1.7	0.862
Mesenteric ischaemia	0.0	0.8	0.6	
Pulmonary	51.9	63.3	60.0	0.159
Pleurisy	7.7	7.0	7.2	
Nodules or cavities	38.5	28.1	31.1	
Other infiltrates	23.1	32.0	29.4	
Endobronchial involvement	3.9	3.1	3.3	
Alveolar haemorrhage	0.0	25.0	17.8	
Respiratory failure	0.0	2.3	1.7	
Renal	28.9	64.1	53.9	<0.001
Haematuria	25.0	28.9	27.8	
Red blood cell casts	3.9	35.9	26.7	
Elevated serum creatinine	3.9	28.1	21.1	
Nervous system	0.0	12.5	8.9	0.017
Meningitis	0.0	0.0	0.0	
Cord lesion	0.0	0.0	0.0	
Stroke	0.0	0.0	0.0	
Cranial nerve palsy	0.0	2.3	1.7	
Sensory peripheral neuropathy	0.0	10.2	7.2	
Motor mononeuritis multiplex	0.0	2.3	1.7	
Other involvement	46.2	39.1	41.1	0.244

* Values are the percentage of patients. BVAS/WG, Birmingham Vasculitis Activity Score for Wegener's granulomatosis.
† Determined by chi-square test or Fisher's exact test for categorical data.
Source: Stone, WGET Research Group (2003).

Table 9.5 Features of major Wegener's granulomatosis cohorts*

Trial/period of collection	WGET/ June 2000–September 2002 (n = 180)	NIH/ 1966–1990 (n = 158)	Lübeck/ 1966–1993 (n = 155)
Mean age at diagnosis, years	47	41	48
Male/female, %	58/42	50/50	49/51
Women with limited disease, %	57.7	NI	NI
Women with severe disease, %	32.8	–	–
Mean follow-up, years	NA	8	7
Total patient-years, no.	381	1229	2144
cANCA positive, no.	73	88	84
Organ involvement ever, %			
Upper respiratory tract	90	92	99
Lung	75	85	66
Kidney	68	77	70
Eye	31	52	61
Heart	3.7	8	25
Skin	38.5	46	33
Gastrointestinal tract	6.8	0	6
Peripheral nerves	14	15	40
Central nervous system	5	8	11
Arthralgias/arthritis	81	67	77

* WGET, Wegener's Granulomatosis Etanercept Trial; cANCA, antineutrophil cytoplasmic antibody (cytoplasmic staining); NI, no information; NA, not applicable.
Source: Stone, WGET Research Group (2003).

that limited Wegener's granulomatosis may have different pathogenetic mechanisms, and therefore prognosis outcome and response to treatment, compared with severe disease, and that it may not be appropriate to manage limited disease in the same way as severe disease.

Comment

The first two small studies suggest that targeting anti-TNF therapy is going to be valuable in patients who have systemic vasculitis but clearly the problem needs to be measured on a much grander scale. The Wegener's Granulomatosis Etanercept Trial (WGET) research group is undertaking a large randomized controlled trial of etanercept versus placebo in patients with Wegener's granulomatosis, and has recently completed the recruitment of 180 patients, of whom approximately 45% represent new disease and 55% relapsing disease. Preliminary analysis suggests that there may be significant differences between the limited and severe Wegener's groups in terms of disease behaviour, and this may be reflected in the overall conclusions once the trial is completed. It is possible that etanercept may have a role in one or other of these disease categories. This highlights the importance of careful clinical characterization of patients in order to plan appropriate therapy.

Conclusion

Many aspects of systemic vasculitis are being actively researched at present. We now have valuable clinical tools for the careful assessment of disease activity and damage and these can be applied in prospective randomized trials of future therapies. Observation of the long-term outcome of such studies and the behaviour of the systemic vasculitides as a result of improvement in mortality is highlighting some of the difficulties that patients face now that they have chronic relapsing diseases over a long period of time. Careful observation of large cohorts of patients with systemic vasculitis will add to our understanding of these unusual but significant diseases.

References

1. Hoffman GS, Kerr GS, Leavitt RY, Hallahan CW, Lebovics RS, Travis WD, Rottem M, Fauci AS. Wegener's granulomatosis: an analysis of 158 patients. *Ann Intern Med* 1992; **116**: 488–98.
2. Gordon M, Luqmani RA, Adu D, Greaves I, Richards N, Michael J, Emery P, Howie AJ, Bacon PA. Relapses in patients with a systemic vasculitis. *Q J Med* 1993; **86**: 779–89.
3. Matteson EL, Gold KN, Bloch DA, Hunder GG. Long-term survival of patients with Wegener's granulomatosis from the American College of Rheumatology Wegener's granulomatosis classification criteria cohort. *Am J Med* 1996; **101**: 129–34.
4. Walton EW. Giant cell granuloma of the respiratory tract (Wegener's granulomatosis). *Br Med J* 1958; **2**: 265–70.
5. Luqmani RA, Bacon PA, Moots RJ, Janssen BA, Pall A, Emery P, Savage C, Adu D. Birmingham Vasculitis Activity Score (BVAS) in systemic necrotizing vasculitis. *Q J Med* 1994; **87**: 671–8.
6. Exley AR, Bacon PA, Luqmani RA, Kitas GD, Gordon C, Savage COS, Adu D. Development and initial validation of the Vasculitis Damage Index (VDI) for the standardized clinical assessment of damage in the systemic vasculitides. *Arthritis Rheum* 1997; **40**: 371–80.
7. Van der Woude FJ, Lobatto S, Permin H. Antibodies against neutrophils and monocytes: tools for diagnosis and marker of disease activity in Wegener's granulomatosis. *Lancet* 1985; **I**: 425–9.

8. Watts RA, Lane SE, Scott DG, Koldingsnes W, Nossent H, Gonzalez-Gay MA, Garcia-Porrua C, Bentham GA. Epidemiology of vasculitis in Europe. *Ann Rheum Dis* 2001; **60**: 1156–7.

9. Myers CM, Seeff LB, Staehman-Breen CO, Hoofnagle JH. Hepatitis-C and renal disease: an update. *Am J Kidney Dis* 2003; **42**: 631–57.

10. Gayraud M, Guillevin L, Le Toumelin P, Cohen P, Lhote F, Casassus P, Jarrouss EB, French Vasculitis Study Group. Long-term follow-up of polyarteritis nodosa, microscopic polyangiitis and Churg–Strauss syndrome; analysis of poor prospective trials including 278 patients. *Arthritis Rheum* 2001; **44**: 666–75.

Acknowledgements

I wish to thank Ms Joan Adams and the Arthritis Research Campaign for secretarial support.

10

Myositis

FREDERICK MILLER

Introduction

The myositis syndromes, also called the idiopathic inflammatory myopathies (IIM), are a heterogeneous group of acquired, systemic connective tissue diseases characterized by chronic muscle inflammation of unknown cause. The rarity and heterogeneity of the IIM has resulted in little progress being made in recent decades in understanding and treating polymyositis (PM), dermatomyositis (DM), inclusion body myositis (IBM) and related conditions, which together comprise the myositis syndromes. Nonetheless, recent developments (relating to increased interest in these diseases, new sources of private support group funding, advances in other areas that have been applied to myositis and increased international collaborations) have all resulted in a faster pace of discovery in this area. This chapter will focus on papers published over the last year, which have advanced our understanding of the diagnosis, possible pathogeneses and treatment of the myositis syndromes and have important implications for the practitioner in this area.

Diagnostic value of MHC class I staining in idiopathic inflammatory myopathies

van der Pas J, Hengstman GJ, ter Laak HJ, Borm GF, van Engelen BG. *J Neurol Neurosurg Psychiatry* 2004; **75**: 136–9

BACKGROUND. The pathological diagnosis of the IIM is often challenging as in many ways these are diagnoses of exclusion and a large number of infectious, metabolic, inherited, environmental, traumatic and other disorders can closely mimic them. The pathology of the IIM includes mononuclear cells surrounding myofibres and vessels, but their presence is often sparse and many biopsies are therefore non-diagnostic. Upregulation of major histocompatibility complex (MHC) class I is known to occur in IIM but not in normal muscle and it is unclear how many other disorders involve increased sarcolemmal class I expression.

INTERPRETATION. A large number (n = 224) of muscle biopsy specimens from subjects with many different myopathies were evaluated in a blinded prospective manner to assess the role of MHC class I staining (Fig 10.1) as an additional clue to the pathological diagnosis of IIM. The sensitivity of the test for diagnosing IIM was 78%

(95% confidence interval [CI] 66–88%), with a specificity of 95% (CI 91–98%) and this was not affected if the biopsy was done within 4 weeks of initiating immunosuppressive therapy. False-positive results were found in only seven subjects (4%), six of whom had a muscular dystrophy, suggesting that the detection of sarcolemmal MHC class I is a useful adjunct for distinguishing IIM from other neuromyopathies.

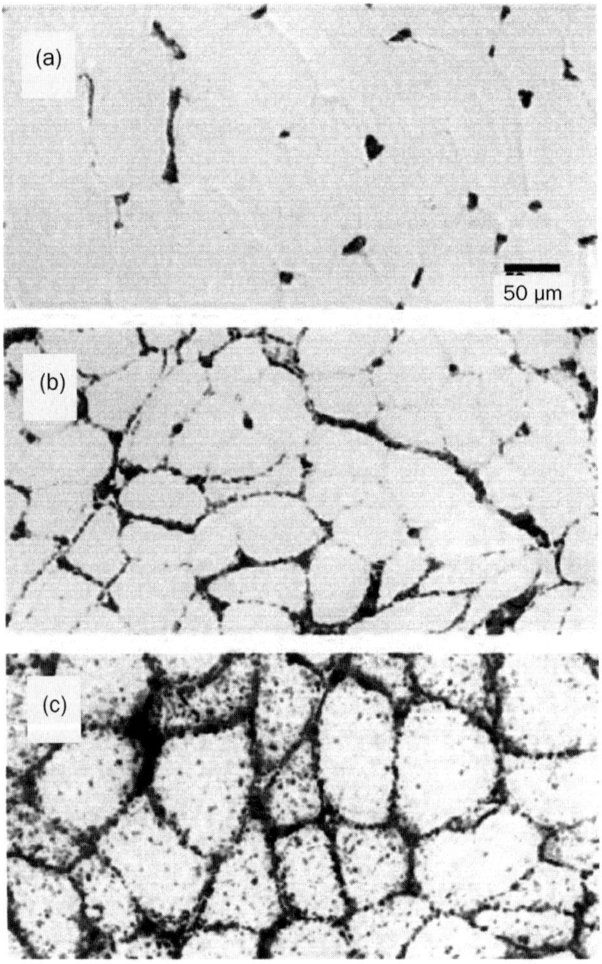

Fig. 10.1 Illustrations of sarcolemmal MHC class I expression in muscle biopsies. (a) Negative: only capillaries stain MHC class I positive. (b) Positive: both capillaries and sarcolemma are MHC class I positive but the capillaries can still be identified easily. (c) Positive: both capillaries and sarcolemma are MHC class I positive but capillaries can no longer be identified. Source: Van Der Pas *et al.* (2004).

Comment

Although the Bohan and Peter criteria (proximal weakness, elevated muscle enzymes, characteristic electromyographic and biopsy findings for PM, with Gottron's papules or heliotrope rashes for DM) remain the gold standard for the diagnosis of PM and DM, they have limitations. As a result, novel serological, radiographic, genetic and pathological methods are being increasingly used to sort out the many other myopathies and neuropathies that can be confused with the myositis syndromes. It has long been known that MHC class I expression is increased on the muscle surface in IIM, and a murine model of myositis has been developed by incorporating a transgenic construct that induced upregulation of class I in muscle. Nonetheless, it has not been clear how many other disorders involve upregulation of class I and if this test could be useful in a clinical setting. This large and careful study from The Netherlands suggests that class I staining is relatively specific for IIM (although it is present in some dystrophy cases) and can be used as an adjunct in confusing or otherwise non-diagnostic cases if the muscle biopsy is done before or soon after the initiation of immunosuppressive therapy.

Muscle-fiber conduction velocity and electromyography as diagnostic tools in patients with suspected inflammatory myopathy: a prospective study

Blijham PJ, Hengstman GJ, ter Laak HJ, van Engelen BG, Zwarts MJ.
Muscle Nerve 2004; **29**: 46–50

Background. As discussed above, diagnostic and classification criteria for the IIM are in need of reassessment and improvement. Electromyography (EMG) and nerve conduction velocity (NCV) studies are useful in the differential diagnosis of a number of neuromuscular disorders. They are especially helpful in distinguishing neuropathies from myopathies and, according to some experts, can help in distinguishing among the myopathies. Nevertheless, false-positive findings are not uncommon, in part due to the subjective nature of the assessment and high interobserver variability. The sensitivity of EMG for the diagnosis of IIM has been estimated to be 80–90%, although this may vary with the stage or severity of the disease and among different muscle groups. In the IIM, NCV are usually normal and the EMG shows a characteristic triad that includes: (i) short, small, low-amplitude polyphasic motor unit potentials; (ii) fibrillation potentials, even at rest; and (iii) bizarre high-frequency repetitive discharges. A new approach that has been suggested to be useful in assessing myopathies is the measurement of muscle-fibre conduction velocity (MFCV). MFCV is an analysis of the propagation velocity of an electrical stimulus along muscle fibres. As both muscle-fibre diameter and sarcolemmal excitability are altered in IIM and influence MFCV, it is reasonable to evaluate MFCV as a way of distinguishing the IIM from other mimics.

Interpretation. A prospective study of 25 patients with suspected IIM were evaluated by both standard EMG and MFCV in a single muscle, using a technique with direct muscle-fibre stimulation and recording (Fig. 10.2). These findings were correlated with other clinical parameters and needle muscle biopsy results. The diagnostic accuracy of combined MFCV and EMG studies was 72%, compared with 60% for EMG alone, as a result of improved specificity. Unfortunately, MFCV did not prove as useful in discriminating IIM from other myopathies, but MFCV findings did correlate with pathological changes in the muscle. These findings suggest that diagnostic accuracy of IIM can be increased if EMG examination is combined with MFCV studies.

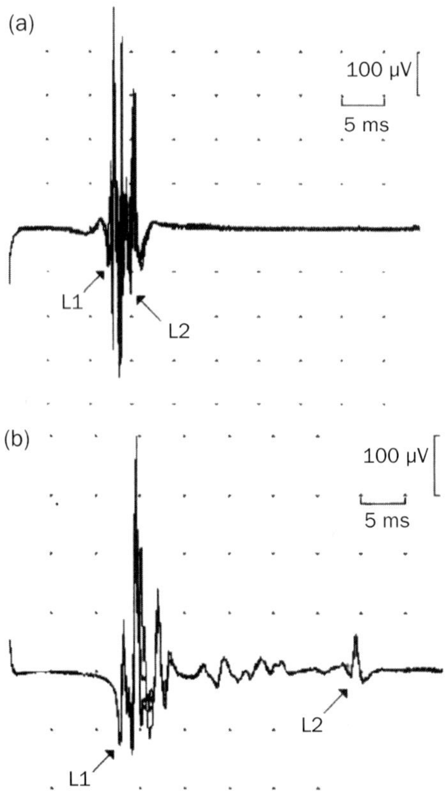

Fig. 10.2 Examples of muscle fibre conduction velocity (MFCV) recording. Five sequential recordings at 1 Hz stimulus interval, superimposed. Markers L1 and L2 indicate latencies of fastest and slowest fibres; distance of stimulus to recording electrode equals 50 mm. (a) Recording in a control subject. Multiple spikes are recorded. MFVC ranges from 4.3 m/s (L1) to 3.3 m/s (L2). (b) Recording in a myositis patient. Several slower spikes follow the normal complex of multiple spikes. MFVC ranges from 4.0 m/s (L1) to 1.5 m/s (L2). Source: Blijham *et al.* (2004).

Comment

Although these findings are preliminary, they add to a growing body of literature that implies that novel combinations of evaluations will enhance our capacity to assess and diagnose IIM and other related conditions. NCV and EMG have been some of the most invasive and painful procedures that myositis patients have been forced to endure. Limiting EMG and the novel MFCV assessments to a single muscle may decrease these undesirable features, and together they may enhance the specificity of the diagnosis. Large prospective studies of sequential patients with weakness or elevated muscle enzymes from a variety of clinics – collecting the same extensive and standardized clinical, laboratory, autoantibody, EMG, and pathological information – are needed to develop new more sensitive and specific criteria for the classification and diagnosis of the IIM.

Inclusion body myositis in connective tissue disorders: case report and review of the literature

Derk CT, Vivino FB, Kenyon L, Mandel S. *Clin Rheumatol* 2003; **22**(4–5): 324–8

Background. The inclusion body myopathies are a heterogeneous group of inflammatory and non-inflammatory myopathies that may occur in a familial or sporadic distribution. Controversy has existed as to whether the inflammatory forms, known as IBM, were considered immune-mediated or other forms of disease, given the relatively few autoantibodies noted in IBM and the poor response to immunosuppressives.

Interpretation. This publication, which is a case report and review of the other published cases of IBM in association with other immune-mediated diseases (mainly lupus, thrombocytopenia and undifferentiated connective tissue disease), suggests that a subset of IBM, as is the case for other IIM, have overlap syndromes. Furthermore, these overlap IBM subjects appear to have more autoantibodies and a better response to immunosuppressive therapy.

Comment

The diverse groups of diseases known as IBM is poorly characterized and few studies have been performed to assess their proper treatment. Early reports in the neurology literature have stated that IBM patients do not respond to treatment, but more recent studies, primarily in the rheumatology literature, imply that a subset may have partial responses to immunosuppressive therapy. Part of the difficulty in assessing these diseases is that of determining the relative contribution of disease activity (due to inflammatory processes that may respond to treatment) and disease damage (fibrotic changes that are almost always present in IBM and may not respond to treatment) in these subjects. A more accurate and standardized assessment of myositis using validated approaches, along with more controlled trials, will ultimately allow for the optimization of the management of IBM.

Magnetic resonance imaging criteria for distinguishing between inclusion body myositis and polymyositis

Dion E, Cherin P, Payan C, *et al. J Rheumatol* 2002; **29**(9): 1897–906

BACKGROUND. Because of its non-invasive nature and ability to evaluate large tissue volumes, magnetic resonance imaging (MRI) is being increasingly used in many areas of medicine. A number of studies over the last decade have shown that MRI is a useful adjunct for determining the degree and location of inflammatory changes in muscle and can help direct muscle biopsies in subjects with undiagnosed weakness and elevated muscle enzymes. Although anecdotes have commented on the different patterns of MRI abnormalities in different IIM subgroups, few studies have carefully defined these differences.

INTERPRETATION. Twenty-five PM and 25 IBM subjects were evaluated by quantitative and qualitative MRI methods in an attempt to define differences in thigh musculature which may be useful in distinguishing these entities. PM was found to significantly ($P \leq 0.05$) differ from IBM in having: (i) less fatty infiltration and atrophy; (ii) more inflammation as the sole abnormality; (iii) more fascial and fewer widespread MRI abnormalities; and (iv) less involvement of the anterior group, less asymmetrical distribution, and less distal predominance (Fig. 10.3). These findings suggest that MRI can help in distinguishing PM from IBM.

Comment

The recently identified entity known as IBM is the most common form of IIM in persons over 50 years of age and remains one of the most underdiagnosed and misdiagnosed subgroups of the myositis syndromes. Although there are many clinical clues that a person may have IBM—an elderly man with slowly progressive and insidious onset of proximal and distal muscle weakness, asymmetric weakness, anterior thigh muscle atrophy, low levels of muscle enzymes, few extramuscular manifestations, and few autoantibodies—the diagnosis rests mainly on the finding of characteristic purplish rimmed vacuoles (the inclusions) in myocytes after trichrome staining or tubulofilaments on electron microscopy. This important study adds clinically useful MRI findings to the list of features, which may distinguish IBM from PM.

Myopathy with antibodies to the signal recognition particle: clinical and pathological features

Miller T, Al-Lozi MT, Lopate G, Pestronk A. *J Neurol Neurosurg Psychiatry* 2002; **73**(4): 420–8

BACKGROUND. Another way of dividing the IIM into more understandable subsets, in addition to the clinical groups of PM, DM and IBM, is through the use of the specific immune responses in myositis patients. These are referred to as myositis-specific

(a)

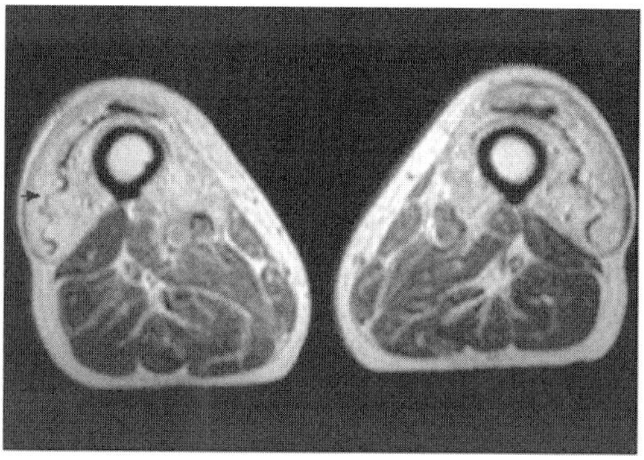

(b)

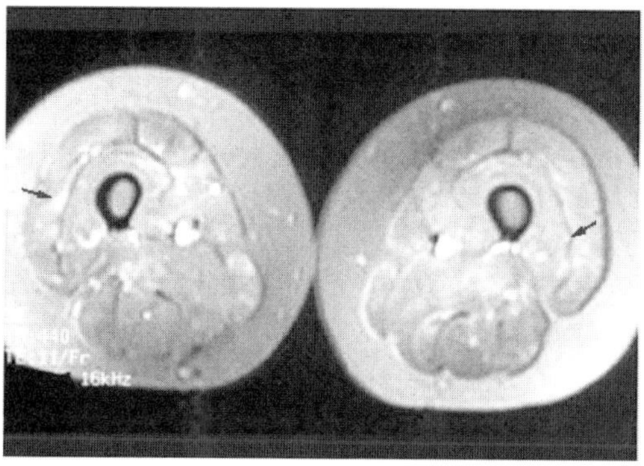

Fig. 10.3 (a) Axial SE T1 weighted image through mid-section of the two thighs in a patient with sIBM. Note diffuse fatty infiltration throughout the quadricepital muscles. The fascia between the vastus intermedius and the vastus lateralis appears as an undulating line (*arrow*). (b) Axial SE T1 weighted image after contrast injection with fat saturation (PM onset 11 months previously). Left: contrast uptake is visible in the quadricepital group (*arrowhead*), muscle volume is preserved and the fascia describes a curved line. Right: slight muscle volume loss is visible and the curve described by the fascia is somewhat irregular. Source: Dion *et al.* (2002).

autoantibodies and exist as three major entities: antisynthetase, anti-Mi-2 and antisignal recognition particle (anti-SRP) antibodies. They are useful because each autoantibody defines a unique group of myositis patients in terms of clinical characteristics, immunogenetics and responses to therapy. These three entities are thus known as the antisynthetase syndrome, the anti-Mi-2 syndrome and the anti-SRP syndrome, respectively. Little is known about the pathological features of each of these groups.

INTERPRETATION. This report confirms information suggested in previous studies and is one of the first careful evaluations of the pathology of the anti-SRP syndrome. This study found that seven patients with anti-SRP autoantibodies developed acute, severe weakness, without a DM rash, but accompanied by very high serum creatine kinase activities (3000–25 000 IU/l), a seasonal disease onset (August to January), and rapid development of disability. All these features of the anti-SRP syndrome had been described before. Novel findings, however, included the muscle pathology of these patients, which showed an active myopathy, with muscle fibre necrosis and regeneration with prominent endomysial fibrosis, hypercontracted muscle fibres with abnormal internal architecture, but little or no inflammation (Fig. 10.4). Of interest, endomysial capillaries were enlarged, reduced in number, and associated with deposits of the terminal components of complement (C5b-9, membrane attack complex). Some patients improved on immunosuppressive therapy.

Comment

Pathological studies of the IIM suggest that each of the major clinical groups, DM, PM and IBM, have both shared and unique features. All clinical groups share a number of non-specific muscle biopsy changes, including variation of myofibre size, muscle cell degeneration and regeneration, increased interstitial space, and fibrosis. In DM, the pathology is primarily a vasculopathy, characterized by vascular wall thickening, a reduction in capillary number, perifascicular atrophy and prominent

(a) (b) (c)

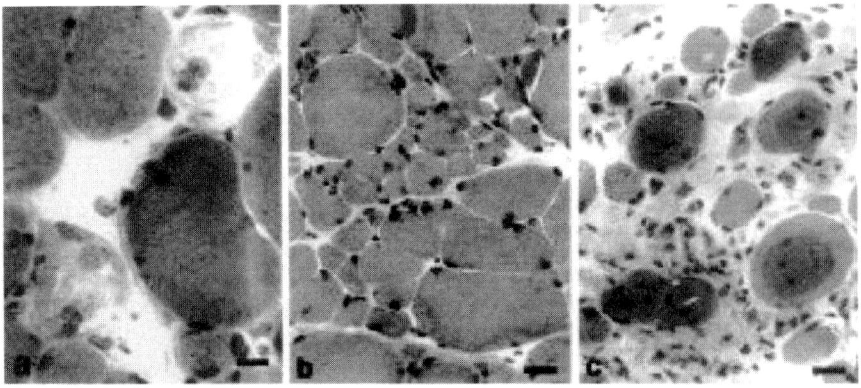

Fig. 10.4 Muscle pathology in patients with myopathy and anti-SRP (signal recognition particle) antibodies. Early changes: (a) Muscle fibre necrosis. Scattered, pale, fragmented muscle fibres, some of which contain cells with large nuclei (macrophages). Haematoxylin and eosin (H & E) stain, bar = 14 μm. (b) Bimodal distribution of fibre sizes. The largest fibres are mildly hypertrophied. There is no inflammation. H & E stain, bar = 18 μm. Late changes: (c) Endomysial connective tissue is increased. Hypercontracted muscle fibres with abnormal internal architecture are present. H & E stain, bar = 18 μm.
Source: Miller *et al.* (2002).

CD4+ T- and B-lymphocyte infiltration associated with vascular endomysial deposits of the terminal components of complement. PM and IBM both show CD8+ T-cell-mediated invasion and destruction of otherwise normal appearing myocytes. IBM is distinguished, however, by eosinophilic lined vacuoles (inclusion bodies) within myocytes and characteristic filaments on electron microscopy. This clinical and pathological study of the anti-SRP syndrome adds a distinctive pathology, combining selected histological aspects of PM and DM, to the other unique features previously described in association with this syndrome. It suggests that just as the IIM clinical groups may differ in pathology, so too may the serological groups. Further careful study of clinical, laboratory, genetic and pathological features of large numbers of IIM subjects, with and without these autoantibodies, are needed to devise more accurate diagnostic and classification criteria and to understand better the pathogenesis of these increasingly recognized syndromes.

Histidyl-tRNA synthetase and asparaginyl-tRNA synthetase, autoantigens in myositis, activate chemokine receptors on T lymphocytes and immature dendritic cells

Howard OM, Dong HF, Yang D, *et al. J Exp Med* 2002; **196**(6): 781–91

Background. The antisynthetase autoantibodies associated with myositis mentioned above are directed at six structurally different enzymes known as aminoacyl-transfer RNA (tRNA) synthetases. These enzymes are important in the cell's protein synthetic machinery and act to bind different amino acids to their cognate tRNAs. The most common of these is called the anti-Jo1 autoantibody and is directed against histidyl-tRNA synthetase. How and why these particular proteins are targeted specifically in myositis patients remains unknown. Both muscle-infiltrating lymphocytes and muscle cells in myositis patients express costimulatory markers and produce several proinflammatory cytokines. Therefore, chemoattractants may contribute to the development or progression of IIM by regulating the influx of inflammatory cells into muscle tissue.

Interpretation. The authors tested the ability of several targets of the antisynthetase autoantibodies (specific aminoacyl-tRNA synthetases) to induce leucocyte migration. They found that histidyl-tRNA synthetase, the target of anti-Jo1 autoantibodies, induced CD4+ and CD8+ lymphocytes, interleukin-2-activated monocytes, and immature dendritic cells to migrate. This activity seemed to be associated with the 48 amino acid NH_2-terminal domain. This enzyme also selectively activated CC chemokine receptor (CCR) 5-transfected cells and monoclonal anti-CCR5 blocked enzyme-induced chemotaxis. Another target of antisynthetase autoantibodies, asparaginyl-tRNA synthetase, also induced migration of lymphocytes, activated monocytes, immature dendritic cells, and CCR3-transfected cells, whereas non-autoantigenic aspartyl-tRNA and lysyl-tRNA synthetases were not chemotactic.

Comment

This is the first paper to show that autoantigenic aminoacyl-tRNA synthetases may perpetuate the development of myositis by recruiting mononuclear cells that induce immune responses. Although these findings do not explain what may have been the initial inducing agent of the myositis, they do propose a mechanism for the perpetuation of the inflammation once it has started. They also suggest a possible reason for why some of the aminoacyl-tRNA synthetases are targeted by autoantibodies and others are not. This may be because the selection of a self molecule as a target for an autoantibody response may be a consequence of the proinflammatory properties of the molecule itself. Understanding these processes could lead to better diagnoses and treatments for myositis in the future.

Global surface ultraviolet radiation intensity may modulate the clinical and immunologic expression of autoimmune muscle disease

Okada S, Weatherhead E, Targoff IN, Wesley R, Miller FW; International Myositis Collaborative Study Group. *Arthritis Rheum* 2003; **48**(8): 2285–93

BACKGROUND. The IIM, like most autoimmune conditions, likely result from chronic immune activation due to exposure to one or more environmental risk factors in genetically susceptible individuals. Although progress has been made in identifying the genetic risk factors for myositis, little understanding exists as to the environmental risk factors for these disorders. Anecdotal reports suggest that certain infections, drugs, vaccines, dietary supplements, collagen and silicone implants, silica, and exposure to ultraviolet radiation (UVR) may play a part in the induction and/or subsequent flares of individual cases of myositis.

INTERPRETATION. This international group of myositis experts used the natural variation of genetic and environmental features around the world to explore possible causes for IIM in the first global study of the ethnogeography of myositis. In a world-wide study of 919 consecutive patients from populations at 15 global locations, they found significant differences in the frequency of DM and PM in different referral populations. The proportion of DM patients seen in Guatemala City (83%), for example, was more than threefold that in Glasgow (27%). To understand these differences, univariate and multivariate analyses were performed and demonstrated that of the 13 geoclimatic variables evaluated, surface UVR intensity (irradiance) most strongly contributed to the relative proportion of DM and was strongly related to the proportion of the DM-associated anti-Mi-2 autoantibodies (weighted $r = 0.939$, $P < 4 \times 10^{-7}$ and weighted $r = 0.69$, $P = 0.02$, respectively) (Fig. 10.5). Immunogenetic allele frequencies imply that the striking differences in the proportion of DM- and the proportion of DM-specific autoantibodies observed around the world are not the result of inherent global variations in known genetic risk factors.

Comment

This worldwide study of myositis is not only the first investigation suggesting that myositis varies in different parts of the world in clinical and autoantibody features, but it is also the first to show that UVR may be the explanation for these differences. The implication is that one can predict the relative proportion of DM and PM, as well

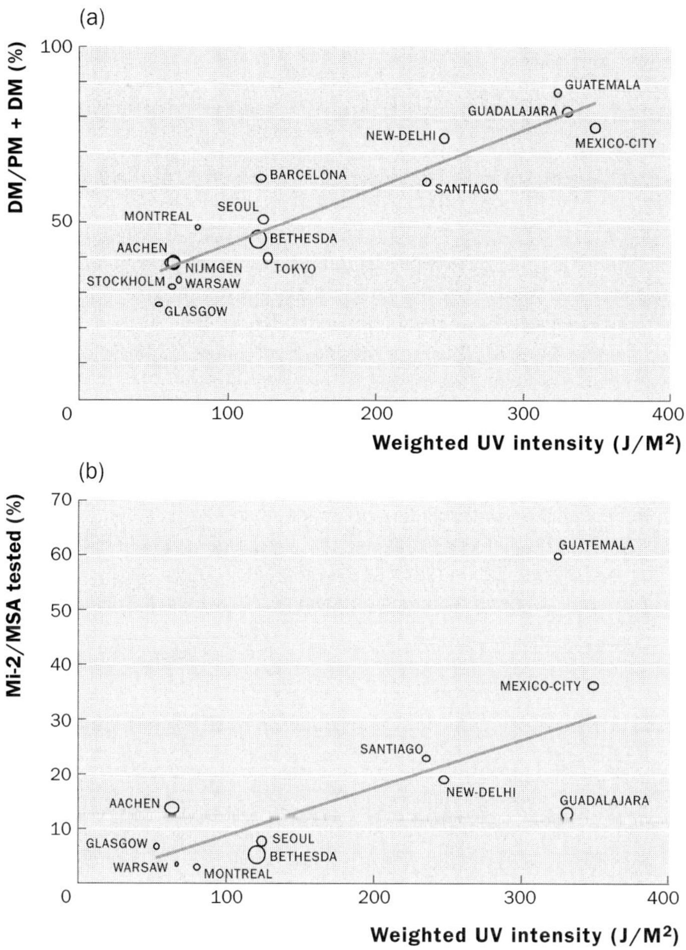

Fig. 10.5 Correlations among the weighted surface UV intensity (irradiance, J/m^2) at each of the global locations, and the proportion of dermatomyositis (DM) patients (a) weighted $r = 0.93$; $P = 7 \times 10^{-7}$) and those with anti-Mi-2 authoantibodies (b) weighted $r = 0.69$; $P = 0.02$) at each centre. The size of the circle representing each site is proprotional to the number of patients evaluated at that location. Source: Okada *et al.* (2003).

as anti-Mi-2 autoantibodies, in any part of the world if one simply knows the UVR levels as measured by satellite data. It remains unclear if UVR induces DM in those who otherwise may not have developed myositis or converts PM cases to DM. Nevertheless, the associations of UVR with DM and a disease-specific autoimmune response directed against an Snf2 family helicase (anti-Mi-2 autoantibodies) have implications for preventative strategies as well as for new avenues of research into the pathogenesis and treatment of inflammatory muscle disease.

Pregnancy outcome in adult-onset idiopathic inflammatory myopathy

Silva CA, Sultan SM, Isenberg DA. *Rheumatology (Oxford)* 2003; **42**(10): 1168–72

Background. The role of pregnancy in many rheumatic diseases remains poorly studied and the data that have been collected on this topic are sometimes contradictory. While pregnancy has been associated with disease improvement in rheumatoid arthritis, disease flares in lupus and with poor outcomes in diffuse scleroderma, little is known about the role of pregnancy in myositis.

Interpretation. This case series and review of the published literature resulted in 33 evaluable patients with 43 pregnancies. Of these, 49% had myositis before becoming pregnant, 35% developed disease during pregnancy, and 16% developed myositis postpartum. Overall, there was little evidence that pregnancy increased the disease activity of PM or DM, yet it may be that pregnancy and the postpartum period are risk factors for the development of myositis. In terms of the pregnancy outcomes, it appeared that the more active the myositis during pregnancy, the greater the chance of fetal loss.

Comment

This study adds useful, albeit preliminary, information to the literature to assist clinicians caring for women with myositis who are invariably asked about how a pregnancy might affect the myositis and how myositis might affect a pregnancy. The suggestion that pregnancy and the postpartum period may be risk factors for the development of myositis is interesting in light of evidence of fetal-to-maternal cell trafficking resulting in higher levels of microchimerism in some connective tissue diseases, especially scleroderma. All pregnancies in myositis patients should be considered high risk and careful and frequent evaluations by appropriate specialists should be undertaken as soon as the woman knows she is pregnant. Pregnancies should be discouraged during periods of increased myositis disease activity. If the myositis is inactive, however, it appears unlikely that either a pregnancy will increase disease activity or that the diagnosis of myositis alone will have a negative impact on the fetus.

Successful treatment of dermatomyositis and polymyositis with anti-tumor-necrosis-factor-alpha: preliminary observations

Hengstman GJ, van den Hoogen FH, Barrera P, *et al. Eur Neurol* 2003; **50**: 10–15

BACKGROUND. Standard approaches to the therapy of myositis include use of corticosteroids, methotrexate, azathioprine, intravenous immunoglobulin, cyclosporin A or cyclophosphamide. In a number of myositis patients, however, these treatments cannot be tolerated or do not result in adequate control of disease activity. Little information is available to address how such patients should be managed. Tumour necrosis factor α (TNF-α) has been found to be increased in expression in the muscles of myositis patients and may play a part in the pathogenesis of IIM.

INTERPRETATION. This publication is a case series of a PM patient and a DM patient successfully treated at disease onset with a chimeric anti-TNF-α monoclonal antibody called infliximab. This treatment was given as a slow intravenous infusion at 10 mg/kg body weight three times, with each dose separated by 2 weeks. Significant clinical and laboratory responses were seen in these two carefully studied patients. These included: decreased pain and feelings of malaise; decreased rash in the DM patient; improved muscle strength that ranged from 33 to 62%; decreased muscle enzyme levels; normalization of electromyographic abnormalities; and decreased infiltrates and necrotic fibres on muscle biopsy. No adverse events were noted.

Comment

These carefully documented cases add to the growing literature suggesting that anti-TNF-α therapies may be useful in the management of IIM. Although much remains to be learned about the advantages and disadvantages of the use of the multiple forms of anti-TNF-α treatments now approved by the FDA and under study, promising case reports and case series have induced the initiation of phase 1–2 clinical trials in myositis patients and results from these studies should be available soon. Many more treatment options are needed to optimize the therapy of IIM.

International consensus outcome measures for patients with idiopathic inflammatory myopathies. Development and initial validation of myositis activity and damage indices in patients with adult onset disease

Isenberg DA, Allen E, Farewell V, *et al. Rheumatology (Oxford)* 2004; **43**: 49–54

BACKGROUND. The treatment of IIM is unsatisfactory, and no agents are currently FDA approved for these diseases. The rarity of IIM has led to a paucity of controlled prospective clinical trials as most publications involve single referral centres reporting

retrospectively on small numbers of patients followed for relatively brief periods of time. Furthermore, the accurate assessment of the effects of therapeutic interventions in IIM patients has been hampered by unreliable and insensitive outcome measures, as well as the challenge of distinguishing active and reversible disease from irreversible damage to muscle. A multispecialty group called the International Myositis Assessment and Clinical Studies Group (IMACS) has been formed to develop such consensus and lay the foundation for large international, multicentred studies. Their accomplishments to date include: development of consensus on core outcome measures and a standardized definition of improvement for all forms of IIM. This paper outlines another IMACS effort relating to the development of novel validated tools to assess comprehensively disease activity and damage.

Interpretation. Through a series of Delphi approaches and nominal group techniques, members of IMACS specializing in adult-onset and paediatric-onset disease achieved consensus on new approaches to evaluate myositis in all age groups. IMACS proposes that myositis disease activity be measured by two tools known as the MITAX (the myositis intention-to-treat index) and MYOACT (the myositis disease activity assessment visual analogue scales). IMACS suggests that the extent and severity of damage developing in different organ systems be assessed by the MDI (the myositis damage index). The systems included in these assessments include constitutional, articular, cardiac, pulmonary, gastrointestinal, cutaneous and skeletal muscle systems. This paper focuses on the results of studies of these tools as applied to adult-onset disease. A series of real patient exercises confirmed that all these tools have good face validity and are comprehensive. The measures' reliability, measured by intraclass correlation coefficients among physicians, and the inter-rater reliability, as assessed by variation in the physicians' ratings of patients, is fair to good for most aspects of the tools.

Comment

The lack of consensus on the conduct and reporting of IIM clinical trials have hampered advances in the treatment of myositis. A long overdue international consensus effort by IMACS has been successful in overcoming a number of prior obstacles relating to the study of myositis. These have included: (i) difficulties in evaluating adequate numbers of subjects at a single institute due to the rarity of these orphan diseases; (ii) greatly different perspectives on myositis by neurologists, rheumatologists, dermatologists and other specialists due to different training and referral biases; and (iii) different biases in paediatric and adult specialists pertaining to juvenile-onset and adult-onset disease. These tools, which are now undergoing further validity testing, should enhance the consistency, comprehensiveness, and reliability of disease activity and damage assessment in patients with myositis.

Conclusion

This report on published findings in the last year that I believe will ultimately have important impacts on how clinicians diagnose, understand and manage myositis is a compilation of diagnostic, pathological, immunological, molecular, therapeutic and epidemiological studies. The IIM do not easily surrender their secrets. That the myositis syndromes are orphan diseases, which generate little interest in and support from governmental, private or pharmaceutical organizations, has greatly inhibited research advances in this field. Further complicating our understanding of myositis is the fact that many different specialists—ranging from rheumatologists to neurologists to dermatologists to others, each with varied training, experiential biases and referral patterns—care for and attempt to study these diseases with little interaction, collaboration or communication. An additional problem is that physicians of all these specialties with adult and paediatric training and expertise care for the adult- and juvenile-onset cases separately and often do not have common meetings or other venues for exchanges of information.

The themes of the papers discussed this year revolve around better understanding of just what the myositis syndromes are: what defines them, how they can be better diagnosed, what are the boundaries between them and other disorders, what causes them and how they can be better assessed and managed.

Our understanding of the IIM today is in many ways similar to that of the other autoimmune diseases. We currently identify all such disorders merely as collections of signs, symptoms and laboratory abnormalities, realizing still that within these indistinct and imperfect borders, great heterogeneity exists yet awaits new insights, technologies and understanding before we can begin to sort these syndromes into more understandable core groups, or what have been referred to as 'elemental disorders'. An elemental disorder in this context is a unique collection of signs, symptoms and laboratory features that results from a distinct pathogenesis after the interaction of the necessary and sufficient genetic and environmental risk factors. While some of the genetic risk factors for myositis and other autoimmune diseases are beginning to be understood, little is known about the environmental risk factors and even less about the gene–environment interactions which are probably the key to a full understanding of the development of these diseases.

Diagnosis, classification and the very definitions of the myositis syndromes are all in need of complete reassessment, and yet few outside the myositis community appreciate how fundamental these problems are, and thus are generally not interested in supporting research in this area. By not having a common definition for these diseases we will end up studying 'apples and oranges' and will not be able to compare results from studies in different fields. Ultimately, deciphering the pathogenetic mechanisms will allow for the true definition of these disorders, but in order to attain this level of understanding, an empiric consensus needs to be achieved as to how they can be best defined and classified today. Fortunately, recent international, multispecialty consortia, organized and initiated by IMACS, have overcome some of these obstacles and have begun to develop and promulgate consensus criteria, new validated tools for assessing disease activity and damage, common definitions of clinical improvement and disease flare and other guidelines for standardizing the conduct and reporting of clinical trials in the IIM. These developments, in addition to increased resources from patient support groups, promise hope that the pace of discovery will quicken and better treatments will soon be available to the tens of thousands who suffer from these diseases.

Part IV

Osteoarthritis

11

Osteoarthritis

ADRIAN JONES

Introduction

Although the commonest condition to affect synovial joints, there remain many unanswered questions regarding the aetiology and epidemiology of osteoarthritis (OA). The best options for management of the symptomatic patient are also not fully established.

As regards aetiology one of the problems in studying OA is in establishing temporal relationships between aetiological factors and the subsequent development of OA. This is because detection of early OA in asymptomatic patients is difficult. The definition of OA remains problematic in spite of many attempts over the last decade to develop generally agreed definitions at all the major joint sites. Genetic influences on the development of OA are more amenable to study as genetic factors are at least stable but several issues remain. The situation is complicated though as it is unlikely that genes involved in OA risk show high degrees of penetrance and there are likely to be complex gene–environment interactions.

As regards the treatment of OA there is still a great deal of uncertainty regarding optimal medical management. Attempts remain ongoing to address this and include both publication of new randomized controlled trials on existing and novel therapies as well as synthesis of current available evidence in the form of structured reviews and meta-analyses.

As always there are far more publications than can be reviewed in an article such as this so I have concentrated on those that I feel have clinical application and that I personally find most interesting.

Aetiology and epidemiology of osteoarthritis

Although many studies have examined the aetiology of OA, most of these have been cross-sectional taking as cases subjects with definite radiographic and/or clinical OA and using community based or other currently non-affected controls. It has been suggested that the risk factors for the incidence of OA are different to the factors that affect progression. The validity of this statement has been difficult to assess as it is unclear whether incidence of radiographic OA is in fact being observed rather than progression of subclinical change.

Development of radiographic changes of osteoarthritis in the 'Chingford knee' reflects progression of disease or non-standardised positioning of the joint rather than incident disease

Mazzuca SA, Brandt KD, German NC, Buckwalter KA, Lane KA, Katz BP.
Ann Rheum Dis 2003; **62**: 1061–5

BACKGROUND. For some years it has been possible to study the progression of OA by examining serial radiographs of subjects. Using this approach some of the factors, such as weight and certain non-steroidal anti-inflammatory drugs (NSAIDs) that can influence radiographic progression of OA have been proposed. In studying factors affecting incidence, the problem has been in identifying cohorts of patients who have no OA, establishing factors that might be associated with incidence and then detecting the onset of OA. As OA is a long-term condition the time and cost constraints of establishing prospective cohorts can be prohibitive. One approach has been to study patients with apparent unilateral OA and study the incidence of OA in the contralateral side [1]. The supposition is that the other joint is at high risk of developing OA within a reasonable time period; incidence of disease in this joint is thus amenable to study and possibly intervention. The concern about this approach has been the suspicion that this does not really represent true incidence but progression of subclinical disease.

INTERPRETATION. One hundred and eighty obese women aged 45–64 years with apparent unilateral knee OA as judged by an anteroposterior radiograph of the tibiofemoral joint were studied. Knee OA was defined using the American College of Rheumatology criteria [2]. The other knee was deemed normal. Additional radiographic views were taken, which included semi-flexed fluoroscopically assisted views and lateral and tangential patellofemoral views. The principal findings were that OA was 'discovered' in 52% of the tibiofemoral joints of the contralateral 'normal' knees. In addition patellofemoral OA was detected in 67% of the contralateral knees. In all only 18% of the normal contralateral knees were truly free of OA using the extended series of radiographs.

Comment

Study of OA incidence requires detection of the true incidence of disease. Previous studies looking at incidence have in general tried to examine development over a relatively short period of say 2 years. The concern has always been that, given what is known about the pathophysiology of OA, this is too short a period and that at the point of recruitment to the study early OA is already present. These findings do, I feel, confirm these suspicions as well as confirming that, in general, OA is a symmetrical disease. It also suggests that studying incidence will require study over much longer time periods and comprehensive imaging of all parts of the joint. The authors do rightly discuss the fact that the 'Chingford knee' still represents an opportunity to examine the impact of early intervention on disease progression.

Weight from birth to 53 years. A longitudinal study of the influence on clinical hand osteoarthritis

Sayer AA, Poole J, Cox V, Kuh D, Hardy R, Wadsworth M, Cooper C. *Arthritis Rheum* 2003; **48**: 1030–3

BACKGROUND. Obesity has been widely regarded as a major risk factor for OA at a number of sites but whether this is simply a mechanical problem (i.e. related to stress on a joint) or is part of a generalized metabolic problem is unclear. One of the problems is that many studies examining this are, by necessity, cross-sectional or at the very least short term. The Framingham Study has examined the effect of weight change in a prospective manner and has demonstrated that subjects that lose weight reduce their risk of the progression of OA [3]. With increasing interest in the effect of early life events on subsequent health and the studies of cohorts established at birth there is an opportunity to examine the effect on OA on apparently non-weight bearing joints such as those of the hands. In this situation it has been speculated that metabolic factors are more important and indeed some of these such as impaired glucose tolerance may also be associated with low birth weight.

INTERPRETATION. This study examined a subset of subjects from the Medical Research Council's National Survey of Health and Development [**4**]. This was a birth cohort established in 1946 and the subjects studied in this paper comprise a living subset of this population who underwent a standardized hand examination to look for features of OA; radiographs were not obtained. Altogether 280 of 1467 men and 458 of 1519 women studied had OA in at least one hand joint. The data were analysed using current weight and birth weight in the model. Height and social class were explored as confounding factors. In men but not women there was association between lower birth weight and higher current birth weight with the presence of hand OA. In particular weight gain in men was associated the development of hand OA (Fig. 11.1). One putative mechanism is that an increased body mass index (BMI) is associated with generalized increased muscle power. However, when grip strength was examined cross-sectionally there was no evidence that the association seen in this study was mediated by increased muscle strength, although it cannot be ruled out that hand OA had not reduced a previously present increased muscle strength.

Comments

Although it may not be possible to alter birth weight significantly it may be possible to influence weight gain throughout life. The increasing prevalence of obesity in the general population gives cause for concern in terms of the future burden of OA. Mechanistically this study adds support to the notion that metabolic or possibly genetic factors are important in the pathogenesis of OA as well as suggesting that it is important to address weight gain during life as one measure to reduce the personal and population burden of OA.

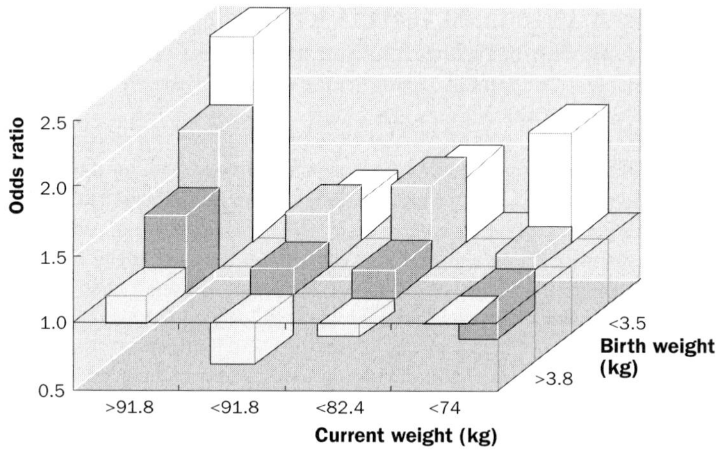

Fig. 11.1 Odds ratio for developing OA in at least one hand joint stratified by current weight and birth weight. Source: Sayer *et al.* (2003).

Osteoarthritis of the knee is associated with vertebral and nonvertebral fractures in the elderly: the Rotterdam study

Bergink AP, van der Klift M, Hofman A, *et al. Arthritis Rheum* 2003; **49**: 648–57

BACKGROUND. For a long time it has been suspected that osteoporosis and OA may be inversely associated, although the relationship is likely to be complex. Most studies suggest that patients with OA may have increased bone mineral density compared with controls. This is not simply related to spinal OA producing spurious bone density measurements. It is also speculated, however, that subchondral bone demonstrates a degree of relative osteopenia. While this is interesting mechanistically what is not clear is whether these findings have clinical relevance in terms of an impact on fracture risk.

INTERPRETATION. The Rotterdam study is a community based cohort study of men and women aged >55 years |**5**|. A sample of 2773 subjects with knee radiographs and no evidence of vertebral fracture were selected as the non-fracture group. A further 1466 patients with known thoracolumbar fractures were selected as the vertebral fracture group. The incidence of non-vertebral fractures was assessed from patient records in a standardized fashion. The non-vertebral fracture group were older (mean age 69.0 years ± SD 7.9) compared with the vertebral fracture group (mean 66.4 years ± SD 6.7). Radiographic OA was defined using the Kellgren and Lawrence grading system, which in this case essentially meant the presence of definite osteophyte in the tibiofemoral joint |**6**|. Even after adjusting for potential confounding factors such as

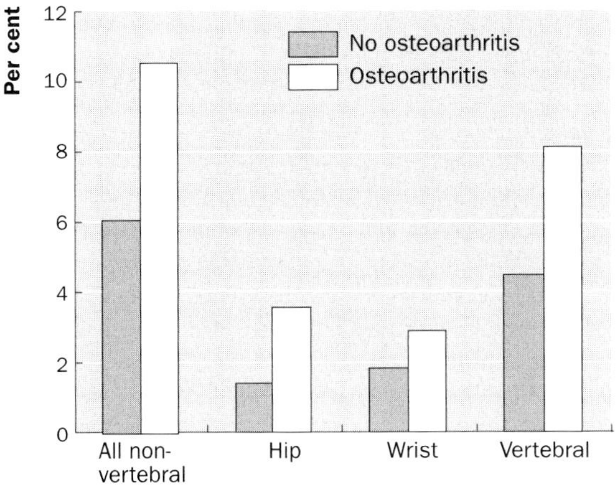

Fig. 11.2 Percentage of patients with fracture depending on the radiographic presence or absence of knee OA. Source: Bergink *et al.* (2003).

age, gender, postural stability, height and weight there was a significant association of fracture with radiographic knee OA (Fig. 11.2). This was true for a number of fracture sites and the association was still apparent after stratifying for bone mineral density.

Comment

Although OA has been fairly convincingly associated with increased bone mineral density the association with fracture has been difficult to establish. This study does, in spite of a low incidence of fracture, demonstrate a link between OA and fracture. In as much as it is possible to adjust for the confounding risks such as bone mineral density and falling (as judged by markers of postural stability) this seems to be an additional independent risk factor. The clinical importance of this will be that attempts to reduce fracture burden in the community could consider subjects with knee OA as a potential target population for targeted strategies such as screening for osteoporosis and adopting preventative strategies.

Physical functioning over three years in knee osteoarthritis

Sharma L, Cahue S, Song J, Hayes K, Pai Y-C, Dunlop D. *Arthritis Rheum* 2003; **48**: 3359–70

Background. Although progression of radiographs is of mechanistic interest, clearly what matters most for the individual with OA is the development of physical impairment.

It is difficult to know how best to approach this. Does one take an inception cohort, studying individuals who present with symptoms in which protopathic bias may exist or a completely asymptomatic prospective cohort in whom the risk of protopathic bias is reduced but for whom the duration of study may be prohibitively expensive? Furthermore, which of these situations is most likely to be applicable clinically?

Interpretation. This prospective study (part of the Mechanical Factors in Arthritis of the Knee study) took volunteer community subjects with symptomatic knee OA and followed them prospectively for 3 years with structured assessments at baseline, 18 months and 3 years. The objective for this study was to assess those factors that predict change in physical function over a 3-year period as assessed by a subscale of the WOMAC (Western Ontario and McMaster Universities Osteoarthritis Index) instrument |**7**|. Factors assessed at baseline included joint laxity, muscle strength, joint alignment, proprioception, BMI, radiographic severity, physical activity, age, knee pain severity, psychological status and self-efficacy. All were assessed using validated instruments; 257 of 285 subjects completed the study of whom 21 underwent total knee replacement and were not included in the analysis. Good outcome was defined by a matrix; a good outcome was when a subject remained in a high functional quintile or improved from baseline; poor outcome was when the subject remained in a poor function group or deteriorated. In univariate analysis a poor functional outcome (WOMAC) at 3 years was statistically associated with the following baseline characteristics: increased BMI, knee pain, valgus/varus joint laxity; decreased mental health score (SF-36), self-efficacy, social support, weekly aerobic exercise. In a multivariate analysis correcting for age, radiographic disease severity and knee pain intensity these relationships remained. Similar results were seen for a functional test (sit-to-stand repetitions) with increased age and decreased muscle strength, proprioception, emotional functioning, self-efficacy and aerobic exercise statistically associated with poorer outcome.

Comment

This study identifies a number of factors at presentation of patients with symptomatic knee OA that might be amenable to intervention in order to improve functional outcome at 3 years. While many of these factors such as BMI, muscle strength, etc. are difficult to address, a large number of studies have demonstrated that both targeted high-intensity programmes and more recently broader low-intensity, high volume community based approaches can successfully do this. Perhaps the most important finding in this study is that self-efficacy is an important factor, particularly as it probably correlates with success in many of the other strategies addressing for example aerobic exercise, muscle strength, BMI and proprioception. Long-term benefits in OA should strongly target improved patient perceived self-efficacy and empowerment.

Treatment of osteoarthritis

Periarticular lesions detected on magnetic resonance imaging

Hill CL, Gale DR, Chaisson CE, *et al. Arthritis Rheum* 2003; **48**: 2836–44

BACKGROUND. The source of pain in OA is still unclear. A treatment study has shown that periarticular injections can relieve some of the symptoms of OA [8]. It is thus possible that periarticular, rather than articular structures are the source of much of the pain in OA. This study attempts to examine this hypothesis by utilizing magnetic resonance imaging (MRI) scanning in a systematic fashion to examine for the presence of periarticular lesions in subjects with or without OA.

INTERPRETATION. Subjects aged >45 years (men) and >50 years (women) were recruited from Veteran Affairs medical centres and from the community. Subjects were asked about knee pain and patients with forms of arthritis other than OA were excluded. Knee pain was defined by asking a simple question about the presence of knee pain in the prior 4 weeks. A subset of patients had the presence of clinical OA confirmed as well as the absence of clinically obvious periarticular sources of pain. All subjects had standardized radiographs of the tibiofemoral and patellofemoral joints as well as an MRI of one, usually the most symptomatic, knee. Clinical examination used a grid to subdivide the knees into specific anatomical areas. Tenderness and pain in these areas were documented by standardized examination. The subjects were divided into three groups. The results are tabulated (Table 11.1). Radiographic OA was associated with fluid in the prepatellar and superficial infrapatellar bursae but interestingly this was not associated with pain. Deep infrapatellar fluid was present in all three groups and was only thought to be symptomatic in three patients, all with knee pain. Other periarticular lesions were common generally in those with pain and on further analysis particularly those with radiographic OA.

Comment

This study has demonstrated that periarticular lesions are common and as such clinical detection of them may be important as it may allow targeted local therapy. There are some caveats to this study. Selection of subjects was not random and the number of asymptomatic subjects relatively small. Furthermore, many of the MRI lesions could not be correlated with local tenderness and symptoms and thus the significance of the observed lesions is hard to interpret. However, in terms of clinical practice this study does mean that we should not just see X-rays in a patient with knee pain and advise blanket treatment—a search for periarticular sources of pain is justified.

Table 11.1 Demographics of study patients and the presence of various periarticular lesions

	Group 1	**Group 2**	**Group 3**
Definitions	KP + OA	No KP + OA	No KP + no OA
n	376	51	24
Male	254	29	17
Mean age	67	66	64
Median tibiofemoral K & L grade (range)	2 (0–4)	0 (0–2)	0 (0–1)
Non-articular lesions (%)			
Prepatellar bursa	3	8	0
Superficial infrapatellar bursa	11	18	0
Deep infrapatellar bursa	52	53	63
Semimembranosus bursa	4	2	0
Anserine bursa	4	3	0
Iliotibial band syndrome	5	0	0
Tibiofibular cyst	4	0	0
Popliteal cyst	33	28	9

KP, knee pain; OA, radiographic osteoarthritis; K & L, Kellgren and Lawrence |**6**|.
Source: Hill *et al.* (2003).

Safety and efficacy of long-term intraarticular steroid injections in osteoarthritis of the knee

Raynauld J-P, Buckland-Wright C, Ward R, *et al. Arthritis Rheum* 2003; **48**: 370–7

BACKGROUND. Intra-articular corticosteroids are widely used in the treatment of OA with proven short-term benefits; probably with a duration of benefit of less than 6 weeks. Concerns have, however, been expressed about possible adverse effects, particularly on OA progression. As a result the recommendation is often made that injections should be used infrequently, e.g. at the knee no more than three to four times per year. In contrast in animal models and *in vitro* potentially beneficial effects of corticosteroids on the OA process have been observed.

INTERPRETATION. This was a double-blind trial involving 68 patients randomized to receive either 3 monthly injections of either triamcinolone acetonide 40 mg or an equivalent volume of saline. Progression of OA was measured using an established radiographic technique to measure joint space loss. Clinical efficacy was assessed using the WOMAC scale |**7**|. Joint space reduction (progression) was compared at 1 year and 2 years using a previously published standardized, digitalized technique |**9**|. Patients were aged 40–80 years and had failed to respond to previous treatment with non-steroidal anti-inflammatory drugs or acetaminophen (paracetamol). Patients had moderate radiographic tibiofemoral OA and were symptomatic. Patients receiving intra-articular steroids went from a mean minimal median joint space of 4.07 mm (SEM 1.01) to 4.02 mm (SEM 1.2) over a 2-year period. Saline-treated knees went from 3.93 mm (0.91) to 3.86 mm (1.2). The difference between the groups was non-significant. There was no significant difference between the groups with regard to clinical and functional outcome. One patient in each group withdrew early on due to lack of efficacy in the saline group and a post-injection flare in the steroid group.

Comment

This paper is reassuring to clinicians who use corticosteroid injections in the management of knee OA and suggests that apart from the known risks of the injection producing a flare or introducing infection we are probably not going to hasten deterioration of the osteoarthritic process at least at the knee. The main implication of this result may not be for the treatment of OA in which corticosteroids are used on an infrequent basis but in inflammatory disease where intra-articular steroid therapy is used more frequently.

Corticosteroid compared with hyaluronic acid injections for the treatment of osteoarthritis of the knee

Leopold SS, Redd BR, Warme WJ, Wehrle PA, Pettis PD, Shott S. *J Bone Jt Surg* 2003; **85A**: 1197–203

Background. Various hyaluronic acids are available for the treatment of osteoarthritis, particularly of the knee. Although efficacy has been suggested by several randomized controlled trials the size of the benefit has commonly been perceived to be relatively low and this is for a product that is relatively expensive both in terms of drug cost and physician time. Multiple injections are also required. There remains debate therefore as to how to position the drug in the treatment of OA particularly in comparison with intra-articular corticosteroids.

Interpretation. One hundred patients were randomized to receive either three injections at weekly intervals of hylan G-F 20 (Synvisc) or a single injection of corticosteroid + local anaesthetic (2 ml betamethasone sodium phosphate/betamethasone acetate + 4 ml bupivicaine + 4 ml lignocaine), with further injections allowable if required. The study had a blinded observer but of course the subjects were not blinded. Although both groups improved from baseline for most of the outcome measures (including pain scores and WOMAC indices) there was no significant difference between the groups. For example in the hyaluronic acid group the median visual analogue pain score went from 70 mm to 52 mm over the 6-month study period compared with a change from 64 mm to 52 mm over the same time period for the corticosteroid-treated group. It should be noted that almost half of the corticosteroid-treated group requested a second injection. This still meant, however, that they only received two injections over the 6-month period rather than three.

Comment

This study adds to knowledge of the relevant benefits of hyaluronic acids and corticosteroids. As with a number of other studies it suggests that the symptomatic benefit of hyaluronic acids is not much greater than that of corticosteroids. It should be noted that this was not simply a comparison of corticosteroid and hyaluronans. The patients were not blinded to the treatment and it is not clear whether the use of multiple injections in the hyaluronan-treated group compared with the corticosteroid-treated group may have affected the outcome. Furthermore, a significant volume of local anaesthetic was used in the corticosteroid treatment and indeed the total volume injected was 10 ml of fluid rather than 2 ml. Again this may have impacted on the results. The overall conclusion from the study is that with no demonstrable benefit for hyaluronan over corticosteroid + local anaesthetic the relative cost of the two preparations and the requirement for multiple injections in the hyaluronan-treated group will be a major factor mitigating against widespread use for symptom relief.

A one-year, randomised, placebo (saline) controlled clinical trial of 500–730 kDa sodium hyaluronate (Hyalgan) on the radiological change in osteoarthritis of the knee

Jubb RW, Piva S, Beinat L, Dacre J, Gishen P. *Int J Clin Pract* 2003; **57**: 467–74

BACKGROUND. If recent studies and meta-analyses suggest that the symptomatic benefits of hyaluronic acids are relatively mild and may be subject to publication bias [10] there have been suggestions that an additional rationale for their use might be their putative disease modification effects. The primary aim of this study was to investigate whether repeated injections of a particular hyaluronan (molecular weight 500–730 kDa, Hyalgan) would result in reduced progression of knee OA as measured by rate of reduction in the medial tibiofemoral joint space of the knee.

INTERPRETATION. Five hundred and thirty-four patients with primary knee OA were screened and 408 patients enrolled in a multicentre randomized, double-blind parallel group trial. The comparator was an equivalent volume of normal saline. The American College of Rheumatology radiographic criteria were used to define knee OA [**2**]; patients with inflammatory joint disease and significant involvement of other joints were excluded. The injection protocol was weekly injections for 3 weeks with repeat course every 4 months (a total of three courses of three injections. Standardized weight bearing tibiofemoral films were analysed digitally and the mean joint space width measured. Eighty-nine patients withdrew from the study and this was similar in both groups; however, only 268 patients had analysable radiographs. Overall the placebo group had a longer duration of symptoms and a trend towards more marked joint space narrowing (4.5 mm [SD 1.6] compared with 4.9 mm [SD 1.5]). Overall there was no significant difference in rate of joint space narrowing between the groups. A subgroup analysis suggested that in the patients with mild joint space loss at recruitment (joint space width ≥4.6 mm) less joint space loss was observed in the hyaluronic acid-treated group. Furthermore, although statistical differences in other outcome measures, e.g. pain on walking, was observed between the two groups, overall the differences were small and not likely to be of great clinical significance.

Comment

This study is intriguing in suggesting a possible disease-modifying role of hyaluronic acids. It should not, however, lead to a wholesale adoption of their use at present. This is because the radiographic technique employed may be subject to an effect of pain on measured joint space width, i.e. modification of pain may result in an apparent increase of joint space width |**11**|. Although this is contested and indeed little symptom difference between the groups was observed in this study it remains a possible confounder. In addition, a simple standing view may not be as effective as a standardized semiflexed view in detecting and assessing tibiofemoral joint space. Although there are major problems with this paper, it is potentially one more step in demonstrating true disease modification in human OA.

Structural and symptomatic efficacy of glucosamine and chondroitin in knee osteoarthritis: a comprehensive meta-analysis

Richy F, Bruyere O, Ethgen O, Cucherat M, Henrotin Y, Reginster J-Y. *Arch Intern Med* 2003; **163**: 1514–22

Background. Although a steady stream of generally positive results has been published regarding glucosamine sulphate and chondroitin sulphate in the management of OA there seems to be a general reluctance by clinicians to take these agents on board in the management of OA. Indeed it has been suggested that double standards of evidence may be being applied |12|. This is particularly interesting in light of a number of studies that suggest that these agents may have structure (disease) modifying properties in OA.

Interpretation. This meta-analysis was performed to synthesize current evidence regarding the efficacy of these two agents for symptom relief and possible disease modification in OA. Using a structured search strategy 15 double-blind, randomized controlled studies of at least 4 weeks' duration and in which analysable outcome measures could be obtained were identified. These comprised 1020 patients treated with glucosamine and 755 with chondroitin sulphate. Both agents produced statistically significant reductions in symptoms compared with placebo with an overall effect size for pain measured on a visual analogue scale of 0.49 (95% confidence interval [CI] 0.31–0.67). Overall, the number needed to treat to produce a clinically significant response (defined in each of the studies themselves) was 4.9. Similar statistically significant effects were seen for Lesquesne index and all components of the WOMAC scales. In terms of an effect of joint space reduction glucosamine sulphate had a statistically significant beneficial effect (effect size 0.41 (95% CI 0.21–0.6). No similar analysis was made for chondroitin sulphate due to the lack of high-quality studies (in general the quality of the studies involving chondroitin sulphate was less than those involving glucosamine sulphate). Examination for publication bias using a funnel plot did suggest that this may have occurred but only to a small degree.

Comment

This meta-analysis confirms earlier reviews suggesting that glucosamine sulphate and chondroitin sulphate have symptomatic benefit in OA. This benefit was apparent after 2 weeks. In addition, glucosamine sulphate may reduce the rate of progression of joint space narrowing. The criticism can again be raised that apparent increases in joint space narrowing may arise because of a reduction in joint pain |**11**|. Nevertheless the evidence is steadily accumulating in favour of these drugs and it is perhaps interesting to speculate why they are not given more prominence by the professional community |**12**|. Clearly in much of the world they are only available as health food products and concerns have been raised as to quality control issues. In view of their apparent safety perhaps we should be more seriously concerned in promoting their use. The results of a large US multicentre trial are awaited with some anticipation.

EULAR recommendations 2003: an evidence based approach to the management of knee osteoarthritis: report of a task force of the standing committee for international clinical studies including therapeutic trials (ESCISIT)

Jordan KM, Arden NK, Doherty M, *et al.* *Ann Rheum Dis* 2003; **62**: 1145–55

Background. Although many papers are continually published regarding the results of clinical trials, systematic reviews and meta-analyses, it can be difficult for a busy clinician to synthesize the evidence and place it in a clinically relevant context. Properly conducted and updated systematic reviews and guidelines can certainly help in this context. In addition, gaps in knowledge can be more readily identified, which can act as a spur to further studies.

Interpretation. This ongoing study uses a systematic search strategy to identify new evidence regarding treatment modalities and questions for OA. Expert opinion is also used to attempt to identify gaps in knowledge about clinically important questions. Subsequent evidence and advice arising from this process is graded according to both the strength of the evidence and expert opinion. In addition, expert opinion was used to assess the 'toxicity' of each treatment. Effect sizes for treatments are calculated where possible. The evidence from this assessment are tabulated (Table 11.2).

Comment

This study is an update of previous guidelines and has tried to take as far as possible an evidence-based approach to their production. This is an important attempt to synthesize the evidence. Some of the final recommendations do, however, move away from the evidence and their strength does appear to have been overwhelmed by expert opinion. A good example of this is acetaminophen where the evidence for benefit is graded at 1B and yet is given a grade A strength of recommendation, presumably because of the offsetting belief that the drug is safe. In addition, as can be seen from some of the other papers presented here, another problem with a committee approach is that it can be overtaken by more recent papers. Nevertheless, this paper is a good basis from which to develop local clinically relevant guidelines.

Table 11.2 Evidence arising from the ESCISIT task force and produced as the EULAR recommendations 2003 for the management of knee OA

Category	Evidence from	Treatments	Effect size
1A	Meta-analysis of RCT	Conventional NSAID	0.47, 0.96
		Topical NSAID	–0.05, 1.03
		Topical capsaicin	0.41, 0.56
		Glucosamine	0.43, 1.02
		Chondroitin	1.23, 1.50
		Education	0.28, 0.35
1B	At least one RCT	Acetaminophen	
		Opioid analgesic	
		Coxibs	0.5
		Antidepressant	
		Diacerein	
		ASU	0.32, 1.72
		Nutrients	0.65
		Herbal remedies	0.23, 1.32
		Minerals/vitamins	
		Exercise	0.57, 1.0
		Telephone	1.09
		Acupuncture	0.25, 1.74
		Laser therapy	0.87
		Pulsed EMF	
		Spa therapy	1.0
		TENS	0.76
		Ultrasound	
		Weight loss	
		Insoles	
		Orthotics	
		Hyaluronic acids	0.0, 0.9
		Corticosteroids	1.27
		Lavage/tidal irrigation	0.84
		Arthroscopy/debridement	
2A	RCT without randomization		
2B	Quasi-experimental study	Sex hormones	
3	Descriptive studies	Osteotomy	
		Unicompartmental knee replacement	
		Total knee replacement	
4	Expert opinion		

RCT, randomized controlled trial(s).
Source: Jordan *et al.* (2003).

Conclusion

Our understanding of the aetiology of OA is still hampered by an incomplete understanding of the time course of the disease. A number of papers published in 2003 have attempted to further this understanding and not only lay important methodological foundations for doing so but have also highlighted areas where intervention may result in a reduced burden of disease.

Treatment progress is still slow and publication bias makes discernment of the true value of a number of treatments difficult. Improved reporting of trials and increased standardization of methodology is certainly improving this. Increased use of systematic reviews and meta-analyses are allowing the clinician to make sense of the ever-burgeoning amounts of information but still must be approached with some caveats. We are also now seeing increased evidence of disease-modifying effects of drugs on the osteoarthritic process—an exciting development that bodes well for the future.

References

1. Spector TD, Hart DJ, Doyle DV. Incidence and progression of osteoarthritis in women with unilateral knee disease in the general population. *Ann Rheum Dis* 1994; **53**: 565–8.
2. Altman R, Asch E, Bloch D, Bole G, Borenstein D, Brandt K, Christy W, Cooke TD, Greenwald R, Hochberg M, Howell D, Kaplan D, Koopman W, Longley S, Mankin H, McShane DJ, Medsger T, Meenen R, Mikklesen W, Moskowitz R, Murphy W, Rothschild B, Segal M, Sokoloff L, Wolfe F. Development of criteria for the classification and reporting of osteoarthritis: classification of osteoarthritis of the knee. *Arthritis Rheum* 1986; **29**: 1039–49.
3. Felson DT, Ahange Y, Anthony JM, Naimark A, Anderson JJ. Weight loss reduces the risk for symptomatic knee osteoarthritis in women. *Ann Intern Med* 1992; **116**: 535–9.
4. Wadsworth ME, Kuh DJ. Childhood influences on adult health: a review of recent work from the British 1946 national birth cohort study, the MRC National Survey of Health and Development. *Paediatr Perinat Epidemiol* 1997; **11**: 2–20.
5. Hofman A, Grobbee DE, de Jong PT, van der Ouweland FA. Determinants of disease and disability in the elderly: the Rotterdam Elderly Study. *Eur J Epidemiol* 1991; **7**: 403–22.
6. Kellgren JH, Ball J. *Atlas of Standard Radiographs of Arthritis.* Vol. 2. *The Epidemiology of Chronic Rheumatism.* Oxford: Blackwell Scientific publications, 1963.
7. Bellamy N, Buchanan WW, Goldsmith CH, Campbell J, Stitt L. Validation study of WOMAC: a health status instrument for measuring clinically important patient-relevant outcomes following total hip or knee arthroplasty in osteoarthritis. *J Orthop Rheum* 1988; **1**: 95–108.

8. Sambrook PN, Champion GD, Browne CD, Cairns D, Cohen ML, Day RO, Graham S, Handel M, Jaworski R, Kempler S, Wacher T. Corticosteroid injection for osteoarthritis of the knee: peripatellar compared with intra-articular route. *Clin Exp Rheumatol* 1989; **7**: 609–13.
9. Buckland-Wright C. Protocols for precise radio-anatomical positioning of the tibiofemoral and patellofemoral compartments of the knee. *Osteoarthritis Cartilage* 1995; **3**: 71–80.
10. Lo GH, LaValley M, McAlindon T, Felson DT. Intra-articular hyaluronic acid in treatment of knee osteoarthritis. A meta-analysis. *JAMA* 2003; **290**: 3115–21.
11. Mazzuca SA, Brandt KD, Lane KA, Katz BP. Knee pain reduces joint space width in conventional standing anteroposterior radiographs of osteoarthritic knees. *Arthritis Rheum* 2002; **46**: 1223–7.
12. Towheed TE. Current status of glucosamine therapy in osteoarthritis. *Arthritis Rheum* 2003; **49**: 601–4.

Part V

Osteoporosis

12

Osteoporosis: assessment, diagnosis and management

HILARY CAPELL, ELAINE MORRISON, WILLIAM FRASER

Introduction

Osteoporosis is a systemic disease that results in an increased risk of fractures due to a reduction in bone mass and quality. The WHO definition of osteoporosis is based on a measurement of bone mineral density (BMD) measured at the lumbar spine, femoral neck or both, with a T-score >2.5 standard deviations (SD) below that of a normal young adult. Using this criterion, it is estimated that 30% of postmenopausal women and 8% of the male population over 50 years old can be classified as having osteoporosis |**1**|. The Z-score reflects the number of SDs by which a patient's BMD differs from that of an individual of the same age (see Table 12.1).

There are significant limitations to this definition of osteoporosis and it has become obvious that while BMD is a major contributor to risk, other factors, including age, body mass index (BMI), falls, bone quality, the rate at which bone is being resorbed by osteoclasts and formed by osteoblasts, play an important part in determining whether a patient will suffer a fracture. The presence of a fragility or minimal trauma fracture (fracture occurring after a fall from a chair or standing) and low bone density (T-score ≤2.5) is classified as severe osteoporosis.

Table 12.1 World Health Organization definitions

Normal	Where an individual has a BMD value between –1SD and +1SD of the young adult mean (T-score –1 to +1)
Osteopenia	Where an individual has a BMD reduced between –1 and –2.5 SDs from the young adult mean (T-score –1 to –2.5)
Osteoporosis	Where an individual has a BMD reduced by equal to or more than –2.5 SDs from the young adult mean (T-score –2.5 or lower)

Source: World Health Organization |**2**|.

Who needs treatment? Assessment of fracture risk to define intervention thresholds

A recent change in the definition of osteoporosis has recognized the need to account for bone quality, rate of bone turnover as well as bone mass (bone strength) when predicting fracture incidence |**3**|. While it is possible to measure bone mass using a number of techniques there is considerable debate regarding the best way to assess bone quality. There has, therefore, been a move to define an absolute fracture risk through assessment of multiple risk factors for each patient that would help to target treatment and optimize management for those who would achieve greatest benefit from therapeutic intervention. Such an approach starts to make a distinction between diagnostic (BMD based) and intervention thresholds.

A new approach to the development of assessment guidelines for osteoporosis

Kanis JA, Black D, Cooper C, *et al.* on behalf of the International Osteoporosis Foundation and the National Osteoporosis Foundation, USA. *Osteoporos Int* 2002; **13**: 527–36

BACKGROUND. The management of osteoporosis has revolved around the use of BMD measurement and application of the WHO criteria. This approach infers that all individuals identified with low BMD are at higher risk of fracture and that those with BMD higher than the diagnostic threshold are at significantly lower risk. It has become clear in recent years that other risk factors provide information on fracture risk over and above that of BMD alone and that intervention thresholds modulated according to risk (absolute risk) would be a better way of deciding who benefits most from treatment. The factors that could contribute to the absolute fracture risk, or more exactly 'long-term probability' of fracture were discussed. Age and secular trends in mortality, choice of fracture end-points, ethnic and geographical variability, gender, prior fracture, BMI, bone turnover, concomitant disease and associated treatments were all highlighted as being important. Any guideline based on risk factor assessment needs to take into account the fact that fracture type and the causative factors vary with age.

INTERPRETATION. The majority of physicians involved in the management of osteoporosis have challenged the simplistic idea that all treatment decisions can be made on the basis of only BMD measurements. While BMD measurement will remain the diagnostic tool, management decisions need to take multiple factors into account.

Comment

This paper is a synthesis of the approach adopted in practice and attempts to refine the possible means to establish guidelines based on absolute risk estimates for fracture. Although no final answer and guideline has been provided, the authors have defined the challenges that exist and thrown down the gauntlet to establish new models of risk prediction and their subsequent independent validation.

The use of risk factors in predicting requirement for treatment

The risk of fracture increases after a previous fracture independently of BMD. Those with a vertebral fracture have a 20% risk of another fracture within 1 year |**4**|. Identifying those individuals most at risk of developing osteoporosis is vital and many articles and textbooks give exhaustive lists of risk factors that are known be important in the pathogenesis of low bone density |**5**|. and therefore associated with osteoporosis and related fractures.

Modifiable risk factors in the prevention of osteoporosis

These include smoking, alcohol consumption, a diet deficient in calcium and vitamin D, lack of exercise (current and past) and low weight (i.e. BMI <19).

Non-modifiable risk factors

These include age, gender, ethnic origin, early menopause and family history of osteoporosis. It is often difficult to decide which of these factors are important in an individual and the strength of the association that exists between the outcome and the risk factor. Recent attempts have utilized large population datasets to define the most important risk factors predicting fractures.

Determinants of incident vertebral fracture in men and women: results from the European Prospective Osteoporosis Study (EPOS)

Roy DK, O'Neill TW, Finn JD, *et al. Osteoporos Int* 2003; **14**: 19–26

BACKGROUND. BMD measurements are widely used to estimate the risk of osteoporotic fractures. In addition, many other risk factors have been identified, some of which are believed to add to the risk independently of BMD measurements. The value of all previously proposed risk factors is a matter for debate. Analysis of data from the European Prospective Osteoporosis Study (EPOS) looking at men and women aged between 50 and 79 years has concluded that none of the life-style factors that they included, such as smoking, alcohol intake, physical activity and milk consumption, demonstrated any consistent associations with incident vertebral fracture. Increasing body weight and BMI were associated with reduced risk of vertebral fracture. Increased age at menarche was associated with increased risk of incident fractures and use of hormone replacement therapy (HRT) protected against fracture.

INTERPRETATION. Modification of life-style factors included in this study would be unlikely to have a major impact on the population occurrence of vertebral fractures.

Relative contributions of bone density, bone turnover, and clinical risk factors to long-term fracture prediction

Melton LJ III, Crowson CS, O'Fallon WM, Wahner HW, Riggs BL. *J Bone Miner Res* 2003; **18**: 312–18

BACKGROUND. This is a prospective study of 225 postmenopausal women from Rochester, Minnesota, USA. These women had baseline data collected in 1980 and have been followed for 3146 person-years. Life-style factors and co-morbidity variables were included in over 100 comparisons and after adjustment for age only a few were associated with fracture risk and some of these could have arisen by chance. Femoral neck BMD predicted osteoporotic fractures. Low dietary protein intake was the only independent life-style predictor of osteoporotic fracture. 'Free oestradiol index' was an independent predictor of both short- and long-term fracture risk with high sex hormone binding globulin and low free oestradiol index associated with increased vertebral, proximal femur, distal forearm and all other osteoporotic fractures.

INTERPRETATION. Femoral neck BMD was the best predictor of overall osteoporotic fracture risk and was as good a predictor after 10 years as was shown in the early years of the study, although the relative hazard was modest (1.37 per SD decrease).

Comment

Both these studies question the relative importance of life-style factors such as smoking, drinking, exercise in the prediction of fractures and the management of osteoporosis. The measurement of femoral neck BMD is less prone to effects from artefacts than other measurements, such as vertebral BMD, and shows good long-term predictive value.

Corticosteroid therapy

Corticosteroids are used to treat a wide variety of medical conditions and their use has been associated with the development of osteoporosis. Particular attention needs to be concentrated on individuals who require corticosteroid therapy for more than 3 months. However, guidelines for the prevention and treatment of osteoporosis in all patients receiving this therapy have been produced |**6**|. Such guidelines are needed as a recent study has shown.

Oral corticosteroid prescribing in women over 50, use of fracture prevention therapy and bone densitometry service

Chantler IW, Davie MWJ, Evans SF, Rees JS. *Ann Rheum Dis* 2003; **62**: 350–2

BACKGROUND. The authors scrutinized general practitioner records from 41 practices and identified 62 230 women aged 50 or more. They assessed incidence of fractures,

duration of corticosteroid use, dose in the study year, the use of fracture prevention therapy and bone densitometry measurements. Overall 3.2% were prescribed corticosteroids and of the group 633 were investigated in detail. The average age was 70 years with a median of 2 years of corticosteroid therapy. Reasons for corticosteroid include asthma/lung disease, rheumatoid arthritis and polymyalgia rheumatica. Between the ages of 70 and 79 years patients with rheumatoid arthritis had significantly more hip fractures than the other groups and corticosteroid prescribing was most common in this group. Bisphosphonates or HRT were used in 48% of the group aged 50–59 but only 32% of the 70–79-year-old age group. Twenty per cent of the entire group had been referred for bone densitometry and 60% had been shown to be osteoporotic. The authors concluded that while the elderly had most prescriptions for corticosteroid treatment, they were least likely to be given effective fracture prevention therapy.

Comment

It is also noteworthy that patients with rheumatoid arthritis sustained more hip fractures than other groups but were the least likely to have effective fracture prevention therapy prescribed.

Falls prevention

Falls prevention is also of considerable importance in reducing the incidence of fragility fractures and will be addressed later.

The importance of prevention and treatment

Osteoporosis is associated with increased mortality and excess mortality is described in patients who develop osteoporotic fractures particularly of the spine and hip [7]. Most deaths occur in the first 3–6 months following a fracture but mortality remains higher than the general population thereafter. Prevention and treatment of osteoporosis and related fractures needs to be justified to those in charge of health budgets in terms of cost-effectiveness and it is important to establish the exact proportion of deaths due to osteoporosis and fracture.

The components of excess mortality after hip fracture

Kanis JA, Oden A, Johnell O, De Laet C, Jonsson B, Oglesby AK. *Bone* 2003; **32**: 468–73

BACKGROUND. The burden of osteoporosis on society relates to the number of fractures and associated morbidity and mortality. Changes in population demographics are resulting in increasing numbers of elderly subjects throughout the world. Predictions on the number of osteoporotic fractures may have become inaccurate so it is important

for resource management to know the outcome of fractures in order to estimate the true benefits of treatment. A total of 158 589 hip fractures were studied in Swedish men and women over 50 years old. It was calculated that, depending on age, causally related deaths (directly or indirectly related to the hip fracture) comprised 17–32% of deaths associated with hip fracture and accounted for more than 1.5% of all deaths in this population. Interestingly, the risk of death was greater for men than women.

Interpretation. This large database permitted robust comparisons to be made between the population mortality statistics and hip fracture-related deaths. The number of deaths due to hip fracture was substantial and greater than those due to stomach or pancreatic cancer. This raises the possibility that treatment for osteoporosis may improve the survival of a high-risk population.

Comment

Interventions designed to decrease fracture should increase survival. However, as the authors point out 2.2 million subjects would need to be included in a clinical trial to prove an effect of treatment assuming a 50% reduction in hip fracture with treatment. Excess mortality is associated with both hip fracture and vertebral fracture but this may be secondary to other medical conditions and general health, so a detailed evaluation of patients at presentation is essential to rule out secondary causes of osteoporosis |**8**|. This evaluation requires radiological, biochemical and haematological investigation of the patient prior to initiation of any therapy. Exclusion of secondary causes of osteoporosis is an essential step in the process of managing any patient with osteoporosis and in the prevention of fractures.

Efficacy of treatment

A number of therapeutic agents are now available for the treatment of osteoporosis. The recent vogue for the practice of evidence-based medicine dictates that systematic reviews using rigorous methods should be employed to present unbiased comprehensive summaries of the available data to help provide the most precise estimates of treatment effects.

Meta-analyses of therapies for postmenopausal osteoporosis

Cranney A, Tugwell P, Wells G, Guyatt G; Osteoporosis Methodology Group and the Osteoporosis Research Advisory Group. *Endocr Rev* 2002; **23**: 496–578

Background. A series of articles were produced that represented a systematic review of the available osteoporosis therapies. State of the art methodologies were employed to provide a clear and accurate characterization of the effectiveness of the

therapies. The meta-analyses have shown that vitamin D (in combination with calcium), calcitonin, raloxifene and the bisphosphonates etidronate, risedronate and alendronate all significantly reduce vertebral fractures. This conclusion was made on the basis of the methodology, quality, magnitude of effect, confidence intervals (CIs) and consistency of study results. A large number of studies were analysed for each intervention and reported in the individual meta-analyses including calcium, vitamin D, calcitonin, raloxifene, HRT, etidronate, risedronate and alendronate. HRT in the meta-analysis did not have a significant effect on vertebral fractures because the pooled estimate from the randomized trials had a wide CI. Only risedronate and alendronate were shown to have convincing evidence for non-vertebral fracture reduction. Minimal data were available for all other treatments and comparators, with the CI overlapping the effect when performing a comparison of the studies. Some treatments may be more effective in subpopulations of patients and the magnitude of effect will be greater in those patients. The evidence for an effect of calcium plus vitamin D in patients who are vitamin D deficient, which can result in secondary hyperparathyroidism, is much stronger than the effect in the overall elderly population. Non-vertebral fracture is significantly reduced in patients who are institutionalized when treated with appropriate doses and of calcium (up to 1500 mg calcium/day) and vitamin D (400–800 IU of vitamin D daily).

Interpretation. The authors avoided commenting on the treatment implication of their results but the analyses point towards the strongest therapeutic effects for alendronate and risedronate. There was recognition that HRT was likely to have an effect on fracture rate but that the CI around the pooled estimate was large and there was also recognition that the Women's Health Initiative (WHI) Trial may clarify this issue. Other treatment options such as vitamin D, raloxifene, etidronate and calcitonin did not meet as stringent criteria as alendronate and risedronate.

Comment

These analyses help provide an evidence-based, rational approach to the management of osteoporosis. In patients at the highest risk of fracture, particularly hip fracture, the best therapies would appear to be either alendronate or risedronate. In patients with milder effects in whom treatment is directed towards preventing vertebral fracture then a wider choice of treatments may be effective. In selected populations, such as the institutionalized elderly, calcium and vitamin D will be effective.

Hormone replacement therapy and fracture efficacy

There has been considerable debate regarding the benefits of HRT in preventing or treating osteoporosis. There have been few randomized controlled trials of HRT with fracture as an outcome measure and those that do exist have insufficient subjects to achieve meaningful results. Although observational, cohort, case–control and comparative studies have suggested that HRT is of benefit the selection bias and inclusion criteria have tended to negate the findings of such studies. The WHI study presented a unique opportunity to answer the questions regarding the benefits of HRT in preventing fractures.

Risks and benefits of estrogen plus progestin in healthy postmenopausal women: principal results from the Women's Health Initiative randomized controlled trial

Rossouw JE, Anderson GL, Prentice RL, *et al. JAMA* 2002; **288**: 321–33

Background. Over 16 000 women in the USA, receiving a continuous combined HRT preparation were studied mainly to investigate the cardiovascular benefits against the adverse outcome, invasive breast cancer. As part of the secondary end-points, hip, vertebral and other osteoporotic fractures were studied and a significant reduction of incidence in all fracture types was observed in the HRT group compared with placebo: hip hazard ratio (HR) 0.66 (95% CI 0.33–1.33), vertebral HR 0.66 (95% CI 0.32–1.34), other fractures HR 0.77 (95% CI 0.63–0.94). The study was terminated at a mean of 5.2 years of follow-up (planned 8.5 years) because the test statistic for invasive breast cancer exceeded the stopping boundary for this adverse event.

Interpretation. The findings were consistent with the previous observational and limited clinical trial data that indicated a beneficial effect of HRT on BMD and subsequent risk of fracture. This study provided definitive data supporting the ability of HRT, when given to postmenopausal women, to prevent fractures at all osteoporotic sites.

Comment

Despite the fact that the women in this trial were in the main at low risk of osteoporosis and subsequent fractures, the study detected a significant reduction of both hip and vertebral fracture in women taking HRT. The WHI study, however, has raised several concerns regarding long-term use of HRT and the commencement of HRT in elderly women. It has been concluded that in the population studied there was a predominance of adverse effects with increased stroke, thrombosis, breast cancer and coronary heart disease over the beneficial effects such as reduction in fractures and colorectal cancer. A statement has therefore been made that the combined preparation of HRT containing 0.625 mg conjugated equine oestrogen and 2.5 mg medroxyprogesterone acetate is not a viable intervention for primary prevention of chronic diseases.

Beyond the Women's Health Initiative trial

As a result of the WHI study there has been considerable reaction against the use of continuous combined HRT for the prevention and treatment of osteoporosis. An important question has also been raised regarding the possible cardiovascular effects of selective oestrogen receptor modulators, such as raloxifene.

Raloxifene and cardiovascular events in osteoporotic postmenopausal women: four-year results from the MORE (Multiple Outcomes of Raloxifene Evaluation) randomized trial

Barrett-Connor E, Grady D, Sashegyi A, *et al.* *JAMA* 2002; **287**: 847–57

BACKGROUND. Raloxifene improves cardiovascular risk factors, but its effect on cardiovascular events is unknown. A secondary analysis of data from the Multiple Outcomes of Raloxifene Evaluation (MORE) randomized, double-blind, placebo-controlled trial has been performed. A total of 7705 osteoporotic postmenopausal women (mean age 67 years) were randomly assigned to receive raloxifene 60 mg/day, or 120 mg/day, or placebo for 4 years. In the overall cohort, there were no significant differences between treatment groups in the number of combined coronary and cerebrovascular events: 96 (3.7%) with placebo, 82 (3.2%) and 94 (3.7%) with 60 or 120 mg/day raloxifene respectively. Relative risks (RRs) were 0.86 (95% CI 0.64–1.15) and 0.98 (95% CI 0.74–1.30) for 60 and 120 mg/day of raloxifene. In the 1035 women with increased cardiovascular risk at baseline, raloxifene had a significantly lower risk of cardiovascular events compared with placebo (RR 0.60; 95% CI 0.38–0.95 for both raloxifene groups). Cardiovascular events during the first year were not significantly different across groups in the overall cohort (*P* = 0.94), or among women at increased cardiovascular risk (*P* = 0.86) or with evidence of established coronary heart disease (*P* = 0.60).

INTERPRETATION. Raloxifene did not significantly affect the risk of cardiovascular events in the overall cohort but significantly reduced the risk of cardiovascular events in the subset of women with increased cardiovascular risk.

Comment

These results give some reassurance that raloxifene use is unlikely to increase cardiovascular events but as was the case with many HRT studies the MORE trial was not designed to look at cardiovascular outcome and the analysis presented is retrospective.

Recent advances in the management of osteoporosis

New therapeutic interventions (e.g. parathyroid hormone 1-34), emerging long-term safety data regarding HRT and bisphosphonates and strategies for falls and fracture prevention will be considered.

Parathyroid hormone

Background

Parathyroid hormone (PTH) stimulates bone formation, especially trabecular bone, when it is administered intermittently. Its anabolic effect contrasts with the anti-resorptive effects of HRT and the bisphosphonates, which have until now been the mainstay of treatment for osteoporosis. Treatment of postmenopausal women with prior vertebral fractures with PTH 1-34 significantly decreased the risk of further vertebral and non-vertebral fractures [9]. Teriparatide (a recombinant version of PTH 1-34) is the latest licensed drug for osteoporosis in postmenopausal women. It is self-administered in a once daily subcutaneous injection for 18 months and is currently targeted at those with severe osteoporosis who already have vertebral fracture. It is an expensive treatment and guidelines for its use are being drawn up nationally and locally.

Parathyroid hormone and bisphosphonate combination therapy

Theoretically the use of PTH, with its anabolic effects, in combination with the antiresorptive effects of a bisphosphonate might confer additional therapeutic benefit to patients with osteoporosis. This hypothesis has been studied in two recent trials.

The effects of parathyroid hormone and alendronate alone or in combination in postmenopausal osteoporosis

Black DM, Greenspan SL, Ensrud KE, *et al.* *N Engl J Med* 2003; **349**: 1207–15

BACKGROUND. Black *et al.* randomly assigned 238 postmenopausal women (who were not using bisphosphonates) with low BMD at the lumbar spine or hip (T-score of <–2.5 or a T-score of <–2 with an additional osteoporotic risk factor) to treatment with PTH (1-84) alone, alendronate alone or combination therapy. The groups were followed for 12 months, the main outcome measures being BMD assessed by dual-energy X-ray absorptiometry (DEXA) and quantitative computed tomography (the latter allowed separate evaluation of trabecular and cortical bone) and biochemical markers of bone turnover. Comparison of the three groups showed that BMD increased in all treatment groups and no significant difference was noted between the group receiving PTH alone and those receiving combination therapy. However, the volumetric density of trabecular bone at the lumbar spine in the PTH group, as measured by quantitative computed tomography, was approximately twice that found in the others. Interestingly, markers of bone formation increased in the PTH group but not in those receiving combination therapy. The authors concluded therefore that there was no evidence to support a synergistic treatment effect between PTH and alendronate in postmenopausal osteoporosis.

The effects of parathyroid hormone, alendronate or both in men with osteoporosis

Finkelstein JS, Hayes A, Hunzelman JL, Wyland JJ, Lee H, Neer RM. *N Engl J Med* 2003; **349**: 1216–26

BACKGROUND. Finkelstein *et al.* reported a similar study to Black *et al.* of 83 men with osteoporosis (here defined as BMD at the lumbar spine or neck of femur at least 2 SDs below that of young normal men). Patients were again randomly assigned to treatment with either PTH alone, alendronate alone or a combination of both. However, in this study alendronate was given for 30 months and PTH was begun at month 6 and continued for 24 months. There was a significant increase in BMD at the lumbar spine and femoral neck in those treated with PTH alone compared with the other groups. Although lumbar spine BMD did increase more in the combination group when compared with the alendronate alone group, once again no additive effect of combination therapy was noted and the authors concluded that alendronate impaired the ability of PTH to increase the BMD at the lumbar spine and femoral neck in men.

Comment

Thus both studies suggest that in terms of the lumbar spine, where trabecular bone predominates, combination therapy is probably better than alendronate alone but that PTH alone is the most effective.

In an accompanying editorial, Khosla [**10**] speculates why this might be so. He reminds us that the classification of drugs as exclusively bone forming or resorptive is rather artificial and may not mirror the *in vivo* situation where there is coupling of bone resorption and formation (e.g. antiresorptive agents eventually reduce bone formation as overall bone turnover decreases).

Khosla suggests that one explanation of the trial findings is that it is not the inhibition of bone resorption *per se* by alendronate but the overall reduction in bone turnover that impairs the effect of PTH, as in conditions of low bone turnover there are fewer osteoblasts to stimulate. Further studies, however, are clearly needed.

Strontium ranelate treatment of osteoporosis

Strontium ranelate is a new compound undergoing trials for the treatment of osteoporosis. It has a unique mode of action simultaneously increasing bone formation and decreasing bone resorption. Two large multicentre trials have recently reported the effects of strontium ranelate, one in the prevention of bone loss in early postmenopausal women (PREVOS) [**11**] and the other in the treatment of postmenopausal vertebral osteoporosis (STRATOS) [**12**].

Strontium ranelate phase 2 dose-ranging studies: PREVOS and STRATOS studies

Reginster JY, Meunier PJ. *Osteoporos Int* 2003; **14**(Suppl 3): S56–65

BACKGROUND. Current treatments for osteoporosis act by inhibiting bone resorption. Strontium ranelate has a unique mode of action simultaneously increasing bone formation and decreasing bone resorption. This paper summarizes the results from two pivotal dose-ranging studies using strontium ranelate: 160 women were studied in PREVOS and 353 in STRATOS.

INTERPRETATION. Strontium ranelate was well tolerated in both studies and a significant dose-dependent increase in BMD was observed. A bone formation marker (bone-specific alkaline phosphatase) increased significantly at all time points in the 2 g/day group and a bone resorption marker (urine N-telopeptide) decreased significantly with 1 and 2 g/day doses at 6 months. A significant reduction in vertebral deformities was noticed in the second year of treatment only in the highest dose group receiving 2 g/day (RR 0.56, 95% CI 0.35–0.89). These results suggested a unique mode of action for strontium ranelate with stimulation of bone formation and inhibition of resorption occurring simultaneously. Theoretically this should result in a sustained, long-term increase in bone mass. The dose of strontium ranelate for prevention of osteoporosis was suggested to be 1 g/day and for treatment 2 g/day.

Comment

It is good to see new treatments being developed for the management of osteoporosis. Not all patients respond well to pure antiresorptive therapies and so treatments with additional anabolic effects are appealing. The relative lack of fracture efficacy in the first year of treatment is a concern when comparison is made with other available treatments and the waning of effect on bone resorption in the second year raises questions about the optimum doses for prevention and treatment.

Statins and bone

Animal studies have suggested that statins can significantly increase bone formation rates by increasing expression of bone morphogenetic protein-2 (BMP-2). These drugs act by inhibiting 3-hydroxy-3-methylglutaryl coenzyme A (HMG-CoA) reductase, an enzyme in the mevalonate pathway, and significantly reduce serum cholesterol by inhibiting hepatic cholesterol biosynthesis. Recent data indicate that *in vitro* the statins also inhibit osteoclast bone resorption and that this is directly related to the level of inhibition of HMG-CoA reductase [**13**]. Concurrently with these findings the mechanism of action of the bisphosphonates has gradually been explained and it is now known that the N_2-containing bisphosphonates cause osteoclast apoptosis due to inhibition of farnesylpyrophosphate synthase and isopentenyl diphosphonate isomerase enzymes also within the mevalonate pathway [**14**]. These two avenues of research have led to the postulate that the statins may have a beneficial effect on bone metabolism in humans preventing deterioration in bone mass. Statins have been widely prescribed throughout the world and large databases have been examined for evidence of an association between statin use and skeletal status. Reviewing the published data the evidence of an association in early reports from observational studies was positive but more recent studies have reported variable effects [**15**].

Statin use, clinical fracture, and bone density in postmenopausal women: results from the Women's Health Initiative Observational Study

LaCroix AZ, Cauley JA, Pettinger M, *et al. Ann Intern Med* 2003; **139**: 97–104

Background. The large number of subjects within the WHI Observational Study presented a unique opportunity to investigate the effects of statin use and bone metabolism. Within the study there were 7846 statin users and 85 870 non-users. Median follow-up was 3.9 years and after adjustment for confounding factors there was no statistically significant difference in fractures at the hip (HR 1.22; 95% CI 0.83–1.81), lower arm or wrist (HR 1.04; CI 0.85–1.27) or other clinical fractures (HR 1.11; CI 1.00–1.22).

Interpretation. No significant difference in BMD was observed between statin users and non-users. Statins with higher potency for reducing cholesterol had no greater effect than weaker agents and duration of use did not reduce the risk of fracture. There was a relatively low prevalence of statin use in this study but the large number of subjects studied should have detected an effect on bone metabolism, in this population, if one existed.

Comment

It is difficult to draw any hard conclusions from the previous and recent studies in this area of osteoporosis management. Too many variables exist in many of the observational and cross-sectional studies to allow definite conclusions. The statins employed in the studies are different, the doses are variable, the length of time on treatment is not consistent, patients have changed the statins they have used within the study period, concomitant medication has varied and the entry criteria into many of the studies were related to cardiovascular criteria not to osteoporosis. Further epidemiology-based studies and cross-sectional data will clearly be of minimal value. While small non-randomized prospective studies have also suggested a beneficial effect of simvastatin the majority of authors conclude that, although the data are tantalizing regarding the effect of statins on bone, until randomized placebo controlled trials have been performed, confirming a statistically significant effect of statins on the skeleton, they should not be advocated for use in the treatment or prevention of osteoporosis.

Other treatment options

Alendronate versus calcitriol for the prevention of bone loss after cardiac transplantation

Shane E, Addesso V, Namerow PB, *et al.* *N Engl J Med* 2004; **350**: 767–76

BACKGROUND. In a study of 149 patients postcardiac transplant, individuals were randomly assigned to receive either alendronate 10 mg daily or calcitriol (0.5 μg/day) for 1 year. The degree of bone loss and rate of fracture did not differ significantly between the two intervention groups. Calcitriol was associated with a higher risk of hypercalcuria—27% of the calcitriol group and 7% of those in the alendronate group.

Comment

The authors concluded that the requirement for monitoring the serum and urinary calcium levels in calcitriol-treated patients makes alendronate a more attractive option for the treatment of bone loss early after cardiac transplantation. However, other treatment options, such as calcitriol, are required if patients cannot tolerate bisphosphonates and there are concerns over HRT use.

Long-term safety issues: practical aspects of prescribing

Hormone replacement therapy

Until recently, HRT was a useful medium- to long-term treatment in postmenopausal women with or at risk of osteoporosis. However, accumulating concerns about increased risk of breast cancer, heart disease, stroke and thromboembolic disease in women taking HRT, combined preparations in particular (both continuous and sequential regimens), has changed therapeutic options dramatically in the last year.

Breast cancer and hormone-replacement therapy in the Million Women Study

Million Women Study Collaborators. *Lancet* 2003; **362**: 419–27

BACKGROUND. The publication of the Million Women Study has altered the perception of the place of HRT in the management of osteoporosis in postmenopausal women. This was a large observational study noting the effects of different types of HRT on the incidence of breast cancer in nearly a million postmenopausal women in the UK over 5 years. The study showed that all types of HRT caused a duration-dependent increase in the risk of breast cancer. The greatest risk related to the use of combined oestrogen/progesterone preparations and this is true of heart disease as well. The risk

begins to decline when HRT is discontinued and by 5 years is at the same level as those who have never taken HRT. The Committee on Safety of Medicines has also provided useful guidance regarding the risks and benefits of HRT [16].

Comment

While it is clear that HRT is of value in osteoporosis, the risks of treatment need to be weighed against possible benefits and this is true even in individuals who do not have a family history of breast cancer. There is a protective effect of HRT in terms of colon cancer but for combination therapy this is outweighed by cardiovascular, stroke and breast cancer risks. The role of HRT at present continues to be debated [17].

However, the decision to prescribe or take HRT is often based on the presence of menopausal symptoms which should not be underestimated. Therefore the benefits versus the risks of therapy need to be carefully balanced even for short term use and treatment reviewed regularly.

Bisphosphonates

Long-term safety data regarding bisphosphonates are important as they are widely used in the treatment of osteoporosis and remain in bone for a long time. In addition, the optimum duration of therapy has been uncertain (Strewler 2004 [18]).

Ten years' experience with alendronate for osteoporosis in postmenopausal women

Bone HG, Hosking D, Devogelaer JP, *et al.*; Alendronate Phase III Osteoporosis Treatment Study Group. *N Engl J Med* 2004; **350**(12): 1189–99

BACKGROUND. In their recent study of 247 postmenopausal women who had taken alendronate for 10 years, Bone *et al.* have shown that the therapeutic effect of alendronate, in terms of BMD, was sustained and the therapy was well tolerated. Discontinuation of alendronate resulted in a gradual loss of effect. There was no demonstrable adverse effect over the prolonged period of follow-up.

Comment

While 10 years of alendronate treatment appear to be safe, the optimal duration of therapy remains uncertain.

Biochemical markers of bone metabolism in the management of osteoporosis

Several interventions have been shown to reduce the incidence of fractures but the optimal response and duration of therapy is still unknown. Few data are available on the rate of adherence to treatment, the rate of response and the potential mechanisms to improve response to interventions. Biochemical markers of bone turnover are available to facilitate follow-up of patients receiving antiresorptive treatments for osteoporosis and they can be used to detect patients who do not adhere or who do not respond to treatment [19]. Markers of resorption are an excellent reflection of osteoclast activity. As the majority of interventions that are being assessed act by affecting osteoclast activity, measurement of resorption markers enables prediction of a reduction in fracture risk. The relative contribution of the decrease in bone turnover or increase in BMD to fracture reduction is of major interest as it is clear that several interventions have a significant effect on fracture rates despite modest increases in BMD.

Changes in bone density and turnover explain the reductions in incidence of non-vertebral fractures that occur during treatment with antiresorptive agents

Hochberg MC, Greenspan S, Wasnich RD, Miller P, Thompson DE, Ross PD. *J Clin Endocrinol Metab* 2002; **87**: 1586–92

BACKGROUND. A meta-analysis was performed to explore the contribution to the reduction in incidence of non-vertebral fractures from BMD and bone turnover assessed by biochemical markers. Eighteen trials with usable data were available for analysis, including a total of 2415 women with incident non-vertebral fractures. Larger increases in BMD or reductions in bone markers were significantly associated with greater reduction in non-vertebral fracture risk. At 1 year a 6% increase in spine BMD reduces non-vertebral fracture by 39%, a 3% increase in hip BMD by 46% and a 70% reduction in resorption or formation markers reduces fracture risk by 40% and 44%, respectively.

INTERPRETATION. These results suggest that changes in BMD and markers provide similar information regarding reductions in non-vertebral fracture risk during treatment. Interestingly, excluding trials using alendronate resulted in loss of significance for all associations.

Comment

The availability of serum markers of bone resorption with significantly reduced biological and measurement variability, compared with urine measurements, make it possible to follow changes with treatment with increasing accuracy. The magnitude and timing of reduction in bone turnover (within weeks) is a significant advantage compared with the slower changes in repeated BMD measurement or awaiting presentation with clinical fracture as an indication of intervention efficacy.

Justifying treatment: costs of osteoporosis

As greater restraint is placed on healthcare resources it has become important to perform outcome and economic studies. Accurate estimates of the costs of osteoporosis are essential to help address the cost/benefit ratio of therapeutic strategies for osteoporosis. Fourteen billion dollars per year was the estimated total cost of osteoporosis to the USA in 1998 [20]. A three- to eightfold increase in costs over a 50-year period is predicted as the elderly population, particularly the over 85 age group, expands. In the UK, the acute and medium term costs are estimated at £1030 million per annum (but a significantly greater cost is liable to accrue in terms of the long-term outcome of osteoporosis [21]. Assuming that the distribution of BMD in the population remains constant and the fracture rates for the population remain the same, the costs for treating osteoporosis related fractures in the UK would increase to £2.1 billion per year by 2010.

The hospital cost of vertebral fractures in the EU: estimates using national datasets

Finnern HW, Sykes DP. *Osteoporos Int* 2003; **14**(5): 429–36

BACKGROUND. While hip fractures are the major contributor to costs, vertebral fractures also account for a significant percentage of total expenditure. The number of patients treated in hospital for vertebral fracture, in the EU, is 25% of those treated with hip fracture. Total hospital costs for vertebral fractures in EU countries have been estimated using national datasets at €377 million per year and the average cost of a vertebral fracture was 63% of that of a hip fracture. Eighty-nine per cent of these vertebral fractures can be attributed to osteoporosis.

INTERPRETATION. Countries throughout the EU had a marked difference in the length of hospital stay following a vertebral fracture ranging from 0.32 days in Austria to 20.2 days in Spain and hospitalization rates differed markedly from 3% in the UK to 18% in Sweden. Men were hospitalized for shorter periods than women in contrast to the opposite effect seen for hip fracture.

Cost-equivalence of different osteoporotic fractures

Melton LJ III, Gabriel SE, Crowson CS, Tosteson AN, Johnell O, Kanis JA. *Osteoporos Int* 2003; **14**(5): 383–8

BACKGROUND. The move to define osteoporosis treatment thresholds on the basis of absolute fracture risk requires an estimate of outcome that combines a number of diverse factors for different fractures. One approach is to quantify all osteoporotic fractures in terms of 'hip fracture equivalents' on the basis of relative morbidity, mortality and cost. In those under 65 years of age hip fractures account for less than 50% of the total morbidity due to osteoporotic fractures. In studies of Olmstead County residents first the direct medical costs attributable to osteoporotic fractures were established and then data were obtained that supported the concept of hip fracture equivalents with incremental costs associated with different types of fracture roughly corresponding to utility loss for these fractures.

INTERPRETATION. There was concordance between the burden of all fractures and hip fractures for both costs and morbidity.

Comment

Having comparative data on costs and being able to provide accurate cost-equivalent data for fractures is essential when attempting to obtain resources for the management of osteoporosis. The data provided in these two studies may help simplify health economic analyses, help set intervention thresholds and improve treatment cost-effectiveness.

Prevention: strategies for preventing falls and fractures and excess mortality from osteoporosis fracture

Background

A recent review |**22**| highlights the well documented importance of reducing the number of falls in preventing fractures. It is also noteworthy that pharmacological treatment is most clinically- and cost-effective when targeted at those who are at highest risk. As previous fracture and low BMD are strong risk factors for future fracture, those at highest risk can be identified by combining these with other risk factors. Reasons for previous falls and unsteadiness in elderly patients should be investigated and treatment of concomitant conditions such as inflammatory joint disease and neurological disease is important, so too is review of any contributing medication.

Two recent studies, one in primary care |**23**|, the other in a subacute hospital setting |**24**| reported that multifactorial risk assessment and management programmes were the most effective strategies in falls prevention.

It is vital when a fracture does occur in older individuals that they are assessed for osteoporosis and receive treatment if required. McLellan *et al.* |**25**| report that prior to the development and introduction of their integrated fracture liaison service very few patients aged 50 years or above presenting with a fracture underwent subsequent evaluation for osteoporosis. During the first 18 months of their service in Glasgow 4600 patients (men and women >50 years) presenting with low trauma fractures were assessed by the fracture liaison service's osteoporosis specialist nurses. Almost three-quarters were considered for BMD testing and of these 82.3% were found to be osteopenic or osteoporotic at the hip or spine.

Excess mortality

Excess mortality is described in patients who develop osteoporotic fractures particularly of the spine and hip. While most deaths occur in the first 3–6 months following a fracture, mortality remains higher than the general population thereafter. As part of the equation of cost-effectiveness of interventions related to osteoporosis it is important to establish what proportion of deaths are due to osteoporosis and fracture.

Conclusion

The approach to the management of patients with osteoporosis needs to be multi-faceted and should include identifying those at risk, modifying their risk factors wherever possible and tailoring treatment interventions to suit individual patients. Significant advances in the management of osteoporosis have taken place in recent years and definition-based management is being replaced by intervention strategies established using very large databases. The major risk factors for fracture have been defined and can be utilized when setting intervention thresholds. Evidence-based guidelines on treatment can now be produced following careful meta-analyses of all the available studies. The WHI study confirmed the efficacy of HRT in reducing fractures but the adverse event profile is likely to inhibit its use.

References

1. Kanis JA, Melton LJ, III, Christiansen C, Johnston CC, Khaltaev N. The diagnosis of osteoporosis. *J Bone Miner Res* 1994; **9**: 1137–41.
2. World Health Organization. *Assessment of fracture risk and its application to screening for postmenopausal osteoporosis.* WHO technical report series 843. Geneva: 1994.
3. NIH Consensus Development Panel on Osteoporosis Prevention, Diagnosis, and Therapy. Osteoporosis prevention, diagnosis, and therapy. *JAMA* 2001; **285**: 785–95.
4. Lindsay R, Silverman SL, Cooper C, Hanley DA, Barton I, Broy SB, Licata A, Benhamou L, Geusens P, Flowers K, Stracke H, Seeman E. Risk of new vertebral fracture in the year following a fracture. *JAMA* 2001; **285**: 320–3.
5. Scottish Intercollegiate Guidelines Network. *71—Management of Osteoporosis, a national clinical guideline.* June 2003.
6. *Glucocorticoid-induced Osteoporosis. Guidelines for prevention and treatment.* London: Bone and Tooth Society of Great Britain, National Osteoporosis Society and Royal College of Physicians, 2002.
7. Center JR, Nguyen TV, Schneider D, Sambrook PN, Eisman JA. Mortality after all major types of osteoporotic fracture in men and women: an observational study. *Lancet* 1999; 353: 878–82.
8. Deutschmann HA, Weger M, Weger W, Kotanko P, Deutschmann MJ, Skrabal F. Search for occult secondary osteoporosis: impact of identified possible risk factors on bone mineral density. *J Intern Med* 2002; **252**: 389–97.
9. Neer RM, Arnauld CD, Zanchetta JR, Prince R, Gaich GA, Reginster J-Y, Hodsman AB, Eriksen EF, Ish-Shalom S, Genant HK, Wang O, Mitlak BH. Effect of parathyroid hormone (1-34) on fractures and bone mineral density in postmenopausal women with osteoporosis. *N Engl J Med* 2001; **344**: 1434–41.

10. Khosla S. Parathyroid hormone plus alendronate—a combination that does not add up. *N Engl J Med* 2003; **349**: 1277–9.

11. Reginster JY, Deroisy R, Dougados M, Jupsin I, Colette J, Roux C. Prevention of early post-menopausal bone loss by strontium ranelate: the randomized, two-year, double-masked, dose-ranging, placebo-controlled PREVOS trial. *Osteoporos Int* 2002; **13**: 925–31.

12. Meunier PJ, Slosman DO, Delmas PD, Sebert JL, Brandi ML, Albanese C, Lorenc R, Pors-Nielsen S, De Vernejoul MC, Roces A, Reginster JY. Strontium ranelate: dose-dependent effects in established post-menopausal vertebral osteoporosis—a 2-year randomized placebo controlled trial. *J Clin Endocrinol Metab* 2002; **87**: 2060–6.

13. Staal A, Frith JC, French MH, Swartz J, Gungor T, Harrity TW, Tamasi J, Rogers MJ, Feyen JH. The ability of statins to inhibit bone resorption is directly related to their inhibitory effect on HMG-CoA reductase activity. *J Bone Miner Res* 2003; **18**: 88–96.

14. Russell RG, Rogers MJ, Frith JC, Luckman SP, Coxon FP, Benford HL, Croucher PI, Shipman C, Fleisch HA. The pharmacology of bisphosphonates and new insights into their mechanisms of action. *J Bone Miner Res* 1999; **14**(Suppl 2): 53–65.

15. Bauer DC. HMG CoA reductase inhibitors and the skeleton: a comprehensive review. *Osteoporos Int* 2003; **14**: 273–82.

16. Committee on Safety of Medicines. HRT: Update on the risk of breast cancer and long-term safety. *Curr Prob Pharmacovigilance* 2003; **29**: 1–3.

17. McPherson K. Where are we now with hormone replacement therapy? *Br Med J* 2004; **328**: 357–8.

18. Strewler GJ. Decimal point—osteoporosis therapy at the 10-year mark. *N Engl J Med* 2004; **350**(12): 1189–99

19. Riggs BL. Are biochemical markers for bone turnover clinically useful for monitoring therapy in individual osteoporotic patients? *Bone* 2000; **26**: 551–2.

20. Eddy D, Johnston C, Cummings SR. Osteoporosis: review of the evidence for prevention, diagnosis and treatment and cost-effectiveness analysis. *Osteoporos Int* 1998; **8**: S1–8.

21. Dolan P, Torgerson DJ. The cost of treating osteoporotic fractures in the United Kingdom female population. *Osteoporos Int* 2000; **11**: 551–2.

22. Woolf AD, Akesson K. Preventing fractures in elderly people. *Br Med J* 2003; **327**: 89–95.

23. Chang JT, Morton SC, Rubenstein LZ, Mojica WA, Maglione M, Suttorp MJ, Roth EA, Shekelle PG. Interventions for the prevention of falls in older adults: a systematic review and meta-analysis of randomised clinical trials. *Br Med J* 2004; **328**: 680–3.

24. Haines TP, Bennell KL, Osbourne RH, Hill KD. Effectiveness of targeted falls prevention programme in subacute hospital setting: randomised controlled trial. *Br Med J* 2004; **328**: 676–9.

25. McLellan AR, Gallacher SJ, Fraser M, McQuillan C. The fracture liaison service: success of a program for the evaluation and management of patients with osteoporotic fracture. *Osteoporosis Int* 2003; **14**: 1028–34.

This chapter is an extension of material by Professor William Fraser which first appeared in the *Year in Post-Menopausal Health 2004*.

List of abbreviations

AAO	American Academy of Opthalmology
ACE	angiotensin-converting enzyme
ACR	American College of Rheumatology
AE	adverse events
AIA	aspirin-induced asthma
AIA	aspirin-intolerant asthma
AIM	ancestry-informative marker
AIMS2	Arthritis Impact Measurement Scales 2
AMI	acute myocardial infarction
ANCA	antineutrophil cytoplasmic antibody
APF	antiperinuclear factor
aPL	antiphospholipid
ARAMIS	Arthritis, Rheumatism, and Aging Medical Information System
ARMADA	Anti-TNF Research study program of the Monoconal antibody Adalimumab in rheumatoid arthritis
AS	ankylosing spondylitis
AUC	area under the curve
BAL	bronchoalveolar lavage
BASDAI	Bath AS Disease Activity Index
BASF1	Bath AS Functional Index
BMD	bone mineral density
BMI	body mass index
BMP	bone morphogenetic protein
BVAS	Birmingham Vasculitis Activity Score
CCR	CC chemokine receptor
CCP	cyclic citrullinated peptide
CHD	coronary heart disease
CI	confidence interval
CLASS	Celecoxib Long-term Arthritis Society Study
COX	cyclooxygenase
CRP	C-reactive protein
CV	cardiovascular
CyA	cyclosporin A
DAS28	disease activity score based on a 28-joint count
DXA	dual-energy X-ray absorptiometry
DL_{CO}	diffusing capacity for carbon monoxide
DM	dermatomyositis
DMARD	disease-modifying antirheumatic drug
DS	damage score
dsDNA	double-stranded DNA
EMG	electromyography
EPOS	European Prospective Osteoporosis Study
ESRD	end-stage renal disease
ET	etanercept
EUVAS	European Vasculitis Study Group
FEV^1	forced expiratory volume
GBM	glomerular basement membrane
Gd	gadolinium
GI	gastrointestinal
HAQ	Health Assessment Questionnaire
HAQ-DI	HAQ Disability Index
HCQ	hydroxychloroquine
HCV	hepatitis C virus
HDCC	high-dose corticosteroids and/or cyclophosphamide
HMG-CoA	3-hydroxy-3-methylglutaryl coenzyme A
HR	hazard ratio
HRT	hormone replacement therapy
HSCT	haematopoietic stem-cell transplantation
HSP	Henoch–Schönlein purpura
IBM	inclusion body myositis

IFN	interferon
IIM	inflammatory myopathies
IL	interleukin
IL-1Ra	interleukin-1 receptor antagonist
IMACS	International Myositis Assessment and Clinical Studies
IN	infliximab
JIA	juvenile idiopathic arthritis
LF	leflunomide
LN	lupus nephritis
LPS	lipopolysaccharide
LTB_4	leukotriene B_4
LTE_4	leukotriene E_4
mAb	monoclonal antibody
MC	mixed cryoglobulinaemia
MDI	myositis damage index
MFCV	muscle-fibre conduction velocity
MHC	major histocompatibility complex
MI	myocardial infarction
MITAX	myositis intention-to-treat index
MORE	Multiple Outcomes of Raloxifene Evaluation
MPA	microscopic polyangiitis
MRI	magnetic resonance imaging
MTX	methotrexate
MYOACT	myositis disease activity assessment
NCV	nerve conduction velocity
NSAID	non-steroidal anti-inflammatory drug
OA	osteoarthritis
OR	odds ratio
OTC	over the counter
PAN	polyarteritis nodosa
PAP	pulmonary artery pressure
PASI	Psoriasis Area and Severity Index
PGE_2	prostaglandin E_2
PHT	pulmonary hypertension
PM	polymyositis
PPD	purified protein derivative
PPI	proton pump inhibitors
PsA	psoriatic arthritis
PsARC	PsA response criteria
PTH	parathyroid hormone
PWA	pulse wave analysis
RA	rheumatoid arthritis
RCT	randomized controlled trial
RF	rheumatoid factor
RLN	recurrent lupus nephritis
ROC	receiver operating characteristic
RP	Raynaud's phenomenon
RR	relative risk
SASP	sulphasalazine
SCORE	Standardized Calculator of Risks for Events
SDI	SLICC Damage Index
SE	shared epitope
SLE	systemic lupus erythematosus
SLEDAI	SLE disease activity index
SLICC	Systemic Lupus International Collaborating Clinics Damage
SPARC	secreted protein, acidic and rich in cysteine
SRP	signal recognition particle
SSc	systemic sclerosis
SScPH	SSC related pulmonary arterial hypertension
SSZ	sulphasalazine
STIR	short tau inversion recovery
SVR	systemic vascular resistance
TB	tuberculosis
TGF	transforming growth factor
Th	T-helper
TNF	tumour necrosis factor
tRNA	transfer RNA
TSE	turbo spin-echo sequence
UA	undifferentiated arthritis
UKFS	UK Schleroderma Functional Score
UVR	ultraviolet radiation
VAS	visual analogue scale
VDI	Vasculitis Damage Index
VU	vertebral unit
WHI	Women's Health Initiative
WOMAC	Western Ontario and McMaster Universities

Index of Papers Reviewed

postmenopausal osteoporosis. *N Engl J Med* 2003; **349**: 1207–15. **232**

Blijham PJ, Hengstman GJ, ter Laak HJ, van Engelen BG, Zwarts MJ. Muscle-fiber conduction velocity and electromyography as diagnostic tools in patients with suspected inflammatory myopathy: a prospective study. *Muscle Nerve* 2004; **29**: 46–50. **189**

Bone HG, Hosking D, Devogelaer JP, Tucci JR,Emkey RD, Tonino RP, Rodriguez-Portales JA, Downs RW, Gupta J, Santora AC, Liberman UA; Alendronate Phase III Osteoporosis Treatment Study Group. Ten years' experience with alendronate for osteoporosis in postmenopausal women. *N Engl J Med* 2004; **350**(12): 1189–99. **237**

Brandt J, Khariouzov A, Listing J, Haibel H, Sorensen H, Grassnickel L, Rudwaleit M, Sieper J, Braun J. Six-month results of a double blind, placebo-controlled trial of etanercept treatment in patients with active ankylosing spondylitis. *Arthritis Rheum* 2003; **48**: 1667–75. **65, 109**

Braun J, Baraliakos X, Golder W, Brandt J, Rudwaleit M, Listing J, Bollow M, Sieper J, Van der Heijde D. Magnetic resonance imaging examinations of the spine in patients with ankylosing spondylitis, before and after successful therapy with infliximab: evaluation of a new scoring system. *Arthritis Rheum* 2003; **48**(4): 1126–36. **67, 112**

Bukhari MA, Wiles NJ, Lunt M, Harrison BJ, Scott DG, Symmons DP, Silman AJ. Influence of disease-modifying therapy on radiographic outcome in inflammatory polyarthritis at five years: results from a large observational inception study. *Arthritis Rheum* 2003; **48**: 46–53. **42**

Carmichael SJ, Beal J, Day RO, Tett SE. Combination therapy with methotrexate and hydroxychloroquine for rheumatoid arthritis increases exposure to methotrexate. *J Rheumatol* 2002; **29**: 2077–83. **34**

Chakravarty EF, Sanchez-Yamamoto D, Bush TM. The use of disease modifying antirheumatic drugs in women with rheumatoid arthritis of childbearing age: a survey of practice patterns and pregnancy outcomes. *J Rheumatol* 2003; **30**(2): 241–6. **39**

Chan FKL, Hung LCT, Suen BY, Wu JC, Lee KC, Leung VK, Hui AJ, To KF, Leung WK, Wong VW, Chung SC, Sung JJ. Celecoxib versus diclofenac and omeprazole in reducing the risk of recurrent ulcer bleeding in patients with arthritis. *N Engl J Med* 2002; **347**: 2104–10. **15**

Chantler IW, Davie MWJ, Evans SF, Rees JS. Oral corticosteroid prescribing in women over 50, use of fracture prevention therapy and bone densitometry service. *Ann Rheum Dis* 2003; **62**: 350–2. **226**

Cranney A, Tugwell P, Wells G, Guyatt G; Osteoporosis Methodology Group and the Osteoporosis Research Advisory Group. Meta-analyses of therapies for post-menopausal osteoporosis. *Endocr Rev* 2002; **23**: 496–578. **228**

Davis JC Jr, Van Der Heijde D, Braun J, Dougados M, Cush J, Clegg DO, Kivitz A, Fleischmann R, Inman R, Tsuji W; Enbrel Ankylosing Spondylitis Study Group. Recombinant human tumour necrosis factor receptor (etanercept) for treating ankylosing spondylitis. *Arthritis Rheum* 2003; **48**: 3230–6. **110**

Deegens JK, Artz MA, Hoitsma AJ, Wetzels JF. Outcome of renal transplantation in patients with pauci-immune small vessel vasculitis or anti-GBM disease. *Clin Nephrol* 2003; **59**: 1–9. **175**

Deegens JK, Artz MA, Hoitsma AJ, Wetzels JFM. Outcome of renal transplantation in patients with systemic lupus erythematosus. *Transplantation Int* 2003; **16**: 411–18. **140**

DeMarco PJ, Weisman MH, Seilbold JR, Furst DE, Wong WK, Hurwitz EL,

Treatment of polyarteritis nodosa and microscopic polyangiitis with poor prognosis factors: a prospective trial comparing glucocorticoids and six or twelve cyclophosphamide pulses in sixty-five patients. *Arthritis Rheum* 2003; **49**: 93–100. **177**

Gyllfors P, Bochenek G, Overholt J, Drupka D, Kumlin M, Sheller J, Nizankowska E, Isakson PC, Mejza F, Lefkowith JB, Dahlen SE, Szczeklik A, Murray JJ, Dahlen B. Biochemical and clinical evidence that aspirin-intolerant asthmatic subjects tolerate the cyclooxygenase-2 selective analgesic drug celecoxib. *J Allergy Clin Immunol* 2003; **111**: 1116–21. **21**

Harrison BJ, Silman AJ, Hider SL, Herrick AL. Cigarette smoking as a significant risk factor for digital vascular disease in patients with systemic sclerosis. *Arthritis Rheum* 2002; **46**: 3312–16. **157**

Hauer HA, Bajema IM, Van Houwelingen HC, Ferrario F, Noel LH, Waldherr R, Jayne DR, Rasmussen N, Bruijn JA, Hagen EC; European Vasculitis Study Group (EUVAS). Determinants of outcome in ANCA-associated glomerulonephritis: a prospective histopathological analysis of 96 patients. *Kidney Int* 2002; **62**: 1732–42. **173**

Hengstman GJ, van den Hoogen FH, Barrera P, Barrera P, Netea MG, Pieterse A, van de Putte LB, van Engelen BG. Successful treatment of dermatomyositis and polymyositis with anti-tumor-necrosis-factor-alpha: preliminary observations. *Eur Neurol* 2003; **50**: 10–15. **199**

Hill CL, Gale DR, Chaisson CE, Skinner K, Kazis L, Gale ME, Felson DT. Periarticular lesions detected on magnetic resonance imaging. *Arthritis Rheum* 2003; **48**: 2836–44. **211**

Hochberg MC, Greenspan S, Wasnich RD, Miller P, Thompson DE, Ross PD. Changes in bone density and turnover explain the reductions in incidence of non-vertebral fractures that occur during treatment with antiresorptive agents. *J Clin Endocrinol Metab* 2002; **87**: 1586–92. **238**

Howard OM, Dong HF, Yang D, Raben N, Nagaraju K, Rosen A, Casciola-Rosen L, Hartlein M, Kron M, Yang D, Yiadom K, Dwivedi S, Plotz PH, Oppenheim JJ. Histidyl-tRNA synthetase and asparaginyl-tRNA synthetase, autoantigens in myositis, activate chemokine receptors on T lymphocytes and immature dendritic cells. *J Exp Med* 2002; **196**(6): 781–91. **195**

Isenberg DA, Allen E, Farewell V, Ehrenstein MR, Hanna MG, Lundberg IE, Oddis C, Pilkington C, Plotz P, Scott D, Vencovský J, Cooper R, Rider L, Miller F; International Myositis and Clinical Studies Group (IMACS). International consensus outcome measures for patients with idiopathic inflammatory myopathies. Development and initial validation of myositis activity and damage indices in patients with adult onset disease. *Rheumatology (Oxford)* 2004; **43**: 49–54. **199**

Jayne D, Rasmussen N, Andrassy K, Bacon P, Tervaert JW, Dadoniene J, Ekstrand A, Gaskin G, Gregorini G, de Groot K, Gross W, Hagen EC, Mirapeix E, Pettersson E, Siegert C, Sinico A, Tesar V, Westman K, Pusey C; European Vasculitis Study Group. A randomized trial of maintenance therapy for vasculitis associated with antineutrophil cytoplasmic autoantibodies. *N Engl J Med* 2003; **349**: 36–44. **176**

Jordan KM, Arden NK, Doherty M, Bannwarth B, Bijlsma JW, Dieppe P, Gunther K, Hauselmann H, Herrero-Beaumont G, Kaklamanis P, Lohmander S, Leeb B, Lequesne M, Mazieres B, Martin-Mola E, Pavelka K, Pendleton A,

General index

KEEPING UP TO DATE IN ONE VOLUME

Subject matters dealt with in previous volume

The Year in Rheumatic Disorders 2003

Degenerative disorders and soft tissue rheumatism
Osteoarthritis: assessment; therapy of osteoarthritis; fibromyalgia: assessment; fibromyalgia: therapy; management of osteoporosis

Mechanisms of allergic disease
Assessment of rheumatoid arthritis; new treatments in rheumatoid arthritis; spondyloarthropathies

Other connective tissue disorders
Antiphospholipid (Hughes) syndrome; management of complex lupus; systemic sclerosis (scleroderma)

Interventions
Pain management; cartilage repair using cell and tissue transplants

---

Atlas Medical Publishing Ltd
Oxford Centre for Innovation
Mill Street
Oxford OX2 0JX, UK

T: +44 1865 811116
F: +44 1865 251550
E: info@clinicalpublishing.co.uk
W: www.clinicalpublishing.co.uk

KEEPING UP TO DATE IN ONE SERIES

"The Year in ..."

EXISTING AND FUTURE VOLUMES

The Year in Allergy 2003	ISBN 1 904392 05 9
The Year in Allergy 2004	ISBN 1 904392 25 3
The Year in Diabetes 2003	ISBN 1 904392 02 4
The Year in Diabetes 2004	ISBN 1 904392 20 2
The Year in Dyslipidaemia 2003	ISBN 1 904392 07 5
The Year in Dyslipidaemia 2004	ISBN 1 904392 21 0
The Year in Gynaecology 2001	ISBN 0 9537339 2 0
The Year in Gynaecology 2002	ISBN 1 904392 01 6
The Year in Gynaecology 2003	ISBN 1 904392 10 5
The Year in Hypertension 2002	ISBN 1 904392 00 8
The Year in Hypertension 2003	ISBN 1 904392 13 X
The Year in Hypertension 2004	ISBN 1 904392 28 8
The Year in Interventional Cardiology 2002	ISBN 0 9537339 7 1
The Year in Interventional Cardiology 2003	ISBN 1 904392 14 8
The Year in Neurology 2003	ISBN 1 904392 03 2
The Year in Neurology 2004	ISBN 1 904392 22 9
The Year in Osteoporosis 2004	ISBN 1 904392 27 X
The Year in Post-Menopausal Health 2004	ISBN 1 904392 23 7
The Year in Respiratory Medicine 2002	ISBN 0 9537339 8 X
The Year in Respiratory Medicine 2004	ISBN 1 904392 31 8
The Year in Rheumatic Disorders 2002	ISBN 0 9537339 9 8
The Year in Rheumatic Disorders 2003	ISBN 1 904392 09 1
The Year in Rheumatic Disorders 2004	ISBN 1 904392 29 6
The Year in Urology 2003	ISBN 1 904392 06 7

To receive more information about these books and future volumes, or to order copies, please contact the address below:

Atlas Medical Publishing Ltd
Oxford Centre for Innovation
Mill Street
Oxford OX2 0JX, UK

T: +44 1865 811116
F: +44 1865 251550
E: info@clinicalpublishing.co.uk
W: www.clinicalpublishing.co.uk